OROFACIAL PAINS
Classification, Diagnosis, Management

THIRD EDITION

OROFACIAL PAINS

Classification, Diagnosis, Management

Third Edition

Welden E. Bell, D.D.S.

Clinical Professor of Oral and Maxillofacial Surgery
Baylor College of Dentistry

Clinical Professor of Oral Surgery
University of Texas Southwestern Medical School
Dallas, Texas

YEAR BOOK MEDICAL PUBLISHERS, INC.
CHICAGO

Copyright © 1985 by Year Book Medical Publishers, Inc. All rights reserved. No part of this publication may be reproduced, stored in a retrieval system, or transmitted, in any form or by any means, electronic, mechanical, photocopying, recording, or otherwise, without prior written permission from the publisher. Printed in the United States of America.

0 9 8 7 6 5 4 3 2 1

Library of Congress Cataloging in Publication Data

Bell, Welden E.
   Orofacial pains.

   Includes bibliographies and index.
   1. Toothache. 2. Facial pain. I. Title. [DNLM: 1. Face. 2. Mouth Diseases--diagnosis. 3. Pain. WU 141 B435o]
RK322.B44   1985   617.6′072   84-20978
ISBN 0-8151-0656-4

Sponsoring editor: Diana L. McAninch
Editing supervisor: Frances M. Perveiler
Production project manager: Sharon W. Pepping
Proofroom supervisor: Shirley E. Taylor

To **LUCY**
--light of my life

Preface to the Third Edition

THE CLINICAL MANAGEMENT of orofacial pain is a primary concern of dentists everywhere. Having been instrumental in the discovery and development of both local and general anesthesia, the dental profession has always been aware of and concerned about patient comfort. The satisfactory management of surgical pain may be considered an accomplished fact. The same, however, cannot be said concerning clinical or pathologic pain.

There are reasons for this. The cause of surgical pain is obvious, and its management consists either of suppressing the passage of nociceptive impulses or of making the patient insensible to them. Therefore, an effective solution lies within the grasp of the doctor. With clinical pain, however, quite different conditions prevail: pain mechanisms are poorly understood; it is not just a matter of identifying and eliminating a cause; and the initiating cause may no longer be present—if, indeed, there was a cause at all. Usually, we do quite well when pain occurs for obvious reasons such as a toothache from pulpitis. But when pain occurs spontaneously or without evidence of structural change, we may become confused and frustrated, and our efforts may prove ineffective.

To cope with clinical pain, we need better understanding of the nature of pain and the mechanisms that generate it. We need that information at the earliest possible period in our professional training.

So we come to the objective of this book. There are numerous sources of available reference material. Many volumes have been written, and worldwide research into pain mechanisms is going on at a feverish pace. For example, a book was published recently in London that lists almost 7,000 titles on back pain alone.* So there is no shortage of information. The challenge is selecting from this mass of data that which has relevance to the orofacial structures and organizing it into a form that can be useful in the clinical management of patients in pain.

This manual is an attempt to do just that: (1) supply sufficient documented information concerning pain behavior that one may better understand what pain is, how it behaves, and what means we have of managing it; (2) develop a more useful classification of orofacial pain syndromes; (3) offer practical diagnostic criteria by which the different pain syndromes can be identified at a clinical level; and (4) suggest

---

*Wyke B.: *A Back Pain Bibliography.* London, Lloyd-Luke Ltd., 1983.

guidelines for the effective management of patients who suffer pain about the mouth and face.

It is with considerable satisfaction and pride that previous editions of this book have been so widely received and used in recent years. The rapid development of new and better information, however, has rendered them obsolete; updating therefore was mandatory. Knowing full well that this too will not be the "final word" in orofacial pain management, it is sincerely hoped that this new third edition will be found to have practical value as a teaching medium at all levels of dental education and as a clinical manual for health care practitioners of all categories who undertake the diagnosis and treatment of patients who suffer pain about the mouth and face.

WELDEN E. BELL
Dallas, Texas

Contents

PREFACE.. vii
LIST OF CASES xiii
DEFINITIONS... xvi

1 / Pain as a Clinical Symptom 1
   Historical Note 2
   Changing Concepts of Pain 3
   Pain as a Symptom 5
   All Pains Are Not Alike 7
   Emergency Nature of Pain 9
   Site of Pain—Source of Pain 10
   Emotional Value of Pain..................................... 11
   Pain Descriptors... 13

2 / Neural Mechanisms of Pain 15
   Phylogenic Considerations.................................. 15
   Neural Structures... 16
   Primary Afferent Neurons................................... 23
   Subnucleus Caudalis 24
   Projection to the Thalamus................................. 25
   Descending Inhibitory System............................. 26
   Neurochemical Effects 26

3 / Peripheral Neural Pathways................................ 32
   Regional Character of Masticatory Function........ 32
   Peripheral Nociceptive Pathways 33
   Somatic Sensory Nerves..................................... 35
   Somatic Motor Nerves....................................... 40
   Visceral Nervous System................................... 41

4 / Pain Modulation 44
   Modulation Concept of Pain 44
   Gate Control Theory 45
   Transcutaneous Electrical Nerve Stimulation....... 53
   Modulating Effect of Nonnoxious Cutaneous Stimulation 54
   Endogenous Antinociceptive System 55
   Acupuncture and Electroacupuncture................. 56
   Psychological Modulating Effects....................... 56

5 / Secondary Effects of Deep Pain 61
   Central Excitatory Effects................................... 61
   Sensory Effects of Deep Pain 64
   Autonomic Effects of Deep Pain 70
   Motor Effects of Deep Pain 70

6 / Genesis of Pain 73
   Pain Induced by Inflammation............................ 73
   Muscular Genesis of Pain 74
   Vascular Genesis of Pain 77
   Neural Genesis of Pain....................................... 78
   Other Causes of Orofacial Pain 83

7 / Classification of Orofacial Pain Syndromes ... 91
Classifications of Pain ... 91
Categories of Orofacial Pain ... 93
Classification of Orofacial Pains ... 100

8 / Cutaneous and Mucogingival Pains ... 102
Cutaneous Pains of the Face ... 102
Mucogingival Pains of the Mouth ... 104
Differential Diagnosis ... 113

9 / Pains of Dental Origin ... 116
Behavior of Dental Pains ... 118
Stimulus-Induced Pulpal Pain ... 120
Pains of Pulpal Origin ... 121
Stimulus-Evoked Periodontal Pain ... 129
Pains of Periodontal Origin ... 130
Secondary Effects of Dental Pain ... 134
Toothaches of Nondental Origin ... 135
Tooth Pain From Secondary Hyperalgesia ... 142

10/ Pains of Muscle Origin ... 144
General Features of Muscle Pain ... 146
Protective Splinting Pain ... 148
Myofascial Trigger Point Pain ... 148
Muscle Spasm Pain ... 160
Muscle Inflammation Pain ... 172
Masticatory Pains of Muscle Origin ... 177

11/ Temporomandibular Joint Pains ... 182
Disc Attachment Pain ... 186
Retrodiscal Pain ... 196
Capsular Pain ... 200
Arthritic Pain ... 205
Differential Diagnosis ... 225

12/ Other Musculoskeletal Pains ... 229
Osseous Pains ... 229
Periosteal Pains ... 232
Soft Connective Tissue Pains ... 233

13/ Vascular Pains ... 236
Behavior of Visceral Pain ... 237
Vascular Pains of the Mouth and Face ... 238
Migrainous Neuralgia ... 243
Atypical Odontalgia ... 252
Common Migraine ... 253
Classic Migraine ... 253
Vascular Inflammation Pain ... 254

14/ Other Visceral Pains ... 257
Primary Pains of Visceral Mucosa ... 257
Pharyngeal Mucosa Pain ... 260
Nasal Mucosa Pain ... 261
Paranasal Sinus Pain ... 264

Contents

    Glandular Pains of the Mouth and Face 266
    Ocular Pains... 266
    Auricular Pains 268

15/ Neurogenous Pains 271
    Neuropathic Pains of the Mouth and Face 271
    Traumatic Neuroma Pain.. 274
    Paroxysmal Neuralgia 279
    Neuritic Neuralgia.. 292
    Deafferentation Pains of the Mouth and Face 301

16/ Chronicity and Psychogenic Pains 311
    Chronic Structural Pain 311
    Chronic Functional Pain 316
    Symptoms of Chronicity... 317
    Chronic Pain Behavior 318
    Conversion Hysteria Pains 320
    Delusional Pains 321

17/ Examination and Diagnosis 325
    Preliminary Interview.. 326
    Charting the Examination 327
    History.. 329
    McGill Pain Questionnaire....................................... 333
    Tentative Clinical Diagnosis 334
    Neurologic Survey... 334
    Psychologic Survey.. 337
    Pain Examination.. 338
    Identifying the Proper Pain Category.............................. 345
    Confirmation of Clinical Diagnosis 348
    Confirmed Working Diagnosis 354

18/ Management of Patients in Pain 356
    Treatment Modalities 357
    Cause-Related Therapy 358
    Sensory Stimulation 359
    Analgesic Blocking 363
    Physiotherapy 365
    Relaxation 366
    Placebo Therapy 369
    Psychotherapy... 369
    Neurosurgery.. 371
    Medicinal Therapy 373
    Dietary Supplement Therapy 379
    Therapeutic Guidelines 380
    Pains of Cutaneous and Mucogingival Origin 381
    Pains of Dental Origin 382
    Pains of Muscle Origin (including masticatory muscle pain) 382
    Temporomandibular Joint Pains.................................. 382
    Other Musculoskeletal Pains (osseous, periosteal, soft ct.) 383
    Vascular Pains 383
    Other Visceral Pains (mucosal, glandular, eye, ear)................ 384

Neurogenous Pains (neuropathy pains, deafferentation pains) 384
Chronic and Psychogenic Pains 385
Masticatory Myalgia 385
Do's and Don'ts of Muscle Exercise Therapy 386

INDEX 393

List of Cases

Case No. 9–1
　Heterotopic pain, felt as toothache, referred from the masseter
　muscle..137
Case No. 9–2
　Heterotopic pain, felt as toothache, referred from the cardiac
　muscle..139
Case No. 10–1
　Masticatory myalgia, expressed as spasm of elevator muscles
　(pain-dysfunction syndrome)..167
Case No. 10–2
　Masticatory myalgia, expressed as spasm of the lateral pterygoid
　muscle (pain-dysfunction syndrome)......................................171
Case No. 10–3
　Masticatory myalgia, expressed as spasm of elevator and lateral
　pterygoid muscles (pain-dysfunction syndrome)..........................173
Case No. 10-4
　Masticatory myalgia, expressed as inflammation of elevator muscles
　(masticatory myositis)..176
Case No. 10-5
　Masticatory myalgia, expressed as inflammation of elevator muscles
　(inflamed myofibrotic contracture).......................................178
Case No. 11-1
　Temporomandibular arthralgia, expressed as disc attachment pain,
　due to acute discitis..191
Case No. 11–2
　Temporomandibular arthralgia, expressed as retrodiscal pain,
　due to trauma..198
Case No. 11–3
　Temporomandibular arthralgia, expressed as capsular pain,
　due to trauma..201
Case No. 11–4
　Temporomandibular arthralgia, expressed as capsular pain,
　due to inflamed capsular fibrosis...204
Case No. 11–5
　Temporomandibular arthralgia, expressed as arthritic pain, due to
　inflammatory degenerative joint disease.................................214
Case No. 11–6
　Temporomandibular arthralgia, expressed as arthritic pain, due to
　hyperuricemia..216
Case No. 11–7
　Temporomandibular arthralgia, expressed as arthritic pain,
　due to inflamed fibrous ankylosis..218
Case No. 11–8
　Temporomandibular arthralgia, expressed as arthritic pain,
　due to an invasive malignant tumor......................................224

xiii

Case No. 13–1
Heterotopic pain, felt as toothache, due to a vascular pain syndrome (migrainous neuralgia)..246

Case No. 13–2
Masticatory myospasm pain (pain-dysfunction syndrome), secondary to deep vascular pain (migrainous neuralgia)..............249

Case No. 13–3
Vascular pain (migrainous neuralgia), mistaken for masticatory pain...251

Case No. 14–1
Heterotopic pain, felt as toothache, referred from inflamed nasal mucosa (so-called sinus headache)....................................264

Case No. 14–2
Heterotopic pain, felt as preauricular pain, referred from inflamed submandibular gland..267

Case No. 14–3
Heterotopic pain, felt as preauricular pain, due to trigger point pain affecting the sternocleidomastoid muscle........................269

Case No. 15–1
Traumatic neuroma pain, located in edentulous mucogingival tissue (postsurgical) 276

Case No. 15–2
Traumatic neuroma pain, located in the temporomandibular joint (posttraumatic)..277

Case No. 15–3
Paroxysmal neuralgia of the auriculotemporal nerve, mistaken for masticatory pain 283

Case No. 15–4
Paroxysmal neuralgia of the maxillary nerve, mistaken for masticatory pain 284

Case No. 15–5
Paroxysmal neuralgia of the mandibular nerve, mistaken for dental pain...285

Case No. 15–6
Paroxysmal neuralgia of the glossopharyngeal nerve, mistaken for masticatory pain 287

Case No. 15–7
Neuritic neuralgia of the superior alveolar nerve, due to maxillary sinusitis, expressed as maxillary toothache 295

Case No. 15–8
Neuritic neuralgia of the inferior alveolar nerve, expressed as mandibular toothache 297

Case No. 15–9
Neuritic neuralgia of the glossopharyngeal nerve, due to fractured styloid process, mistaken for masticatory pain........................299

Case No. 15–10
Herpes zoster involving the mandibular nerve, expressed intraorally..302
Case No. 15–11
Deafferentation syndrome, expressed as sensory aberrations (postsurgical) 304
Case No. 15–12
Deafferentation syndrome, expressed as mandibular toothache (posttraumatic)...307
Case No. 15–13
Deafferentation syndrome, expressed as reflex sympathetic dystrophy, mistaken for masticatory pain (postsurgical)...............308
Case No. 16–1
Psychogenic pain, expressed as conversion hysteria, mistaken for structural masticatory pain 322

Definitions

TERMS THAT COMPRISE the language of pain should be defined precisely enough to prevent ambiguity and misunderstandings. Many of the definitions listed below are based on terminology proposed by the Subcommittee on Taxonomy of the International Association for the Study of Pain.[1,2] Some are from a standard medical dictionary.[3] A few are specially defined to express precise meaning by the author. The reader is urged to become familiar with these definitions.

ALLODYNIA—Pain that occurs *without noxious stimulation* at the site of pain.
[Note: This term applies broadly to all painful sensations regardless of location that occur in the absence of noxious simulation at the site of pain. This would apply therefore to spontaneous pain regardless of etiology and to pain evoked by nonnoxious stimulation.]

ANALGESIA—Absence of sensibility to pain.
[Note: Other sensibilities may remain present.]

ANESTHESIA—Absence of all sensation.

ANESTHESIA DOLOROSA—Pain in an area that is anesthetic as the result of deafferentation.

CAUSALGIA—A syndrome of unremitting, burning pain as the result of deafferentation. Reflex sympathetic dystrophy.

CENTRAL PAIN—Pain associated with a lesion of the CNS.

DEAFFERENTATION—The effect of eliminating afferent neural activity due to interrupted neurons.

DENERVATION—Resection of or removal of the nerves to an organ or part.

DYSESTHESIA—An *unpleasant* abnormal sensation.
[Note: Paresthesia is an abnormal sensation whether unpleasant or not. Paresthesia includes dysesthesia, but not vice versa.]

HETEROTOPIC PAIN—A general term to designate pain that is felt in an area other than its true site of origin.
[Note: Peripheral heterotopic pain may be felt as projected pain, referred pain, or secondary hyperalgesia.]

HYPALGESIA—Diminished sensitivity to stimulation-evoked pain.

HYPERALGESIA—Increased sensitivity to stimulation-evoked pain.
[Note: *Primary* hyperalgesia is stimulation-evoked primary pain due to lowered local pain threshold. *Secondary* hyperalgesia is stimulation-evoked heterotopic pain that occurs without appreciable change in local pain threshold.]

HYPERESTHESIA—Increased sensitivity to stimulation.
[Note: When sensation is painful, the terms *allodynia* and *hyperalgesia* are appropriate.]

HYPOESTHESIA—Diminished sensitivity to stimulation.
[Note: When sensation is painful, the terms *hypalgesia* and *analgesia* are appropriate.]

INFLAMMATORY PAIN—Pain that emanates from tissue that is inflamed.

MUSCULOSKELETAL PAIN—Deep somatic pain that originates in skeletal muscles, fascial sheaths, and tendons (myogenous pain); in bones and periosteum (osseous pain); in joints, joint capsules, and ligaments (arthralgic pain); and in soft connective tissues (soft connective tissue pain).

MYALGIA—Pain that is *felt* in muscle tissue.
[Note: If such site of pain represents the source, the myalgia would be myogenous; otherwise, it would be heterotopic.]

MYOFASCIAL TRIGGER POINT—A hyperirritable spot, usually within a taut band of skeletal muscle or in the muscle fascia, that is painful on compression and that can give rise to characteristic referred pain, tenderness (secondary hyperalgesia), and autonomic phenomena.[4]

MYOGENOUS PAIN—Deep somatic musculoskeletal pain that originates in skeletal muscles, fascial sheaths, or tendons.
[Note: Several types of myogenous pain are identifiable clinically: (1) protective muscle splinting pain, (2) myofascial trigger point pain, (3) muscle spasm pain, and (4) muscle inflammation pain.]

NEURALGIA—Neurogenous pain felt along the peripheral distribution of a nerve trunk.
[Note: Paroxysmal neuralgia consists of sudden bursts of burning pain. Neuritic neuralgia is persistent, unremitting burning pain.]

NEUROGENOUS PAIN—Pain that is generated within the nervous system due to some abnormality of neural structures.

NEUROPATHY—A general term used to designate an abnormality or pathologic change in a peripheral nerve.

NOCICEPTIVE PATHWAY—An afferent neural pathway that mediates pain impulses.

NOCICEPTOR—A sensory receptor preferentially sensitive to noxious or potentially noxious stimuli.

NOXIOUS STIMULUS—A tissue-damaging stimulus.

ODONTALGIA—Pain that is *felt* in a tooth.
[Note: If the tooth is the source of the pain, the odontalgia would be odontogenous; if not, it would be heterotopic.]

ODONTOGENOUS PAIN—Deep somatic pain that originates in dental pulps, periodontal ligaments, or both.

PAIN—An unpleasant sensory and emotional experience associated with actual or potential tissue damage, or described in terms of such damage.
[Note: Pain is always subjective. If the subject reports his experience as pain, it should be accepted as pain.]

PAIN THRESHOLD—The least stimulus intensity at which a subject perceives pain.

PAIN TOLERANCE LEVEL—The greatest stimulus intensity that a subject is prepared to tolerate.

PARESTHESIA—An abnormal sensation, whether spontaneous or evoked. [Note: If an abnormal sensation is unpleasant, the term *dysesthesia* is appropriate.]

PERIODONTAL PAIN—Odontogenous pain that emanates from the periodontal ligaments.

PRIMARY PAIN—Pain that identifies the true source of nociceptive input.

PROJECTED PAIN—Heterotopic pain that is felt in the anatomical peripheral distribution of the same nerve that mediates the primary pain.

PULPAL PAIN—Odontogenous pain that emanates from the dental pulps.

REFERRED PAIN—Heterotopic pain that is felt in an area that is innervated by a nerve different from the one that mediates the primary pain. [Note: The term *referred pain* implies that it occurs without provocation at the site of pain.]

REFLEX SYMPATHETIC DYSTROPHY—A syndrome of unremitting, burning pain as the result of deafferentation. Causalgia.

SECONDARY HYPERALGESIA—Heterotopic pain that is evoked by stimulation at the site of pain.

SECONDARY PAIN—Heterotopic referred pain and/or secondary hyperalgesia induced by deep somatic pain as a central excitatory effect.

SITE OF PAIN—The anatomical site where pain is *felt*.

VASCULAR PAIN—A type of deep somatic pain of visceral origin that emanates from the afferent nerves that innervate blood vessels. [Note: Inflammatory vascular pain should be designated as vasculitis (arteritis, phlebitis.)]

VISCERAL PAIN—Deep somatic pain that originates in visceral structures such as mucosal linings, walls of hollow viscera, parenchyma of organs, glands, dental pulps, and vascular structures.

REFERENCES

1. Merskey H.: Pain terms: A list with definitions and notes on usage. *Pain* 6:249, 1979.
2. Merskey H.: Pain terms: A supplementary note. *Pain* 14:205, 1982.
3. *Dorland's Illustrated Medical Dictionary*, ed. 26. Philadelphia, W.B. Saunders Co., 1981.
4. Travell J.G., Simons D.G.: *Myofascial Pain and Dysfunction.* Baltimore, Williams & Wilkins Co., 1983.

1

Pain as a Clinical Symptom

PAIN IS AN EXPERIENCE that cannot be shared; it is wholly personal, belonging to the sufferer alone. Different individuals sensing identical noxious stimulation feel pain in different ways and react at different levels of suffering. It is impossible for one person to sense exactly what another feels. Therefore, the examiner, knowing only how his own pain feels and what such suffering means to him, is faced with the task of securing from the patient enough information to help him imagine how the pain feels to that person and what meaning it has for him. The ability to diagnose and treat a person afflicted with pain rests largely on a knowledge of the mechanisms and behavioral characteristics of pain in its various manifestations.

Upon the dentist rests a great burden of responsibility for the proper management of pains in and about the mouth, face, and neck. He must therefore be competent to differentiate between pains that stem from dental, oral, and masticatory sources and those that emanate elsewhere. He must become expert in pain diagnosis so as to choose the complaints that are manageable by dental methods and techniques and should be approached on a dental level. He must be able to positively identify complaints that may relate to oral and masticatory functioning but which in fact stem from causes that cannot reasonably be resolved by dental procedures. Such complaints require treatment on a medical level.

The dentist's responsibility in managing pain problems of the mouth and face is twofold. His initial responsibility is diagnostic. He should identify those complaints that are correctable by dental therapy. To do this, he must have accurate knowledge of pain problems arising from other than oral and masticatory sources. If he cannot make a proper diagnosis, it becomes his responsibility to refer the patient to someone he thinks competent in that field of practice.

The second responsibility of the dentist relates to therapy. Once the pain complaint is correctly identified as a condition amenable to dental therapy, treatment by the dentist is in order. Whether consultation with another practitioner is needed should be considered in the treatment planning. If therapy at any point does not prove effective as planned, it becomes the dentist's responsibility to seek the cause of failure, using, if needed, the aid of colleagues. If the condition presented is clearly one that would not be amenable to dental therapy, the patient should be referred to the appropriate medical practitioner.

Many pain problems are such that interdisciplinary management is needed. Such problems require a good working relationship between the doctors represented. It is important that the dentist understand what his responsibilities are in the case so that he can conduct his portion of the therapy effectively. He should exercise care not to attempt more than his fraction of responsibility calls for; nor should he relinquish what should legitimately be his. A positive, confident competence tempered by a reasonable and cooperative attitude should properly equip him to work effectively in any multidisciplinary environment, whether it be wholly dental or dental and medical combined.

HISTORICAL NOTE

Merskey[1] has reviewed some of the historical background of modern pain concepts. In ancient times, Homer thought that pain was due to arrows shot by the gods. The feeling that pain is inflicted from without seems to be a primitive instinct that has persisted to some degree down through the ages. Aristotle, who probably was the first to distinguish the five physical senses, considered pain to be a "passion of the soul" that somehow resulted from the intensification of other sensory experience. Plato contended that pain and pleasure arose from within the body, an idea that perhaps gave birth to the concept that pain is an emotional experience more than a localized body disturbance.

The Bible makes reference to pain not only in relationship to injury and illness but also as anguish of the soul. Hebrew words used to express grief, sorrow, and pain are used rather interchangeably in the old scriptures.[2] This implies that the early Hebrews considered pain to be a manifestation of concerns that lead also to grief and sorrow. As knowledge of anatomy and physiology increased, however, it became possible to distinguish between pains due to physical and emotional causes.

During the 19th century the developing knowledge of neurology fostered the concept that pain was mediated by specific pain pathways and not simply due to excessive stimulation of the special senses.

More recently, it has come to be known that strict specificity of neural structures for the mediation of pain impulses is not present. Freud developed the idea that physical symptoms could result from thought processes. He considered that such symptoms as pain could develop as a solution to emotional conflicts.

It can be seen therefore that, until very recent years, concepts concerning pain have changed but little since ancient times.

CHANGING CONCEPTS OF PAIN

The definition of pain found in the medical dictionary summarizes very well the traditional understanding of what pain is like: "A more or less localized sensation of discomfort, distress, or agony, resulting from the stimulation of specialized nerve endings. It serves as a protective mechanism insofar as it induces the sufferer to remove or withdraw from the source."[3] This definition identifies pain as a localized sensation that occurs as the result of stimulation—noxious stimulation. It is mediated by way of specialized neural structures that are made for that purpose. It serves as a protective mechanism against injury; being external to the body, the presumed noxious agent could be avoided by proper evasive action. Such definition actually describes only one type of pain: superficial somatic pain—that which occurs as the result of noxious stimulation of cutaneous structures by an environmentally located agent that affects the exteroceptive nociceptors.

During recent years, quite a different concept of pain has evolved. Although the usefulness of pain as a protective mechanism is recognized with regard to purely exteroceptive noxious stimulation, most pain occurs *too late* to have much protective value. It has to do with events that have already taken place.

Pain now is considered to be more than a sensation. It constitutes an experience that involves both sensation and emotion. The sensory dimension registers the nature of the stimulus; the emotional property disrupts ongoing behavior and drives the subject into activities to alleviate it. Pain also involves neocortical processes (attention, anxiety, suggestion) that provide control over both systems.[4] This is considerably more complex than pure sensation such as touch. It is more akin to need-states such as hunger and thirst; it initiates a drive for action. Pain cannot be sensed in a detached manner; it comes in combination with dislike, anxiety, fear, and urgency.[5] Although pain does result from noxious stimulation, it occurs also from nonnoxious stimuli, as well as spontaneously when there is no stimulus at all. The source of stimulation need not be external to the body.

The newer concept of what constitutes pain is expressed in the definition proposed by the Subcommittee on Taxonomy of the International Association For the Study of Pain: "An unpleasant sensory and emotional experience associated with actual or potential tissue damage, or described in terms of such damage."[6] By this definition, pain is understood to represent a subjective psychological state rather than an activity that is induced solely by noxious stimulation. It should be noted that, if the subject regards his experience as pain, it should be accepted as pain.

More precisely, pain as presently conceived has a sensory-discriminative dimension to identify the form of energy (thermal, mechanical, chemical) and the spatial, temporal, and intensive aspects of the stimulus. It also has a motivational-affective property by which the consequences of the experience become manifest as escape and avoidance behavior which includes reflex somatic and autonomic motor responses.[7]

When identifiable cause can be established for pain, management usually entails measures to eliminate such cause if possible. Some pains, however, are behavioral and therefore are *learned*. Such pains may confuse the doctor who is stimulus-response oriented and thinks in terms of cause. Many times, however, the consequences of the experience become the paramount issue in managing the pain problem. In such cases the proper manipulation of various environmental factors may help the patient *unlearn* his pain behavior.[8]

It is interesting to note that the more severe the pain and the more distressed the patient, the more emotional are his responses and the greater the impact on his ability to function.[9] The pressure to seek aid for a pain problem increases when the patient is under greater than usual stress. It seems to be more reasonable to assume that subjects try to escape from stress by using illness behavior than that the stress causes such behavior. It seems that those who find their life situation satisfactory tend to ignore symptoms.[10]

It has also been observed that the intensity of pain from physical injury relates to the attention given at the time. Pain and injury are coincident only when attention is directed specifically to the injury. If one's attention is fully absorbed at the time of injury, no pain at all may be felt. The subject may remain relatively free of pain if he is distracted by events having to do with self-preservation, fighting back, escaping, or obtaining aid. Pain may not become an issue until the consequences of the injury induce feelings of concern and anxiety that relate more to therapy and recovery processes than to the injury itself.[11]

With the changing concepts of pain represented in body, mind, and person, the diagnosis and management of such problems require a broad understanding of people on the part of the attending doctor.

Good therapy begins with an attitude of *caring*—concern for the person more than for his body. Human beings are more than patients that have to be treated.[12] Loren Pilling has said, "I don't treat pain. I treat people."

PAIN AS A SYMPTOM

Pain Intensity

Severity of pain is more a measure of the suffering it induces than the actual perception of noxious stimulation. This is referable more to the meaning the sensation has for the sufferer than a true indication of its seriousness. Low-intensity pain may stem from very serious causes, whereas maximum-intensity pain such as tic douloureux may arise from imperceptible causes. Although pain intensity relates to the urgency for instituting therapy, it should not be taken as an accurate measure of the seriousness of its cause.

Pain may be judged subjectively or objectively. Subjective evaluation depends on the patient's description of the complaint and reflects the examiner's ability to conduct a proper interview. Objective evaluation relates to what the pain does to the patient physically, as manifested by changes in the vital signs, skin color, pupil size, gland effects, and muscle effects. This reflects the accuracy of the examiner's clinical examination. Pain intensity may be classified as mild if evident only subjectively. Objective evidence of pain should cause the intensity to be classified as severe.

It should be noted that there is a definite relationship between intensity and duration of pain. The higher the intensity, the shorter the period it can be tolerated by the sufferer. Low-intensity pain can be sustained for up to seven hours, whereas maximum-intensity pain can be tolerated for no more than a few seconds. The higher the intensity, the more likely it is that the pain will be intermittent. Only low-intensity pain can be protracted. Intractable pain, regardless of the patient's contention to the contrary, must be either periodic or of extremely low intensity. In fact, intractable pain may not be pain at all but simply an unpleasant or unwanted sensation.[13, 14]

Temporal Behavior

The onset of pain is described as spontaneous, induced, or triggered. It is classed as *spontaneous* when the pain occurs without being provoked. It is *induced* when some particular provocation causes the painful sensation. Pain is said to be *triggered* when the evoked response is out of proportion to the stimulus.

The manner of onset has diagnostic value and forms part of the behavioral characteristics of certain pain syndromes. The manner of onset should not be confused with conditions that increase or decrease the painful sensation after it is started.

A single *episode* or period of painful experience may last from a few moments to many weeks or months, during which time the pains occur at sufficient frequency to establish a temporal relationship. During such an episode, the individual pains that make up the episode are either intermittent or continuous. Pains of short duration and separated by wholly pain-free periods are described as *intermittent*. Pains of longer duration, even though of variable intensity, are called *continuous*. Classifying pain in this manner implies of course the true nature of the pain, not influenced by medications or conditions that normally increase or decrease pain severity. A painful episode that lasts for several days or more is usually described as *protracted*. Pain that does not respond to therapy is called *intractable*. Two or more similar episodes of pain are termed *recurrent*. The pain-free interval between recurring episodes is called a *remission*. Pain that is characterized by regularly recurring episodes is said to be *periodic*.

Quality of Sensation

Apart from intensity and temporal behavior of pain are other qualities that help to describe them. The terms *steady* and *paroxysmal* relate to the quality of the painful sensation that makes up an individual pain. A *steady* pain flows as an unpleasant sensation, in contrast to *paroxysmal* pain, which is a volley of jabs. *Bright* pain has a stimulating quality, whereas *dull* pain is depressing. Either may be punctuated by sharp, lancinating, or radiating exacerbations. Pain may also be described as spreading, enlarging or migrating as it concerns the area where the sensation is felt.

The character of painful sensation may be classified as itching, pricking, stinging, burning, aching, or throbbing. *Itching* is subthreshold pain and usually is not described as pain at all. It may have a warm or even burning quality and can become intractable. When induced by light superficial movement, this sensation is usually called *tickle*. *Pricking* pain has a sharp intermittent character of short duration like pin pricking the skin. Sustained pricking sensation occurs as when one's leg "goes to sleep." *Stinging* pain has a more continuous, higher-intensity smarting quality. *Burning* pain connotes a feeling of warmth or heat like "pepper in the tissues." When short and intense, it may have an electric shock feeling. *Aching* is the usual "garden variety" painful sensation and is the descriptive term most frequently used unless the pain is overshadowed by one of the other characteristic sensations. *Throbbing* or *pulsatile* pain is timed to the cardiac systoles.

ALL PAINS ARE NOT ALIKE

Clinical vs. Experimental Pain

Beecher[15] has pointed out that pain as presented by patients, so-called clinical or pathologic pain, is different from experimental pain induced and studied in the laboratory. The difference is illustrated in the capacity of morphine to give relief. A large dose of morphine does not significantly alter the brief jabs of experimental pain, while a much smaller dose consistently reduces pain that has meaning to the patient. The difference is also borne out in placebo effects. Beecher determined that the average effectiveness of placebos when dealing with clinical pain was about 35%, whereas it was only 3.2% with experimental pain. Nyquist and Eriksson,[16] in commenting on this problem, said, "We interpret our findings to suggest that clinical and experimental pain are explained by different mechansims and that direct correlations cannot be drawn between them."

It seems likely that the emotional significance embodied in clinical pain is the real determinant. Indeed, the purpose of the signal detection (sensory decision) theory for determining the effectiveness of analgesic medications is to minimize this bias factor.[17,18]

Acute vs. Chronic Pain

As the duration of pain input continues, the level of suffering increases even though the intensity of input remains the same. In fact, protracted input may sustain a high level of discomfort although the intensity decreases or disappears altogether. It follows that a sustained level of discomfort may remain after the initiating cause has regressed or resolved. With chronicity, all pains regardless of initial type or origin seem to take on the clinical characteristics of psychogenic intensification. As such, well-established chronic orofacial pain syndromes display features suggestive of depressive illness. Treatment measures effective for alleviating acute pain are no longer applicable. As pain becomes chronic, management options shift from local to systemic modalities. Pain that initially could be managed on a purely dental level may require extensive and coordinated interdisciplinary therapy when it becomes chronic.

Somatic vs. Neurogenous Pain

Pain emanating from a particular area may result from noxious stimulation of the somatic structures, the nociceptive impulses being received and transmitted by normal components of the sensory nervous system. Such pain is referred to as *somatic pain*. It presents clinical characteristics that relate to the effect of stimulation of normal neural structures. Quite a different type of pain, however, may emanate from the same area due, not to abnormality in the structures that comprise the area, but to abnormality in the neural components that innervate the area. Such pain is termed *neurogenous*. It presents clinical characteristics that relate to the type and location of neural abnormality rather than to noxious stimulation as such.

Superficial vs. Deep Somatic Pain

Pains emanating from the cutaneous and mucogingival tissues present clinical characteristics that are similar to other exteroceptive sensations. They are precisely localizable and relate faithfully to provocation in timing, location, and intensity. In contrast, pains due to stimulation of deeper somatic and visceral structures resemble other proprioceptive and interoceptive sensations. As such, they are more diffusely felt, are less faithfully responsive to provocation, and frequently initiate secondary effects such as referred pain and muscle spasm activity.

Primary vs. Secondary Pain

The site where pain is felt may or may not identify the location of the source of pain. If the pain does in fact emanate from the structures that hurt, it constitutes a primary nociceptive input. If, however, the true source of pain is located elsewhere, and the heterotopic referred pain or secondary hyperalgesia is felt in otherwise normal structures, the area of discomfort represents secondary pain, a manifestation of deep somatic pain input.

Musculoskeletal vs. Visceral Pain

All deep somatic pains are not alike. That which emanates from muscles, bones, joints, tendons, ligaments, and soft connective tissue bears a close relationship to the demands of biomechanical function. Such pain also yields a graduated response to noxious stimulation. Visceral structures, however, are innervated by high-threshold receptors so that pain usually is not felt until threshold level is reached. Such pains therefore do not ordinarily yield a graduated response to noxious stimulation and are not responsive to biomechanical function.

Inflammatory vs. Noninflammatory Pain

Tissue injury and healing are attended by an inflammatory reaction that includes pain. Such pain relates to the location, type, and phase of the inflammatory process that prevails. Inflammatory pains therefore display a clinical time frame that relates to the inflammatory curve and symptoms that relate to the confinement of inflammatory exudate. Noninflammatory pains do not display this type of pain behavior.

Stimulus-Evoked vs. Spontaneous Pain

Most primary somatic pain results from stimulation of neural structures that innervate the site. The actual stimulus may be obscure and positive identification difficult, but the clinical characteristics displayed by stimulus-evoked pain relate to the location, timing, and intensity of such stimulus. Some pains, however, occur spontaneously and do not require a stimulating force. Neurogenous pain may be felt spontaneously along the peripheral distribution of the affected nerve, while referred pains may occur spontaneously as far as the site of pain is concerned.

EMERGENCY NATURE OF PAIN

Pain creates for the patient an emergency and therefore becomes a prime motivating cause for seeking aid. When the suffering occurs in and about the mouth, the dentist is usually the first to be called. When it occurs about the ears, face, head, or neck, a physician may be consulted. The actual location of the symptom may well determine who

ence therefore has deep religious and moral roots that affect human attitudes even today.

Depending on past emotional experience, especially from childhood, one may use pain to gain attention, substitute for other forms of aggression, or express grief.[20] We may recognize in a demanding patient his frustration that the pain has not gained for him as much attention as he needs.

The emotional significance of oral and facial pain has important implications, especially in relation to concepts of body image. Distortion of this image due to injury or surgery may initiate pain that persists long after the cause has ceased, and such factors must be considered when these pains are evaluated. Pain induced by emotions tends to become chronic. If it persists as long as six months, it may become too "valuable" to give up.

Pain has other emotional values. It commonly excuses one from carrying out an unpleasant task. Headaches have been used frequently as socially acceptable excuses. Pain may serve as a means of avoiding responsibilities, the actual physical pain being the lesser of the two forms of suffering. To be the "center of attention" may in some cases be ego-building. Pain, as with other illness, can be used as a weapon or threat against those over whom the subject would have his way. Thus the "victim" not only becomes defenseless against his pain-ridden aggressor but frequently is made to suffer with him.

Pain may become a dependable crutch to sustain the subject in a variety of emotional situations, many of which he may be responding to wholly subconsciously. It may be a form of malingering to avoid duty. Sometimes it represents justification for addiction to narcotic drugs.

Early in the management of a patient with a pain complaint, the doctor must ask himself several questions, and effective treatment may depend much on the answers he is able to find:

1. Does the patient really hurt? Is this real pain or simply an unpleasant, unwanted sensation?
2. Is the suffering bona fide, occurring realistically in response to the noxious stimulation that initiates it? Or does the suffering serve the patient in some beneficial way, conscious or subconscious? If the benefit appears to be conscious, is it a "game" or is it malingering? If the benefit is subconscious, does the patient need medical consultation on an emotional level?
3. Does the patient want *relief* from his suffering or does he seek only attention and sympathy?

PAIN DESCRIPTORS

Words used by patients to describe their pains have been studied and classified by Melzack.[21] This work has led to the McGill Pain Questionnaire, which may be used to help evaluate pain. Formerly, most measurement of pain dealt only with intensity. It is evident that pain has other qualities that enter into a judgment concerning its true meaning to patients. These can be described subjectively if the patient has at his disposal the proper means of communication.

The descriptors used in the McGill Pain Questionaire are organized and arranged in such a manner as to be useful in obtaining information that is accurate. These descriptors are arranged in classes composed of several groups. Each group is arranged in a series in the order of increasing intensity. The descriptors are classified as sensory, affective, evaluative, and miscellaneous. In each series only one word is chosen, the word that *best* describes the complaint. If none in a series is truly applicable, none should be selected.

By using such lists of descriptors a patient is able to communicate important subjective information to the doctor. Thus, intensity levels can be estimated more accurately. It also helps to determine the effectiveness of therapy and the general progress of pain management.

REFERENCES

1. Merskey H.: Some features of the history of the idea of pain. *Pain* 9:3, 1980.
2. Strong J.: *Strong's Exhaustive Concordance of the Bible.* Grand Rapids, Mich., Associated Publishers and Authors, Inc.
3. *Dorland's Illustrated Medical Dictionary,* ed. 26. Philadelphia, W.B. Saunders Co., 1981.
4. Melzack R.: Psychological concepts and methods for the control of pain, in Bonica J.J. (ed.): *Advances in Neurology.* New York, Raven Press, 1974, vol. 4, pp. 275–280.
5. Wall P.D.: Why do we not understand pain? in Duncan R., Weston-Smith M. (eds.): *The Encyclopaedia of Ignorance.* Oxford, Pergamon Press, 1977, pp. 361—368.
6. Merskey H.: Pain terms: A list with definitions and notes on usage. *Pain* 6:249–252, 1979.
7. Price D.D., Dubner R.: Neurons that subserve the sensory-discriminative aspects of pain. *Pain* 3:307–338, 1977.
8. Fordyce W.E.: Pain viewed as learned behavior, in Bonica J.J. (ed.): *Advances in Neurology.* New York, Raven Press, 1974, vol. 4, pp. 415–422.
9. Lipton J.A., Marbach J.J.: Components of the response to pain and variables influencing the response in three groups of facial pain patients. *Pain* 16:343–359, 1983.

10. Marbach J.J., Lipton J.A.: Aspects of illness behavior in patients with facial pain. *J.A.D.A.* 96:630, 1976.
11. Wall P.D.: On the relation of injury to pain. *Pain* 6:253–264, 1979.
12. Degenaar J.J.: Some philosophical considerations on pain. *Pain* 7:281–304, 1979.
13. Dalessio D.J.: *Wolff's Headache and Other Head Pain*, ed. 3. New York, Oxford University Press, 1972.
14. Wolff H.G., Wolf S.: *Pain*, ed. 2. Springfield, Ill., Charles C Thomas, Publisher, 1958.
15. Beecher H.K.: The use of chemical agents in the control of pain, in Knighton R.S., Dumke P.R. (eds.): *Pain*. Boston, Little, Brown & Co., 1966, pp. 221–239.
16. Nyquist J.K., Eriksson M.B.E.: Effects of pain treatment procedures on thermal sensibility in chronic pain patients. *Pain*, suppl. 1, 1981, p. S91.
17. Chapman C.R.: An alternative to threshold assessment in the study of human pain, in Bonica J.J. (ed.): *Advances in Neurology*. New York, Raven Press, 1974, vol. 4, pp. 115–121.
18. Clark W.D.: Pain sensitivity and the report of pain: An introduction to sensory decision theory. *Anesthesiology* 40:171, 1974.
19. Bonica J.J.: *The Management of Pain*. Philadelphia, Lea & Febiger, 1953.
20. Pilling L.F.: Psychosomatic aspects of facial pain, in Alling C.C., Mahan P.E. (eds.): *Facial Pain*, ed. 2 Philadelphia, Lea & Febiger, 1977, pp. 213–226.
21. Melzack R.: The McGill Pain Questionnaire: Major properties and scoring methods. *Pain* 1:277–299, 1975.

2

Neural Mechanisms of Pain

THE CENTRAL AND PERIPHERAL MECHANISMS of nociception are extremely complex and only partially understood. It is known that about half the fibers of dorsal (sensory) and a significant number (perhaps as many as 20%) of the fibers of ventral (motor) spinal roots are nociceptive. Most nociceptors are polymodal, transmitting encoded information on stimulus intensity. There is no "pain center" in the central nervous system (CNS) as with the special senses. Motor and sympathetic reflex responses occur in the spinal cord. The limbic system has to do with emotional reactions. The neocortex controls the cognitive components of pain behavior. Zimmermann[1] states: "We are far from having a coherent picture of central pain physiology."

PHYLOGENIC CONSIDERATIONS

Man has what amounts to three brains: (1) the old reptilian brain constituting the spinal cord and medulla, (2) the primitive mammalian brain constituting the limbic structures, and (3) the neocortex of primates, which is phylogenetically more recent. The cord and medulla facilitate automatic function and reflex activities. This has influence on pain reaction in that nociceptive input may be reacted to reflexly. The limbic structures function especially with regard to instinctive and emotional responses to noxious input. Primates, however, are endowed with neocortical structures that account for such mental processes as thought, concepts, judgment, and decision making.

Man reacts to pain on a reflex and emotional level. But, in addition, he reacts in accordance with what he considers to be the consequences of the pain. The significance he attaches to the painful experience will color and change his whole reactive behavior. Consequences induce marked facilitory and inhibitory influence on the experience of pain and may become the dominant determinant in total suffering and reactive behavior.

NEURAL STRUCTURES

Nerve Cell or Neuron

A nerve is a cordlike structure that conveys nervous impulses. It consists of a connective tissue sheath called *epineurium*, which encloses bundles (fasciculi) of nerve fibers, each bundle being surrounded by its own connective tissue sheath called *perineurium*. Within each bundle the nerve fibers are separated by interstitial connective tissue called *endoneurium*.

An individual nerve fiber consists of a central bundle of neurofibrils in a matrix of nerve protoplasm called *axoplasm* and enclosed in a thin nerve tissue plasma membrane called *axolemma*. Each peripheral nerve fiber is covered by a cellular nerve tissue sheath called *neurolemma* (primary sheath or sheath of Schwann). Some of these fibers also have a layer of fatty nerve tissue called the *myelin sheath* (medullary sheath or white substance of Schwann). Fibers with myelin sheaths form the "white nerves," those without myelin sheaths the "gray nerves." Constrictions called nodes of Ranvier occur in myelinated nerves at intervals of about 1 mm. These nodes are caused by the absence of myelin material so that only neurolemma covers the nerve fiber. Nerve fibers in the CNS have no neurolemma. Those situated in the white substance are myelinated, whereas those in the gray substance are nonmyelinated. The ultrastructure of the primary trigeminal neuron is now well known,[2] thanks to the use of electron microscopic techniques.

The structural unit of the nervous system is the nerve cell or neuron. It is composed of a mass of protoplasm termed the nerve cell body (perikaryon), which contains a spherical nucleus (karyon) and gives off one or more processes. The nerve cell body with its nucleus is located within the gray substance of the CNS or peripherally within a nerve ganglion. The term *nucleus* as applied to the gross structure of the CNS is used to designate a group of nerve cells that bear a direct relationship to the fibers of a particular nerve. Protoplasmic processes from the nerve cell body are called *dendrites* and *axons*. A dendrite (from the Greek word *dendron*, meaning tree) is a branched arborizing process that conducts impulses toward the cell body. An axon (from the Greek word *axon*, meaning axle or axis) or axis-cylinder is the central core that forms the essential conducting part of a nerve fiber and is an extension of cytoplasm from a nerve cell.

Depending on the number of axons present, a nerve cell is unipolar, bipolar, or multipolar. Peripheral sensory neurons are unipolar. The single axon leaves the nerve cell body located in the posterior root ganglion and branches into two parts: a peripheral branch that extends to terminate in a sensory receptor and a central branch that passes through the root of the nerve to terminate in the gray substance of the central nervous system.

Depending on their location and function, neurons are designated by different terms. An *afferent* neuron conducts the nervous impulse toward the CNS, whereas an *efferent* neuron conducts it peripherally. *Internuncial* neurons or *interneurons* lie wholly within the CNS. *Sensory* or *receptor* neurons, afferent in type, receive and convey impulses from receptor organs. The first sensory neuron is called the primary or first-order neuron. Second- and third-order sensory neurons are internuncial. *Motor* or *effector* neurons are efferent and convey nervous impulses to produce muscular or secretory effects. A *preganglionic* neuron is an autonomic efferent neuron whose nerve cell body is located in the CNS and terminates in an autonomic ganglion; a *postganglionic* neuron has its nerve cell body in the ganglion and terminates peripherally.

Nervous impulses are transmitted from one neuron to another only at a *synaptic junction* or *synapse* where the processes of two neurons are in close proximity. All afferent synapses are located within the gray substance of the central nervous system. Most of the primary synapses of nerve fibers that mediate pain are located in the substantia gelatinosa of the cord and brain stem, the ultrastructure of which is now known.[3] It should be noted that the only synapses that normally occur outside the CNS are those of the efferent preganglionic and postganglionic autonomic fibers, and these are located in the sympathetic ganglia. This indicates that there are no anatomical peripheral connections between sensory fibers. All connections are within the CNS, and the peripheral transmission of a sensory impulse from one fiber to another is abnormal. Any artificial or false peripheral synapse, called an *ephapse*, must signify pathologic change.[4]

Some neural circuits are simple, an impulse from a sensory receptor being conveyed by the primary afferent neuron to synapse in the CNS with a secondary internuncial neuron, which in turn synapses with a third efferent motor neuron, which conducts the impulse peripherally to an effector organ such as a muscle. A circuit formed by a chain of neurons in such a way that stimulation is followed by an immediate and automatic response is called a reflex arc.

Most neural circuits are much more complex, involving several and sometimes vast numbers of internuncial neurons, with many possible responses.

There are more primary pain-conducting axons in the posterior roots than there are secondary neurons in the spinothalamic tracts of the spinal cord.[5] It therefore follows that primary sensory neurons must connect with more than single secondary neurons. The synapsing of a neuron with several others is known as *convergence*.

At the synapse there may be a cumulative effect, called *summation*. Such summation may be spatial or temporal referring, respectively, to quantification and timing of the accumulated impulses.

Intensification of response is known as *facilitation*; suppression of response is called *inhibition*.

Classification of Axons by Size

It has long been known that a relationship exists between the diameter of nerve fibers and their conduction velocities,[6-8] the large fibers conducting impulses more rapidly than the smaller ones. This relationship can be summarized as follows (Gasser and Erlanger[7]):

Type A Fibers
1. Alpha fibers: size 13–22 μ in diameter velocity 70–120 m/sec
2. Beta fibers: size 8–13 μ in diameter velocity 40–70 m/sec
3. Gamma fibers: size 4–8 μ in diameter velocity 15–40 m/sec
4. Delta fibers: size 1–4 μ in diameter velocity 5–15 m/sec

Type B Fibers size 1–3 μ in diameter velocity 3–14 m/sec

Type C Fibers size 0.5–1 μ in diameter velocity 0.5–2 m/sec

There appears also to be some relationship between fiber size and the type of impulse transmitted, although strict specificity has not been proved. It appears to be generally agreed that the fast conducting A-alpha, beta, and gamma fibers carry impulses that induce tactile and proprioceptive responses but not pain. It seems that pain is conducted by A-delta and C fibers, but these are not specific for pain only.

It is recognized that there are two types of cutaneous pain sensation: pricking pain, which is rapidly felt, and burning pain, which is slightly delayed. It is thought by some investigators that these sensations are mediated by different fibers, the pricking sensation by A-delta, the burning sensation by C fibers.[9] It is known, however, that A-delta fibers also conduct touch, warmth, and cold, whereas C fibers also conduct itch, warmth, and cold.[10-12]

There is no general agreement among investigators as to the specificity of function as related to fiber size. It has been demonstrated[13] that the fine peripheral nerve fibers that innervate the cornea are able to convey touch, pain, warmth, and cold. It seems fairly certain that the larger peripheral nerve fibers have specificity of function that excludes pain and that, although small fibers are activated by nonpainful stimuli, the activation of small fibers is necessary for the organism to appreciate pain.[14,15]

Sensory Receptors

Distal terminals of sensory nerves that respond to physical stimuli and convert them into nervous impulses for conduction toward the CNS are called *sensor-transducers* or *receptors*. Sensory receptors are classified in three main groups, namely, exteroceptors, interoceptors, and proprioceptors.[16]

Exteroceptors are stimulated by the immediate external environment and are appropriately fashioned and located so as to become exposed to the organism's environment. Most impulses arising from these receptors are sensed at conscious levels. Some examples of this type of receptor are as follows:
 1. Merkel's corpuscles: tactile receptors in submucosa of tongue and oral mucosa.
 2. Meissner's corpuscles: tactile receptors in skin.
 3. Ruffini's corpuscles: pressure and warmth receptors.
 4. Krause's corpuscles or end-bulbs: cold receptors.
 5. Free nerve endings: perceive superficial pain and tactile.

Interoceptors are located in and transmit impulses from the cavities of the body. Sensation from these receptors for the most part is involved in the involuntary functioning of the body and as such is below conscious levels. Some examples of this type of receptor include the following:
 1. Pacinian corpuscles: concerned in perception of pressure.
 2. Free nerve endings: perceive visceral pain and other sensations.

Proprioceptors give information concerning the presence, position, and movement of the body and are involved chiefly in automatic functioning. For the most part, sensations conducted from proprioceptors are below conscious levels even though many such sensations can be brought into consciousness voluntarily. Some examples of this type of receptor are as follows:

1. Muscle spindles: mechanoreceptors found between the skeletal muscle fibers, which respond to passive stretch of the muscle, thus signaling muscle length; they are responsible for the myotatic reflex.
2. Golgi tendon organs: mechanoreceptors in tendons of muscles, which signal muscle tension both in contraction and stretching; they are probably responsible for nociceptive and inverse stretch reflexes.
3. Pacinian corpuscles: receptors concerned in perception of pressure.
4. Periodontal mechanoreceptors that respond to biomechanical stimuli.
5. Free nerve endings: perceive deep somatic pain and other sensations.

The more highly specialized receptor organs are complex and admirably designed to receive a particular type of stimulus. The neuromuscular endings or muscle spindles have their own sensory and motor innervation comprising a monosynaptic reflex system known as the *myotatic* or *stretch reflex*. When muscle spindles are elongated due to passive stretching of the muscle, reflex contraction occurs. This appears to function not only to oppose the forces of gravity but function also during reflex and voluntary contraction of muscles, both flexor and extensor. It is noteworthy that few if any muscle spindles have been found in the lateral pterygoid muscles, which function so importantly when the mandible is elevated against the resistance of food during mastication. This holding action of the lateral pterygoids until intercuspation of teeth induces stretching of these muscles, and it has been postulated that the extensor stress for which these muscles are so well structured requires the *absence of myotatic reflection* in order to prevent antagonistic and disruptive shortening of the muscle at its most critical phase of functioning.[16]

It should also be noted that neurotendinous receptors called Golgi tendon organs respond to tendon stretch and muscle contraction. When these receptors are stimulated, an inhibitory reflex occurs that limits contraction and thus protects the muscle from disruption or detachment. The reflex mechanism involved in this activity is called the *nociceptive reflex* and is a polysynaptic relay that involves concurrently the contraction of flexor and inhibition of extensor muscles, resulting in withdrawal of the part stimulated.[16]

When a muscle is maximally stretched, stimulation of Golgi tendon organs induces a reflex that causes contraction to cease and the muscle to relax. This reflex is usually called the *inverse stretch reflex*. It should be noted that occasional stretching of a muscle that induces this reflex activity is necessary for the muscle to maintain its normal resting length. If conditions prevent normal operation of this reflex, muscular contracture may occur, causing the muscle to become permanently shortened.[17] Therefore, contracture of elevator masticatory muscles may occur when conditions prevent the full opening of the mouth for extended periods. This phenomenon is also seen involving the lateral pterygoid muscles in edentulous patients, causing progressive shift of the mandibular position anteriorly. It results from lack of the inverse stretch reflex in the lateral pterygoid muscles, and they fail to maintain their full resting length. The full intercuspation of natural teeth satisfactorily stimulates the Golgi tendon organs, but artificial dentures do not—due to the resiliency of the interposed underlying soft tissues.

The simplest type of receptor is the nonencapsulated branching of the axon called the *free nerve ending*. These terminations are usually described as naked, and they form a network that is especially dense in the cutaneous layers, mucous membranes, and periodontium. In deeper tissues the ramification is neither as widely spread nor as dense. The simple free nerve endings are no doubt the receptors for pain, but they are not specific for pain only.

Theories as to the mechanisms of stimulation of pain receptors are presently little more than speculative.[18] It has been established that they are both *chemoceptive* and *nociceptive*.[19] It should be noted that free nerve endings are not required for the reception of noxious stimulation, since the nerve fiber itself has the same propensity, and the evoked response is similar to that initiated by receptors.

Associated with all vascular tissue, including the endocardium, is a remarkable sensory network derived from myelinated nerve fibers called the *end-net*.[20]

Transmission of Afferent Impulses

Myelination alters impulse generation in that resting and action potentials are generated only at the nodes of Ranvier where fiber is not covered by myelin sheath. Impulses travel from node to node in myelinated nerves;[21] since the amount of charge is greatly reduced at the nodes, it requires less time for an action potential to depolarize an adjacent inactive node region. Thus myelination increases the conduction velocity of the fiber.

Pain sensation from the face and mouth is mediated centrally by way of afferent primary neurons that pass through the posterior roots of the fifth, seventh, ninth, and tenth cranial nerves and the first, second, and third cervical spinal nerves and by way of visceral afferents that descend through the cervical sympathetic chain to pass through the posterior roots of the upper thoracic spinal nerves. The nerve cell bodies of the primary sensory neurons are located in the posterior root ganglion of the nerve through which they pass—except for the proprioceptive fibers of the fifth cranial nerve, which are located in the mesencephalic nucleus in the midbrain.[22]

The pain fibers from the maxillofacial area terminate in the nucleus caudalis, which is the lower caudal portion of the massive trigeminal spinal tract nucleus. The initial synapses occur in the substantia gelatinosa of the nucleus caudalis where the secondary medullary (second-order) trigeminal neurons begin and considerable convergence takes place.

The secondary medullary trigeminal neurons project to the thalamus where they terminate in several nuclei, and synapse occurs with third-order trigeminal neurons in which greater convergence takes place as they project to the cerebral cortex.

Prerequisite to the perception of facial pain sensation is the convergence of peripheral nocifensor impulses, other somatosensory inputs, and especially impulses descending from cortical structures that inhibit the sensory afferents.[23] It should be noted that pain is not a simple conduction of noxious impulses from the receptor through the primary peripheral neuron to synapse in the nucleus caudalis with the secondary medullary neuron, which in turn synapses in a thalamic nucleus with a third neuron that projects to the cerebral cortex, where it is sensed and acted upon.

What is sensed as pain does not necessarily arise from noxious stimulation of peripheral receptors or fibers. *Normal ongoing somatosensory input that ordinarily would not be perceived at all, or not as painful sensation, may be sensed as pain if certain centrally initiated inhibitory influences are not effective.* Conversely, the overactivity of such inhibitory influence may cause the subject not to perceive as pain noxious stimulation that would under other circumstances unquestionably cause pain. Also, the general intensity of suffering relates to preconditioning experience, attention, attitude, and temperament of the subject, all of which no doubt exert certain presynaptic inhibitory influences on the painful impulses that reach the nucleus caudalis. This phenomenon of central inhibition requires the organic presence of *efferent neural circuits* extending from the higher centers to cause a presynaptic inhibitory effect on the pain impulses that reach the nucleus caudalis. Such circuits have been identified.[24]

The central inhibitory mechanism is extremely complex.

Endogenous analgesic effects appear to relate to the level of certain antinociceptive morphinelike substances in the cerebrospinal fluid. These *endorphins* simulate the action of morphine when administered to laboratory animals, and this effect is neutralized by morphine antagonists.[25]

Other factors relating to the noxious stimulus per se are known to modulate the experience of pain. It appears that such factors as modality, location, intensity, and duration of the physical characteristics of the stimulus itself have bearing on the suffering that occurs. This implies that the higher centers receive accurate information concerning the stimulus and act on it by way of efferent neural circuits to produce presynaptic effects before the actual pain impulse reaches the initial synapse in the nucleus caudalis. This phenomenon presupposes the organic presence of bypass circuits in the brain stem that permit direct cerebral evaluation of the impulse before it arrives at the nucleus caudalis with efferent relays back to the nucleus. Such circuits involving the lemniscal system have been identified.[26]

Transmission of painful impulses from the mouth and face is not a simple thing. At least four cranial nerves, three cervical spinal nerves, and one or two thoracic spinal nerves take part in primary neuron conduction. The upper cord and brain-stem transmission is extremely complex, actively incorporating bypass and efferent inhibitory circuits as well as the better-known projections through second- and third-order trigeminal neurons. A basic comprehension of this complexity, even though not fully understood, is essential to the understanding, diagnosis, and management of oral and facial pains at a clinical level.

PRIMARY AFFERENT NEURONS

The nerve cell body (soma) of the primary neuron located in the gasserian ganglion produces peptides and proteins that are moved to the distal terminal by an axon transport system thought to be via microtubules or microfilaments in the axon. The velocity of this transport system does not seem to vary appreciably between myelinated and nonmyelinated fibers. Some transport substances likely serve as primary afferent neurotransmitters and therefore are essential to the transmission of pain information. There is ample evidence that antidromic activity takes place in primary neurons. Likely, the axon transport system is involved in this complex neurochemical process. Substance P is thought to be a neurotransmitter released at the central terminal of nociceptive primary neurons. This substance is found also at the distal terminals, having reached there no doubt by way of the axon transport system.[27] Thus, sensory information may be signaled very rapidly to the CNS by transmission of nerve impulses, or more slowly by way of neurochemical substances conducted through the axon transport system.[28]

Wall and Devor[29] have recently determined that the peripheral receptor is not alone in the inception of afferent impulses. The dorsal root ganglion cells also initiate sensory impulses. They form a tonic, low-level, spontaneous background discharge that is propagated orthodromically into the root and antidromically into the peripheral nerve. This newly discovered source of afferent input may account for nociceptive impulses persisting after peripheral anesthesia.

Nociceptive neurons range from high-threshold mechanosensitive and mechanothermoreceptive afferents to slowly adapting low-threshold polymodal afferents. Although a significant proportion of afferent fibers enter the CNS through the dorsal root entry zone of the brain stem at the level of the pons, a good number travel in the ventral root. About 20% of the fibers in the motor root are unmyelinated. Since no autonomic efferents are present in the trigeminal motor root, it is likely that these are sensory and potentially nociceptive afferents.[27]

The complexity of the human nervous system is truly astronomical.[30] For example, a large nerve may contain as many as 30,000 C fibers per square millimeter.[31] The somatic afferent and visceral efferent unmyelinated fibers are indistinguishable from each other and are not compartmentalized. Since such C fibers are closely intermixed within nerve fascicles, it is postulated that some ephaptic transfer of signals (called "cross talk") may take place.[31] There is definitely some coupling of outgrowing sprouts from the cut end of peripheral axons, especially in traumatic neuromas.[28]

Perl[32] has determined that nociceptors seem to be distinct from other afferent organs in that they are specific in function and in their central connections. Neither are all nociceptors alike. Some differ in receptive characteristics and probably also in their central connections. It appears that nociceptive information conveyed by different types of nociceptors is to some extent kept segregated in the central projections.[32]

SUBNUCLEUS CAUDALIS

Rexed[33,34] described the lamination of the spinal cord gray substance in terms of distinctive groups of cell bodies. Subsequent modifications have been made by Gobel,[35] Kerr,[36] and others. Lamina I (marginal zone) is the most superficial layer of the dorsal horn. Laminae II and III comprise the substantia gelatinosa, which receives nociceptive A-delta and C-fiber neurons. It has been reported that there are several classes of gelatinosa neurons in which noxious and nonnoxious input produces inhibition of spontaneous activity. The cells inhibited by nonnoxious stimuli were excited by noxious input, while the cells inhibited by noxious stimuli were excited by nonnoxious input.[37] Laminae IV, V, and VI comprise the nucleus proprius. There is progressive convergence from superficial to deeper layers.

There is sufficient evidence that facial nociceptive afferents project to the subnucleus caudalis of the massive trigeminal spinal tract nucleus.[38] Evidence at this time supports the concept that the subnucleus caudalis is homologous to the substantia gelatinosa of the spinal dorsal horn.[39] Therefore, information concerning dorsal horn structure can safely be extrapolated and applied to the subnucleus caudalis. The marginal rim of the nucleus corresponds to lamina I of the dorsal horn. The structure of laminae II and III, comprising the substantia gelatinosa of the dorsal horn, should represent the cellular arrangement present in the subnucleus caudalis.

PROJECTION TO THE THALAMUS

The direct spinothalamic system has two phylogenetically different components. The paleospinothalamic tract is the older structure common to all mammals. It projects to the midline-intralaminar thalamic regions. The phylogenetically newer neospinothalamic tract is found in primates especially. These *direct* pathways, however, conduct numerically few nociceptive interneurons. Actually, the majority of ascending fibers in the anterolateral quadrant of the cord belong to neither category. Presumably, most go by way of the spinoreticulothalamic system, sending fibers throughout the brain stem reticular formation. The more intense the ongoing pain, the wider the anatomical spread.[40] Other routes of projection of ascending nociceptive neurons include postsynaptic fibers of dorsal lateral columns, the spinocervical tract, and gray columns.[41]

There are significant differences in CNS organization in lower animals and man. This is especially so with nociceptive pathways. Extrapolation of information is hazardous, and great caution is needed. Experimental information obtained from animal studies must be tested in higher primates and, if possible, in man.[36] The possible elaboration of impulses in the human brain is enormous. It is thought that in some parts of the brain a single neuron may have synaptic terminals numbering as many as 400,000.[30]

DESCENDING INHIBITORY SYSTEM

The nociceptive messages ascending the neuraxis are modified by facilitory and inhibitory influences at virtually every synapse in the ascending pathway. This modulating system changes the message by (1) altering the modalities to which the neuron responds, (2) altering the characteristics of its receptive field, or (3) altering the temporal character of the evoked discharge.[27]

Afferent input may activate these neural systems that descend from supraspinal centers. It appears that monoamines play an important role; their depletion decreases stimulation-produced analgesia. Dopamine is necessary to the induction of such analgesia, while norepinephrine reduces its activity. Several structures are known to be involved in this inhibitory mechanism: (1) the periaqueductal gray matter (PAG), (2) the periventricular structures, and (3) the medullary raphe nuclei. It appears that morphine also may act at least in part through activation of the descending pain inhibitory system.[42]

The descending inhibitory system has been thought to represent a specific intrinsic analgesic mechanism. Actually, it may have other, more important functions during normal activities, such as sensory inhibition during sleep or selective attention. It is likely that motor and autonomic, as well as sensory, neurons are regulated in an integrated behavioral mechanism.[43]

NEUROCHEMICAL EFFECTS

The biochemical basis of nociception is becoming better understood. Several chemicals play important roles in the neural mechanisms of pain. Some of these act principally as algogenic agents; some act centrally as neurotransmitters; some act in both capacities.

Prostaglandins

The prostaglandins are a group of chemically related long-chain hydroxy fatty acids. There are six types, each designated by a suffix letter. Subscript numerals indicate the degree of saturation of the side chain. Prostaglandin E_2 is metabolized from arachidonic acid through action of an enzyme cyclo-oxygenase. This occurs in conjunction with an inflammatory process.

Prostaglandins do not seem to be algogenic substances per se. They sensitize nociceptive nerve endings to different types of stimuli, thus lowering their pain thresholds to all kinds of stimulation.[44] Prostaglandins are required for bradykinin to act[45]; bradykinin in turn stimulates the release of prostaglandins.[46] The two therefore are mutually potentiating. Prostaglandin E also increases the response of slowly adapting A-delta mechanoreceptors to nonnoxious stimuli.[47] There is evidence that a prostaglandinslike substance is released in the CNS during an inflammatory reaction that induces prostaglandin hyperalgesia.[48]

Bradykinin

Bradykinin is an endogenous polypeptide consisting of a chain of nine amino acids. It is released as part of an inflammatory reaction. It is a powerful vasodilator and causes increased capillary permeability. With few exceptions, bradykinin acts as an algogenic agent that excites all types of receptors. It sensitizes some high-threshold receptors so that they respond to otherwise innocuous stimuli such as occur during normal activities.[49] Bradykinin requires the presence of prostaglandins to act.[45] It is also released during ischemic episodes.[50]

Serotonin

Serotonin is a monoamine released by blood platelets. It is synthesized in the CNS from L-tryptophan, a dietary essential amino acid.[51] It is released when the nucleus raphe magnus in the brain stem is stimulated by sensory input.[52] Peripherally, serotonin is an algogenic agent[53] and is thought to relate especially to vascular pain syndromes. In the CNS, serotonin is an important element in the endogenous antinociceptive mechanism.[54] Central serotonin is thought to potentiate endorphin analgesia.[51] It reduces stimulation-evoked excitation of nociceptive dorsal horn interneurons.[55] The activation of serotoninergic pathways in the brain stem by tricyclic antidepressants yields paralleling analgesic effects along with its action on depressive states.[56]

Substance P

Substance P is a polypeptide composed of 11 amino acids. It is released at the central terminals of primary nociceptive neurons and acts as a transport substance, being found at the distal terminals as well.[27] Centrally, it acts as an excitatory neurotransmitter for nociceptive impulses.[1] It is released from spinal cord cells by the stimulation of A-delta and C-fiber afferents and excites neurons in the dorsal horn that are activated by noxious stimuli.[57] Its modulating action on pain is both rapid and short-lived.[58] Substance P is thought by some to be an algogenic substance.[59] Others have not found evidence to confirm this.[27]

Histamine

Histamine is a vasoactive amine that derives from the amino acid histadine. It is a vasodilator and increases small-vessel permeability. It causes contraction of smooth muscle in the lung. Although histamine is considered to be an algogenic substance, there are no clinical indications that antihistamines have appreciable analgesic value. It has been postulated that histamine also serves as a CNS neurotransmitter.

Other Agents

A number of other substances are considered to be algogenic. These include potassium[60] and acetylcholine[27] as well as a variety of extraneous toxic substances.[61]

REFERENCES

1. Zimmermann M.: Peripheral and central nervous mechanisms of nociception, pain, and pain therapy: Facts and hypotheses, in Bonica J.J., Liebeskind J.C., Albe-Fessard D.G. (eds.): *Advances in Pain Research and Therapy.* New York, Raven Press, 1979, vol. 3, pp. 3–32.
2. Kerr F.W.L.: Fine structure and functional characteristics of the primary trigeminal neuron, in Hassler R., Walker A.E. (eds.): *Trigeminal Neuralgia.* Stuttgart, Georg Thieme Verlag, 1970, pp. 11–21.
3. Hassler R., Bak I.J.: The fine structure of different types of synapses and circuit arrangement in the substantia gelatinosa trigemini, in Hassler R., Walker A.E. (eds.): *Trigeminal Neuralgia.* Stuttgart, Georg Thieme Verlag, 1970, pp. 50–58.
4. Gardner W.J.: Trigeminal neuralgia, in Hassler R., Walker A.E. (eds.): *Trigeminal Neuralgia.* Stuttgart, Georg Thieme Verlag, 1970, pp. 153–174.
5. Ruch T.C.: Visceral sensation and referred pain, in Fulton J.F. (ed.): *A Textbook of Physiology,* ed. 16. Philadelphia, W.B. Saunders Co., 1947, chap. 19.
6. Clark D., Hughes J., Gasser H.S.: Afferent function in the group of nerves of slowest conduction velocity. *Am. J. Physiol.* 114:69, 1935.
7. Gasser H.S., Erlanger J.: The role played by sizes of constituent fibers of a nerve trunk in determining the form of its action potential wave. *Am. J. Physiol.* 80:522, 1927.

8. Gasser H.S.: Conduction in nerves and relation to fiber types. *Assoc. Res. Nerv. Dis. Proc.* 15:35, 1934.
9. Hallin R.G., Wiesenfeld Z., Persson A.: Do large diameter cutaneous afferents have a role in the transmission of nociceptive information? *Pain*, suppl. 1, 1981, p. S90.
10. Bishop G.H.: Neural mechanism of cutaneous nerves. *Physiol. Rev.* 26:77, 1946.
11. Bishop G.H.: The relationship between nerve fiber size and sensory modality: Phylogenetic implications of the afferent innervation of cortex. *J. Nerv. Mental Dis.* 128:89, 1959.
12. Bishop G.H.: Fiber size and myelinization in afferent systems, in Knighton R.S., Dumke P.R. (eds.): *Pain*. Boston, Little, Brown & Co., 1966, pp. 83–89.
13. Lele P.P., Weddell G.: The relationship between neurohistology and coronal sensibility. *Brain* 79:119, 1956.
14. Collins W.F., Nulsen F.E., Shealy C.N.: Electrophysiological studies of peripheral and central pathways conducting pain, in Knighton R.S., Dumke P.R. (eds.): *Pain*. Boston, Little, Brown & Co., 1966, pp. 33–45.
15. Ochoa J.L., Torebjork H.E.: Pain from skin and muscle. *Pain*, suppl. 1, 1981, p. S87.
16. Ramfjord S.P., Ash M.M.: *Occlusion*. Philadelphia, W.B. Saunders Co., 1966.
17. Bechtol C.O.: Muscle physiology, in *The Amer. Acad. Orthoped. Surg. Instructional Course Lectures*. St. Louis, C.V. Mosby Co., 1948, vol. 5, chap. 11.
18. Nichols W.A.: Physiology of facial pain, in Alling C.C. (ed.): *Facial Pain*. Philadelphia, Lea & Febiger, 1968, pp. 21–32.
19. Lim R.K.S.: Pharmacologic viewpoint of pain and analgesia, in Way E.L. (ed.): *New Concepts in Pain*. Philadelphia, F.A. Davis Co., 1967, pp. 33–47.
20. Miller M.R.: Pain: Morphologic aspects, in Way E.L. (ed.): *New Concepts in Pain*. Philadelphia, F.A. Davis Co., 1967, pp. 7–12.
21. Kramer H.S., Schmidt W.H.: Regional anesthesia of the maxillofacial region, in Alling C.C., Mahan P.E. (eds.): *Facial Pain*, ed. 2. Philadelphia, Lea & Febiger, 1977, pp. 237–256.
22. DuBrul E.L.: *Sicher's Oral Anatomy*, ed. 7. St. Louis, C.V. Mosby Co., 1980.
23. Hassler R.: Dichotomy of facial pain conduction in the diencephalon, in Hassler R., Walker A.E. (eds.): *Trigeminal Neuralgia*. Stuttgart, Georg Thieme Verlag, 1970, pp. 123–138.
24. Wiesendanger M., Hammer B., Hepp-Reymond M.C.: Corticofugal control mechanisms of somatosensory transmission in the spinal trigeminal nucleus of the cat, in Hassler R., Walker A.E. (eds.): *Trigeminal Neuralgia*. Stuttgart, Georg Thieme Verlag, 1970, pp. 86–89.
25. Seltzer S.: *Pain Control in Dentistry*. Philadelphia, J.B. Lippincott Co., 1978.
26. Darian-Smith I.: The neural coding of tactile stimulus parameters in different trigeminal nuclei, in Hassler R., Walker A.E. (eds.): *Trigeminal Neuralgia*. Stuttgart, Georg Thieme Verlag, 1970, pp. 59–72.
27. Yaksh T.L., Hammond D.L.: Peripheral and central substrates involved in the rostral transmission of nociceptive information. *Pain* 13:1-85, 1982.

28. Wall P.D.: Mechanisms of acute and chronic pain, in Kruger L., Liebeskind J.C. (eds.): *Advances in Pain Research and Therapy.* New York, Raven Press, 1984, vol. 6, pp. 95–104.
29. Wall P.D., Devor M.: Sensory afferent impulses originate from dorsal root ganglia as well as from the periphery in normal and nerve injured rats. *Pain* 17:321-339, 1983.
30. Melzack R.: Neuropsychological basis of pain measurement, in Kruger L., Liebeskind J.C. (eds.): *Advances in Pain Research and Therapy.* New York, Raven Press, 1984, vol. 6, pp. 323–339.
31. Ochoa J.: Peripheral unmyelinated units in man: Structure, function, disorder, and role in sensation, in Kruger L., Liebeskind J.C. (eds.): *Advances in Pain Research and Therapy.* New York, Raven Press, 1984, vol. 6, pp. 53–68.
32. Perl E.R.: Characterization of nociceptors and their activation of neurons in the superficial dorsal horn: First steps for the sensation of pain, in Kruger L., Liebeskind J.C. (eds.): *Advances in Pain Research and Therapy.* New York, Raven Press, 1984, vol. 6, pp. 23–51.
33. Rexed B.: The cytoarchitectonic organization of the spinal cord in the cat. *J. Comp. Neurol.* 96:415, 1952.
34. Rexed B.: Cytoarchitectonic atlas of the spinal cord in the cat. *J. Comp. Neurol.* 100:297, 1954.
35. Gobel S.: Neural circuitry in the substantia gelatinosa of Rolando: Anatomical insights, in Bonica J.J., Liebeskind J.C., Albe-Fessard D.G. (eds.): *Advances in Pain Research and Therapy.* New York, Raven Press, 1979, vol. 3, pp. 175–195.
36. Kerr F.W.L.: Neuroanatomical substrates of nociception in the spinal cord. *Pain* 1:325-356, 1975.
37. Cervero F., Molony V., Iggo A.: Supraspinal linkage of substantia gelatinosa neurons: Effects of descending impulses. *Brain Res.* 175: 351-355, 1979.
38. Henry J.L., Sessle B.J., Lucier G.E., et al: Effects of substance P on nociceptive and nonnociceptive trigeminal brain-stem neurons. *Pain* 8:33–45, 1980.
39. Shigenaga Y., Nakatani J.: Distribution of trigeminothalamic projection cells in the caudal medulla of the cat, in Matthew B., Hill R.G. (eds.): *Anatomied, Physiological and Pharmacological Aspects of Trigeminal Pain.* Amsterdam, Elsevier Biomedical Press, 1982, pp. 163–174.
40. Bowsher D.: Role of the reticular formation in response to noxious stimulation. *Pain* 2:361-378, 1976.
41. Dennis S.G., Melzack R.: Pain-signaling system in the dorsal and ventral spinal cord. *Pain* 4:97, 1977.
42. Mayer D.J., Price D.D.: Central nervous system mechanisms of analgesia. *Pain* 2:379-404, 1976.
43. Willis W.D. Jr.: Modulation of primate spinothalamic tract discharges, in Kruger L., Liebeskind J.C. (eds.): *Advances in Pain Research and Therapy.* New York, Raven Press, 1984, vol. 6, pp. 217–240.
44. Higgs G.H., Moncada S.: Interactions of arachidonate products with other pain mediators, in Bonica J.J., Lindblom U., Iggo A. (eds.): *Advances in Pain Research and Therapy.* New York, Raven Press, 1983, vol. 5, pp. 617–626.

45. Chahl L.A., Iggo A.: The effects of bradykinin and prostaglandin E_1 on rat cutaneous afferent nerve activity. *Br. J. Pharmacol.* 59:343-347, 1977.
46. Greenberg S., Palmer G.C.: Biochemical basis of analgesia: Metabolism, storage, regulation, and actions. *Dent. Clin. North Am.* 22:31-46, 1978.
47. Pateromichelakis S., Rood J.P.: Effects of prostaglandin E on A-beta and A-delta mechanoreceptor responses. *Pain*, suppl. 1, 1981, p. S203.
48. Ferreira S.H.: Prostaglandins: Peripheral and central analgesia, in Bonica J.J., Lindblom U., Igga A. (eds.): *Advances in Pain Research and Therapy.* New York, Raven Press, 1983, vol. 5, pp. 627–634.
49. Mense S., Meyer H.: Bradykinin-induced sensitization of high-threshold muscle receptors with slowly conducting afferent fibers. *Pain*, suppl. 1, 1981, p. S204.
50. Foreman R.D., Blair R.W., Weber R.N.: Effects on T3 to T5 primate spinothalamic tract cells of injecting bradykinin into the heart. *Pain*, suppl. 1, 1981, p. S212.
51. Seltzer S., Marcus R., Stoch R.: Perspectives in the control of chronic pain by nutritional manipulation. *Pain* 11:141-148, 1981.
52. Basbaum A.T.: Brainstem control of nociception: The contribution of the monoamines. *Pain*, suppl. 1, 1981, p. S231.
53. Beck P.W., Handwerker H.O.: Bradykinin and serotonin effects on various types of cutaneous nerve fibers. *Pflugers Arch. Ges. Physiol.* 347: 209-222, 1974.
54. Messing R.B., Lytle L.D.: Serotonin-containing neurons: Their possible role in pain and analgesia. *Pain* 4:1-21, 1977.
55. Belcher G., Ryall R.W., Schaffner R.: The differential effects of 5-hydroxytryptamine, noradrenalin, and raphe stimulation on nociceptive and nonnociceptive dorsal horn interneurons in the cat. *Brain Res.* 151:307-321, 1978.
56. Ward N.G., Bloom V.L., Friedel R.O.: The effectiveness of tricyclic antidepressants in the treatment of coexisting pain and depression. *Pain* 7:331–341, 1979.
57. Lembeck F., Donnerer J., Colpaert F.C.: Increase of substance P in primary afferent nerves during chronic pain. *Neuropeptides* 1:175, 1981.
58. Yasphal K., Wright D.M., Henry J.L.: Substance P reduces tail-flick latency: Implications for chronic pain syndromes. *Pain* 14:155-167, 1982.
59. Hosobuchi Y: Elevated CSF level of substance P in arachnoiditis is reduced by systemic administration of morphine. *Pain*, suppl. 1, 1981, p. S257.
60. Keele K.D.: A physician looks at pain, in Weisenberg M. (ed.): *Pain: Clinical and Experimental Perspectives.* St. Louis, C.V. Mosby Co., 1975, pp. 45–55.
61. Chahl L.A., Kirk E.J.: Toxins which produce pain. *Pain* 1:3-49, 1975.

3

Peripheral Neural Pathways

AN UNDERSTANDING OF THE NEURAL SYSTEM involved in the sensory and motor innervation of structures of the mouth and face is essential to the effective management of nociceptive activity in that region. A somewhat wider area than just the face, however, is implicated in masticatory function.

REGIONAL CHARACTER OF MASTICATORY FUNCTION

Masticatory functioning involves a regional system of muscles that broadly cuts across neurologic boundaries. Not only the chief masticatory muscles (masseters, temporals, medial pterygoids, and lateral pterygoids) along with the second masticatory muscles (mylohyoids and digastrics especially) but also the muscles of the lips, cheeks, tongue, floor of mouth, neck, palate, and pharynx are involved. Muscular coordination and reciprocal reflexes must be accurately timed. Involved in this function are bilateral motor structures innervated by many paired nerves: fifth, seventh, ninth, tenth, eleventh, and twelfth cranial nerves plus several cervical spinal nerves. These muscles are under reflex feedback control as well as conscious volition involving bilaterally the sensory elements of many paired nerves: fifth, seventh, ninth, and tenth cranial nerves and at least the upper three cervical spinal nerves.

Orofacial functioning is necessary to the normal life of the organism, and the neurologic system that integrates it is complex indeed. Painful sensation in any part of this regional system may be sensed as a threat to the entire system; hence, the complexity of pain behavior in this area. The frequent reference of pain across neurologic boundaries and the tendency for secondary painful muscle involvement to become widely spread testify to the need for considering masticatory function a regional system not confined to the oral cavity. The intimate neurologic relationship of their afferent and efferent neuron terminations in the upper cord and brain stem is further testimony to the regional character of the masticatory system.

A good understanding of the sensory and motor innervation of these structures is prerequisite to effective management of masticatory problems including pain.

It would not be appropriate in a text of this type to include the descriptive anatomy of the structures involved. The student is referred to standard textbooks on human anatomy for that information. Attention should be directed especially toward *Sicher's Oral Anatomy*[1] for details of the oral and masticatory structures.

PERIPHERAL NOCICEPTIVE PATHWAYS

Pains arising from peripheral sources are mediated by anatomical structures of the nervous system, namely, sensory receptors and primary sensory neurons. These structures constitute the peripheral pain pathways. In the light of currently held concepts regarding the mechanisms of pain, the clinician must be well informed concerning all the sensory pathways that exist. The brain is constantly receiving a voluminous input of sensory impulses initiated by stimulation of sensory receptors of all types: exteroceptive, proprioceptive, and interoceptive. Of this volume, only a fraction is ordinarily perceived at conscious levels. Most of this ongoing sensory input is for reflective and regulatory purposes to control automatic body functioning. Formerly, the significance of such sensation in pain processes appears not to have been fully appreciated. It is important to be aware of the various routes by which such sensation is conducted. This includes both somatic and visceral pathways.

Dentists traditionally have received excellent instruction concerning the trigeminal pathways, which are of great significance in oral and facial pain complaints. Unfortunately the impression is sometimes gained that the trigeminal pathways are exclusively responsible for the mediation of painful sensation from this region. This impression is a fundamental error and may account for some of the confusion that exists in the clinical management of pain complaints. For example, it is a common notion that surgical interruption of the posterior root of the trigeminal nerve will assuredly arrest oral and facial pain, and great consternation may follow failure of such an operation to be effective.

It should be noted that the oral and masticatory region is innervated by at least six major sensory somatic nerve trunks other than the trigeminal, namely, the seventh, ninth, and tenth cranial nerves and the first, second, and third cervical spinal nerves. It should also be well understood that the visceral nerves actively participate in the mediation of painful sensations. It has been established that all sympathetic afferents and at least the sacral parasympathetic afferents mediate pain at conscious levels.[2] Hannington-Kiff[3] strongly believes that cranial parasympathetic afferent fibers mediate pain, especially that of migrainous neuralgia. An understanding of the anatomy of these pathways is important in the management of oral and facial pains. Vast numbers of impulses are conducted to the central nervous system (CNS) by afferent visceral nerves. Such ongoing sensory input is normally below conscious levels.

It should be noted that *all cranial parasympathetics*, although carried in the sheaths of trigeminal branches for peripheral distribution, *leave the trigeminal before entering the CNS, and none of them passes through the posterior root of the fifth cranial nerve.* The parasympathetic afferents in the trigeminal region enter the CNS by way of the seventh and ninth cranial nerves. It should also be noted that *all sympathetic afferents of the head regions*, although carried in the sheaths of various cranial nerves including the trigeminal for peripheral distribution, *leave these cranial nerves and join the cervical portion of the sympathetic chain and finally enter the cord by way of the posterior roots of the upper thoracic spinal nerves.*

It has long been known that the afferent as well as the efferent limb of the myotatic reflex is mediated by motor nerves.[4] In 1975 Coggeshall et al[5] reported that approximately one fourth of the population of neural fibers in human motor roots of spinal nerves were unmyelinated axons. In 1978 Young[6] observed that approximately 20% of the fibers of the human trigeminal motor root were unmyelinated. Since there are no autonomic efferents in the trigeminal root, these axons suggest an afferent population. In 1980 Hosobuchi[7] reported several cases of hyperesthesia following rhizotomy that were relieved by dorsal ganglionectomy, presumably by destroying unmyelinated fibers from the ganglion that passed through the ventral instead of the dorsal root. Since there is ample evidence of the presence of many afferent fibers in the trigeminal motor root, the motor nerves should be included among nociceptive pathways. It is quite certain that motor nerves mediate normal sensory impulses from the skeletal musculature. This phenomenon may explain why noxious stimulation of motor trunks elicits deep somatic pain felt diffusely in the muscles innervated by those nerves.[8]

It should be evident that painful sensations from the mouth and face can be mediated by many pathways other than the familiar trigeminal route. For this reason, pain from the facial region may not necessarily be arrested by division of the trigeminal sensory root. Such operation would not affect the mediation of nociceptive sensation conducted by (1) afferents of the seventh, ninth, and tenth cranial nerves or the first, second and third cervical nerves, (2) afferent neurons carried by motor elements of the trigeminal as well as other cranial and upper cervical nerves, and (3) afferent visceral nerves of the sympathetic and parasympathetic systems (Figs. 3–1 and 3–2).

SOMATIC SENSORY NERVES

The peripheral nervous system has two major parts, the somatic and the visceral. The *somatic nervous system* has afferent fibers that receive exteroceptive and proprioceptive stimuli, much of which accounts for consciousness. Somatic efferent fibers mediate neural impulses to the skeletal muscles.

The *visceral nervous system* is composed of two divisions, the craniosacral portion known as the parasympathetics and the thoracolumbar portion known as the sympathetics. The afferent elements of these nerves receive interoceptive stimuli that normally do not reach the level of consciousness. Under unusual or abnormal conditions, however, such stimuli may be perceived as pain. The efferent elements of these nerves comprise the *autonomic nervous system,* the activities of which are relatively independent of volition. The craniosacral visceral efferents constitute the parasympathetic autonomics; the thoracolumbar visceral efferents constitute the sympathetic autonomics.

TRIGEMINAL NERVE.—The chief mediator of somatic sensation from the mouth and face is the fifth cranial nerve, which innervates the face superficially in the region forward of a line drawn vertically from the ears across the top of the head and superior to the level of the lower border of the mandible. The ophthalmic division supplies the parietal and frontal areas as well as the upper eyelid and nasal bridge down to the tip of the nose. The maxillary division supplies the anterior portion of the temple, malar, and maxillary areas including the lower eyelid, ala of the nose, and upper lip. The mandibular division supplies the posterior temple, tragus, and preauricular area, masseter area, and mandibular region down to the lower border of the mandible, excluding the mandibular angle area. This includes the lower lip and a portion of the auricle and external auditory canal (Fig 3–3).

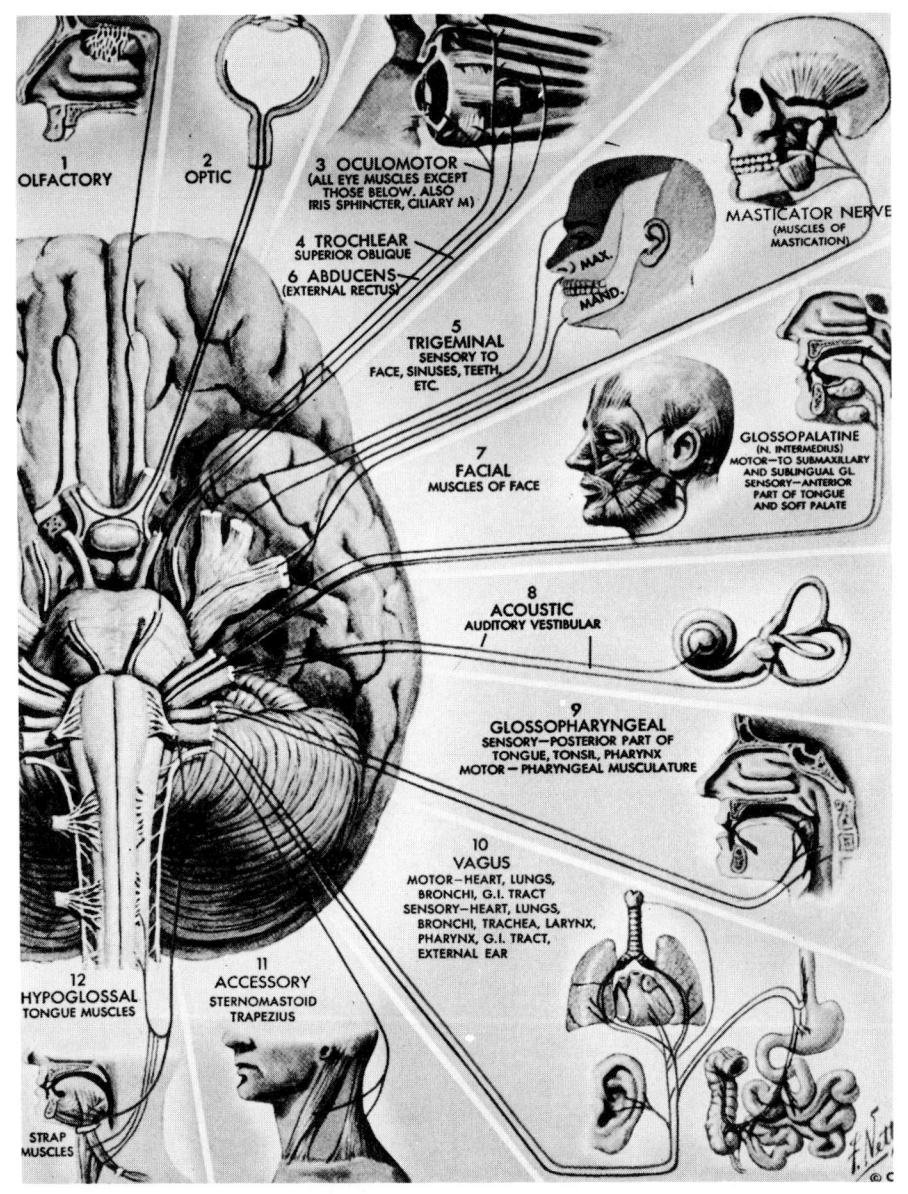

Fig 3–1.—Diagrammatic representation of the cranial nerves and the structures each subserves. (Copyright 1953, 1972 CIBA Pharmaceutical Company, Division of CIBA-GEIGY Corporation. Reproduced with permission from *The CIBA Collection of Medical Illustrations* by Frank H. Netter, M.D. All rights reserved.)

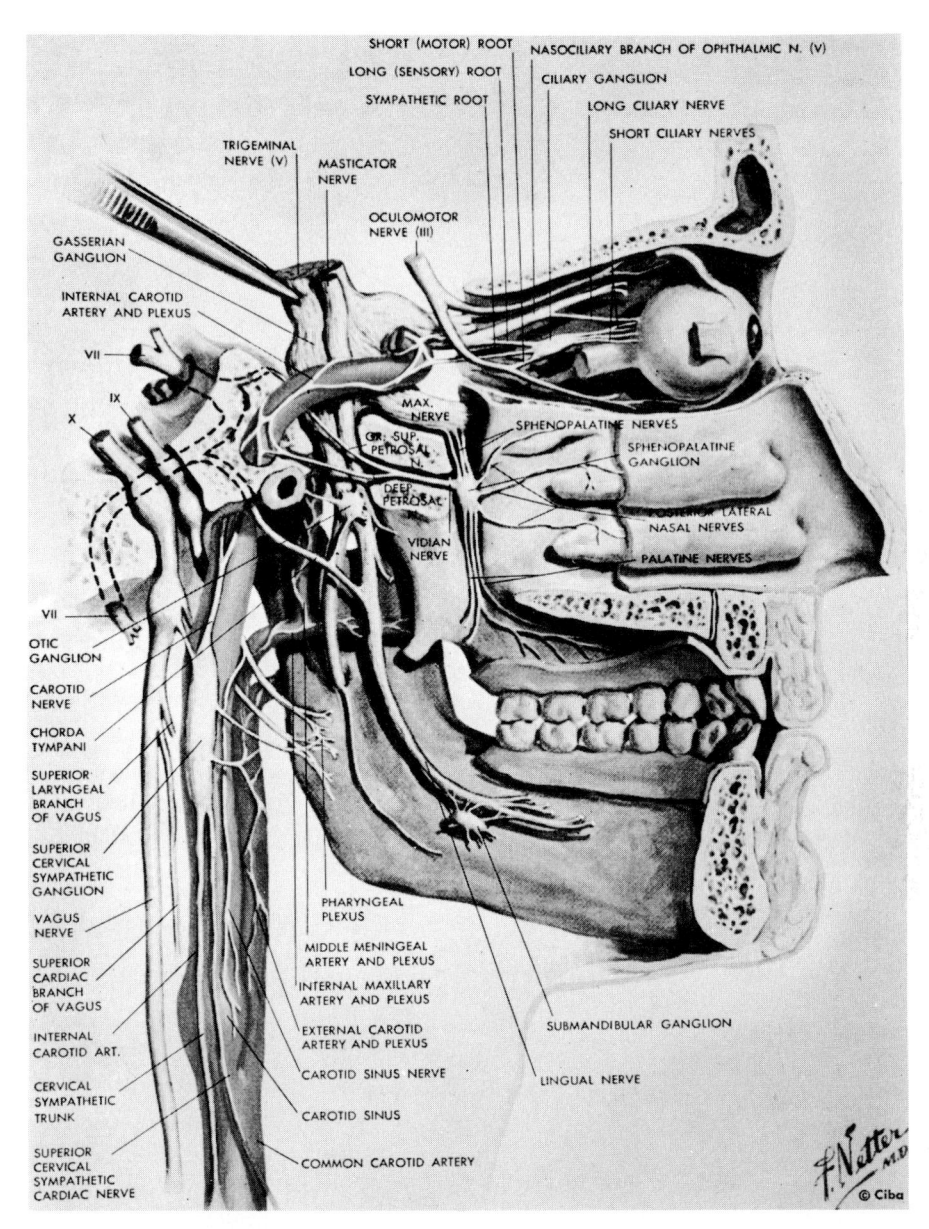

Fig 3–2.—Diagrammatic representation of the autonomic nerves of the head. (Copyright 1953, 1972 CIBA Pharmaceutical Company, Division of CIBA-GEIGY Corporation. Reproduced with permission from *The CIBA Collection of Medical Illustrations* by Frank H. Netter, M.D. All rights reserved.)

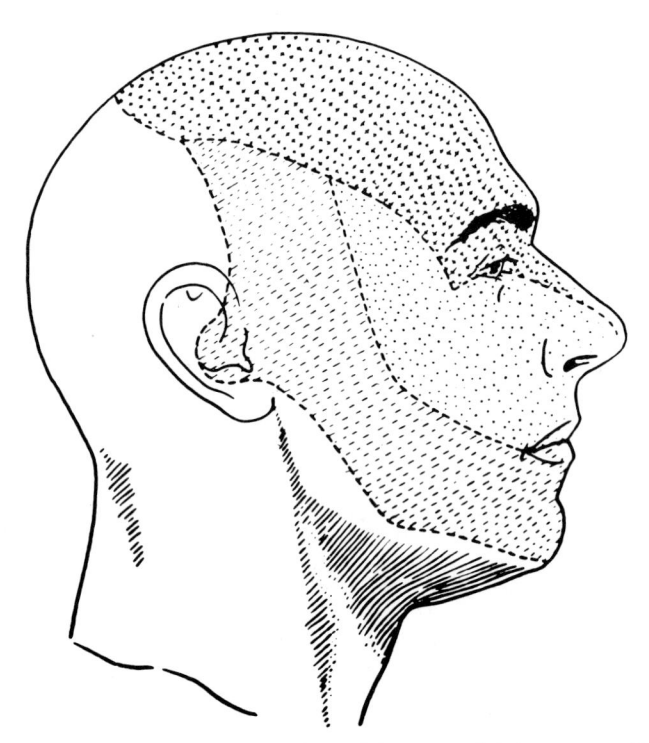

Fig 3–3.—Diagrammatic representation of the superficial sensory distribution of the trigeminal and upper cervical nerves. *Crosses,* first division; *stippled,* second division; *broken lines,* third division; *blank areas,* upper cervical nerves. (From Sicher H., DuBrul E.L.: *Oral Anatomy,* ed. 5. St. Louis, C.V. Mosby Co., 1970. Reproduced with permission.)

The deeper structures of the orofacial region are innervated by branches of the same cranial nerve. The ophthalmic division supplies the orbit and upper part of the nasal cavity. The maxillary division supplies a major portion of the nasal cavity; the palate; the maxillary antrum; the maxillary alveolar process along with the teeth, periodontium and overlying gingiva; and a small portion of the buccal mucosa in the posterior oral vestibule. The mandibular division supplies the anterior two thirds of the tongue; the mandible along with the teeth, periodontium, and overlying gingiva; the mucosa of the floor of the mouth and most of the oral vestibule; and the temporomandibular joint. This division also contains proprioceptive sensory fibers that serve the deep sensibility of the mandibular muscles (masseter, temporal, medial pterygoid, lateral pterygoid, mylohyoid, anterior digastric) and tensor palati and tensor tympani muscles.

Each of the three divisions gives off sensory branches that pass intracranially to supply structures above the tentorium cerebelli.

FACIAL NERVE.—The intermediate nerve of Wrisberg (nervus intermedius) contains proprioceptive sensory fibers that serve the deep sensibility of the face except the muscles innervated by the fifth cranial nerve (mandibular muscles, tensor palati, and tensor tympani) and the 12th cranial nerve (tongue muscles). These fibers also serve the deep sensibility of the platysma, stylohyoid, and posterior digastric muscles that are innervated by the seventh nerve. According to Wolff[9] and Finneson,[10] this nerve contains sensory fibers that supply superficial sensation to the tympanic membrane and part of the external auditory canal.

The facial nerve contains taste fibers to the anterior two thirds of the tongue. These fibers form part of the chorda tympani nerve that is carried in the terminal areas within the sheath of the lingual branch of the trigeminal nerve.

GLOSSOPHARYNGEAL NERVE.—Sensory fibers of the ninth cranial nerve innervate the base of the tongue, pharynx, and most of the ear and tympanic membrane. There is considerable overlapping of trigeminal and glossopharyngeal terminal afferent fibers in the throat area so that pain arising from the deeper recesses of the oral cavity may be mediated by either or both nerve trunks. This nerve also contains the taste fibers to the posterior one third of the tongue. Some intracranial fibers of this nerve mediate sensation below the level of the tentorium cerebelli.

The glossopharyngeal nerve contains proprioceptive sensory fibers that serve the deep sensibility of the pharyngeal area.

VAGUS NERVE.—Sensory fibers of the tenth cranial nerve innervate the lower part of the pharynx, larynx, posterior part of the external auditory canal, and skin immediately behind the auricle. It also contains taste fibers to the region of the epiglottis.

CERVICAL SPINAL NERVES.—The upper three cervical spinal nerves mediate sensory impulses from the superficial structures of the head and face posterior to the trigeminal area and below the lower border of the mandible, including the mandibular angle. This includes most of the auricle as well as the postauricular region except for the skin immediately posterior to the auricle, which is supplied by the vagus nerve. In about 8% of cases, the sensory root of the first cervical nerve is missing.

The upper cervical spinal nerves contain proprioceptive sensory fibers that serve the deep sensibility of the cervical areas except those muscles innervated by other nerves (mylohyoid and anterior digastric by the fifth cranial nerve; platysma, stylohyoid, and posterior digastric by the seventh cranial nerve; tongue muscles by the 12th cranial nerve). Although parts of the sternocleidomastoid and trapezius muscles are innervated by the 11th cranial nerve, actually these fibers arise from the upper cervical segments. These muscles may be considered to be innervated by cervical spinal nerves.

SOMATIC MOTOR NERVES

OCULOMOTOR, TROCHLEAR, AND ABDUCENT NERVES.—The third, fourth, and sixth cranial nerves contain somatic motor fibers to the ocular muscles and the levator of the upper eyelid.

TRIGEMINAL NERVE.—The fifth cranial nerve contains somatic motor fibers that innervate the masseter, temporal, medial pterygoid, lateral pterygoid, mylohyoid, anterior digastric, tensor palati, and tensor tympani muscles. All these motor fibers are part of the mandibular division of this nerve.

FACIAL NERVE.—The seventh cranial nerve contains somatic motor fibers that innervate the muscles of facial expression including the occipitofrontal scalp muscles, the muscles of the auricle, and the platysma. They also supply the stapedius, stylohyoid, and posterior digastric muscles.

GLOSSOPHARYNGEAL NERVE.—The ninth cranial nerve contains somatic motor fibers that innervate the stylopharyngeal muscle and along with the vagus supply the constrictor muscles of the pharynx and palatopharyngeal muscle.

VAGUS NERVE.—The tenth cranial nerve contains somatic motor fibers that innervate musculature of the pharynx and larynx.

ACCESSORY NERVE.—The 11th cranial nerve contains somatic motor fibers of both cranial and cervical origin. Those of cranial origin innervate muscles of the larynx and pharynx as branches of the vagus nerve. Those of cervical origin arise from several of the upper cervical segments and innervate parts of the sternocleidomastoid and trapezius muscles.

HYPOGLOSSAL NERVE.—The 12th cranial nerve contains somatic motor fibers that innervate the intrinsic and extrinsic muscles of the tongue. This nerve also contains motor fibers of cervical origin that innervate some of the hyoid muscles, including the geniohyoid muscle.

CERVICAL SPINAL NERVES.—The upper cervical spinal nerves contain somatic motor fibers that supply the cervical and hyoid muscles, directly as well as indirectly, via the 11th and 12th cranial nerves, as noted above. It should be remembered that the mylohyoid and anterior digastric muscles are innervated by the fifth cranial nerve and the platysma, posterior digastric, and stylohyoid muscles by the seventh cranial nerve.

VISCERAL NERVOUS SYSTEM

PARASYMPATHETIC AFFERENTS.—The oral and facial structures are supplied with parasympathetic visceral afferents that are carried within the trigeminal sheath but exit by way of the sensory roots of the seventh and ninth cranial nerves rather than the fifth. The fibers from the lacrimal, submandibular, and sublingual glands leave the fifth nerve and join with the seventh, whereas those from the parotid gland leave the fifth and join with the ninth.

PARASYMPATHETIC EFFERENTS.—The sphincter of the pupil, the ciliary muscle of accommodation, the lacrimal gland, and all the salivary glands receive parasympathetic autonomic efferent fibers that are incorporated in the oculomotor, facial, and glossopharyngeal nerves. The preganglionic fibers in the oculomotor nerve leave it to synapse with postganglionic fibers in the ciliary ganglion and henceforth are contained within the trigeminal sheath to supply the sphincter of the pupil and the ciliary muscle. The preganglionic fibers in the facial nerve leave it to synapse with postganglionic fibers in the pterygopalatine and submandibular ganglia and henceforth are contained within the trigeminal sheath. Those from the pterygopalatine ganglion supply the lacrimal gland, and those from the submandibular ganglion supply the submandibular and sublingual glands. The preganglionic fibers in the glossopharyngeal nerve leave it to synapse with postganglionic fibers in the otic ganglion and henceforth are contained within the trigeminal sheath to supply the parotid gland. None of the parasympathetic efferents of the vagus nerve supply structures in the masticatory area.

SYMPATHETIC AFFERENTS.—The oral and facial structures are supplied with sympathetic visceral afferents that are carried within the sheaths of the fifth, seventh, and ninth cranial nerves. All the sympathetic fibers leave these vehicular nerve trunks and pass to the cervical sympathetic chain and enter the CNS through the sensory roots of the upper thoracic spinal nerves.

Afferent nerves from blood vessels arise from receptors called endnets.[11] The fibers that carry these sensory impulses may be either somatic or visceral.[6,12] This may explain the clinical observation that some vascular pains of the head can be interrupted by rhizotomy, whereas others require sympathectomy.[13]

SYMPATHETIC EFFERENTS.—The dilator of the pupil, the tarsal and orbital muscles and the salivary glands, as well as the blood vessels and skin, receive sympathetic autonomic efferents. All sympathetic efferents to the head are postganglionic. The preganglionic fibers are contained within the upper thoracic spinal nerves, from which they take leave to join the sympathetic chain at about the level of the stellate ganglion and synapse with the cranial postganglionic fibers in the superior cervical ganglion. These fibers follow the external and internal carotid arteries. Those that follow the internal carotid artery form the internal carotid nerve, which becomes a loose plexus from which fibers join several cranial nerves for terminal distribution to the pupil and orbital muscles as well as to the glands of the nasal cavity, palate, and pharynx. The fibers that follow the external carotid artery supply the smooth muscle of blood vessels and skin as well as the cutaneous glands and large salivary glands.

REFERENCES

1. DuBrul E.L.: *Sicher's Oral Anatomy*, ed. 7. St. Louis, C.V. Mosby Co., 1980.
2. Wolff H.G., Wolf S.: *Pain*, ed. 2. Springfield, Ill., Charles C Thomas, Publisher, 1958.
3. Hannington-Kiff J.G.: *Pain Relief*. Philadelphia, J.B. Lippincott Co., 1974.
4. McIntyre A.K.: Afferent limb of the myotatic reflex arc. *Nature* 168: 168, 1951.
5. Coggeshall R.E., Applebaum M.L., Fazen M., et al.: Unmyelinated axons in human ventral roots, a possible explanation for the failure of dorsal rhizotomy to relieve pain. *Brain* 98:157-166, 1975.
6. Young R.F.: Unmyelinated fibers in the trigeminal motor root: Possible relationship to the results of trigeminal rhizotomy. *J. Neurosurg.* 49:538-543, 1978.
7. Hosobuchi Y.: The majority of unmyelinated afferent axons in human ventral roots probably conduct pain. *Pain* 8:167, 1980.
8. Cailliet R.: *Neck and Arm Pain*. Philadelphia, F.A. Davis Co., 1964.
9. Dalessio D.J.: *Wolff's Headache and Other Head Pain*, ed. 3. New York, Oxford University Press, 1972.

10. Finneson B.E.: *Diagnosis and Management of Pain Syndromes*, ed. 2. Philadelphia, W.B. Saunders Co., 1969.
11. Collins W.F., Nulsen F.E., Shealy C.N.: Electrophysiological studies of peripheral and central pathways conducting pain, in Knighton R.S., Dumke P.R. (eds.): *Pain*. Boston, Little, Brown & Co., 1966, pp. 33–45.
12. Gross D.: Pain and autonomic nervous system, in Bonica J.J. (ed.): *Advances in Neurology*. New York, Raven Press, 1974, vol. 4, pp. 93–103.
13. D'Errico A.: Personal communication.

4

Pain Modulation

UNTIL RECENTLY, HUMAN PAIN was conceived as a sensory experience evoked by noxious stimulation of neural structures. The impulses thus generated were thought to be transmitted to the central nervous system (CNS) where they were perceived as pain and reacted to. The reaction was thought to comprise extensive behavior on the part of many body systems. The dominant factors in pain reaction were thought to be on a mentation level such as prior conditioning, evaluative significance of the pain, memory, and emotional response. This perception-reaction hypothesis was originated in the 19th century by Marshall[1] and Strong.[2] It was recognized that great difference in pain reaction was commonplace. Maurice concluded: "The exaggerated reaction is due to psychic factors and is termed *psychoneurotic pain*."[3] It became popular to think in terms of human suffering as being *organic* or *psychogenic*—organic constituting pain behavior that could be accounted for on the basis of structural conditions, while psychogenic labeled everything else.

During the second half of the 20th century, clinical and experimental evidence accumulated that gave reason to question the validity of the perception-reaction concept of pain. Thus, the currently held concept of pain modulation evolved.

MODULATION CONCEPT OF PAIN

Pain is now considered to be more than the noxious stimulation of neural structures. It is more than systemic reaction to unpleasant signals received by the brain. It is more than a choice between organic and psychogenic. Pain comprises all these features in a unified sensory and emotional experience that is "organic" all the way. The concept of pain modulation is based on documented experimental evidence that neural impulses are altered, changed, and modulated as they travel up the neuroaxis to the higher centers. Excitatory and inhibitory influences bear on the impulses at various levels in the CNS so that perception and reaction become merely facets of the same mechanism rather than separate components of it.

Whether pain is generated by noxious stimulation of tissues or occurs spontaneously is no longer of great concern. Whether pain is the result of injury or of mentation processes is of little significance. It is more important to consider the various factors that influence the inhibition and excitation of painful experience. In recent years, worldwide research into pain mechanisms has brought to light much information relative to these factors. A door has been opened, and the study of human suffering has come out of the area of philosophy and has entered the scientific community.

GATE CONTROL THEORY

In 1965 Melzack and Wall[4] proposed a new theory to help explain, and serve as a model to visualize, pain modulation. This they termed the *gate control theory*. Although the neurophysiologic mechanisms are still under debate and many uncertainties remain, the theory has served to bridge us from the former perception-reaction concept. Theory it was and theory it remains; however, an understanding of it is needed to gain better insight into the modulation concept of pain. Total validity is not the issue.

Noxious stimulation of skin evokes nerve impulses that are conducted to three spinal cord systems:
1. Cells of the substantia gelatinosa situated in the dorsal horn.
2. Dorsal column fibers that project toward the brain.
3. First central transmission cells in the dorsal horn.

The new theory proposes that the substantia gelatinosa functions as a gate control system that modulates the afferent patterns before they influence the transmission cells. The afferent patterns in the dorsal column system act in part at least as a central control trigger, which activates selective brain processes that influence the modulating properties of the gate control system. The transmission cells activate neural mechanisms that comprise the *action system* responsible for response and perception. *Each of these systems receives nerve impulses initiated by noxious stimulation of skin* (Fig 4-1).

Gate Control System

When skin is noxiously stimulated, the impulses thus generated are transmitted centrally by both large A-delta and small C fibers. The

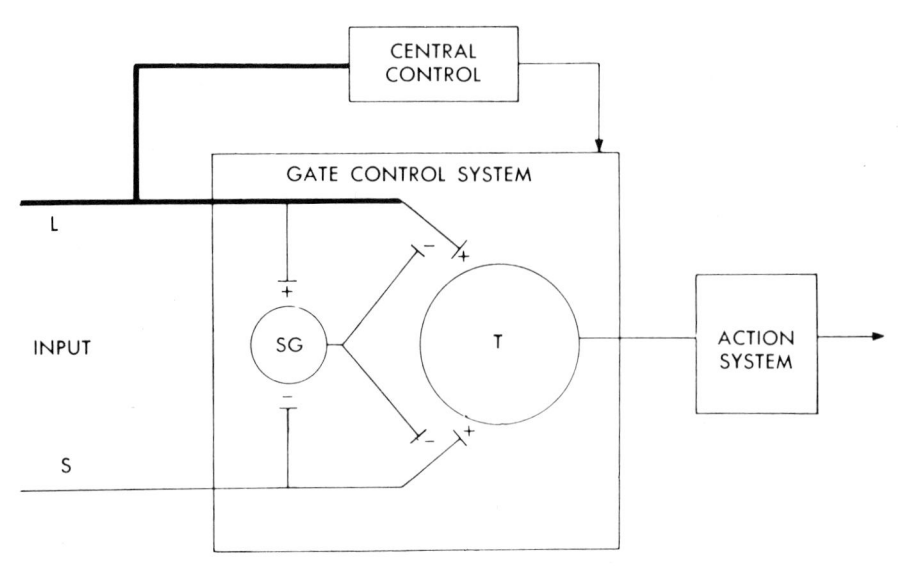

Fig 4-1.—Schematic diagram of the gate control theory of pain mechanisms: *L*, the large-diameter fibers; *S*, the small-diameter fibers. The fibers project to the substantia gelatinosa (*SG*) and first central transmission (*T*) cells. The inhibitory effect exerted by *SG* on the afferent fiber terminals is increased by activity in *L* fibers and decreased by activity in *S* fibers. The central control trigger is represented by a line running from the large-fiber system to the central control mechanisms; these mechanisms, in turn, project back to the gate control system. The *T* cells project to the entry cells of the action system. +, Excitation; −, inhibition. (From Melzack R., Wall P.D.: Pain mechanisms: A new theory. *Science* 150:971–978, 1965, p. 975. Copyright 1965 by the American Association for the Advancement of Science. Reproduced with permission.)

large fibers have a much higher conduction rate than the small fibers. The nerve impulses via larger fibers arrive at the substantia gelatinosa well ahead of those transmitted by small fibers. Volleys of nerve impulses in large fibers are extremely effective in activating the transmission cells initially, but these impulses also activate a *negative* feedback mechanism, which reduces their effect on the transmission cells. These cells must be stimulated before the sensation is either perceived or acted upon. Volleys of nerve impulses in small fibers activate a *positive* feedback mechanism, which exaggerates the effect of arriving impulses on the transmission cells. The effect of large-fiber activity is to "close the gate," whereas that of small-fiber activity is to "open the gate" for the passage of impulses to the transmission cells, the gate being the initial synapses between peripheral neurons and secondary medullary neurons.

Three features of afferent sensory input are significant:
1. Ongoing activity that precedes the stimulus.
2. Stimulus-evoked activity itself.
3. Relative balance of activity of the large fibers related to that of the small fibers.

Presetting The Gate

There is a continuous, unceasing, ongoing bombardment by afferent nerve impulses, most of which is well below conscious levels. This activity, although perceived and acted on by the brain, is not ordinarily perceived consciously as suffering or acted on as painful sensation. Such sensation is conducted chiefly by the small fibers, which tend to be tonically active and to adapt slowly—thus holding the gate in a relatively open position. This ongoing activity of course precedes the noxious stimulus and presets the gate before such noxious stimulation occurs. The presetting of the gate for a particular individual at a particular time depends in part on the intensity of prior ongoing activity in the small fibers. *If such activity is accentuated for example by sustained hyperemia or inflammation in the area to be noxiously stimulated, then the presetting of the gate is already wide, and any stimulus that follows will more effectively stimulate the transmission cells and be perceived as pain. In fact, if the ongoing activity is sufficiently great, that sensation itself may stimulate transmission cells as pain of a spontaneous, nonprovoked type.*

Resetting The Gate

Next to be considered is the stimulus-evoked activity itself. The noxious stimulus increases immediately the activity of nerve impulses in both large and small fibers, the number of receptor fiber units thus affected being disproportionately that of large over small fibers because many large fibers are normally inactive in the absence of stimulation, whereas many small fibers are already engaged in the continuous ongoing activity described above. As a result, some transmission cells are fired, and the stimulus is received as pain. But the predominant large-fiber activity also partially closes the synaptic gate due to the effect of its negative feedback mechanism, thus shortening the barrage on the transmission cells. *In effect, the perception of and reaction to the noxious stimulus is shortened and reduced (modulated) as the stimulus disproportionately affects the large fibers over the small.*

The synaptic gate that permits the nerve impulses of the primary afferent neurons to fire the secondary transmission cells is affected or reset by the noxious stimulus itself, depending on the total number of active fibers involved, frequency of the nerve impulses and balance of activity in large and small fibers. As a stimulus is increased, more receptor fiber units are recruited, and the firing frequency of the active units is increased. This results in positive and negative effects that are counteractive, and the output of transmission cells slowly rises. *In effect, as the noxious stimulus is increased, pain perception and reaction slowly increase. But still other factors act to modulate the increase so that it is not necessarily proportionate to its cause.*

If the stimulation is prolonged, the large fibers begin to adapt, decreasing large-fiber activity. This results in a shift of balance in favor of small-fiber activity with the effect of opening the gate more widely. Even though the intensity of the noxious stimulation may not increase, the simple fact of its continuation tends to gradually increase the perception of and reaction to the stimulus. It should be readily seen that high-intensity stimulation cannot be tolerated for long periods because the suffering would soon become wholly unbearable. In effect, *the duration of pain normally increases its intensity.*

Critical Firing Level

Another feature of the gate control system concerns the critical level to which the output of the transmission cells must rise before the action system is fired and pain perception and reaction occur. Until this firing takes place, there is neither perception of pain nor any reaction to it. This critical level is affected by the balance of peripheral fiber activity in that the critical firing level is lowered by large-fiber activity. This means that large-fiber activity keeps the passage of impulses across the synaptic gate more faithfully perceived and reacted to, so that the subject feels more proportionately the true intensity and duration of the noxious stimulation. Decreased large-fiber activity increases this critical level, the attainment of which is not graduated but is an all-or-none effect. When the critical level is high, the pain is not perceived until the firing level is reached, thus causing a delay between stimulus and perception. This is known as *temporal summation*. When the critical level is finally reached, the barrage on the transmission cells may occur explosively, causing pain that is wholly disproportionate to the intensity of the stimulus. This is known as *spatial summation*. In effect, the lack of large-fiber activity elevates the critical firing level of the gate control system and produces summation effects. In addition, as we have already seen, lack of large-fiber activity also opens the gate so that lower-intensity stimulation is perceived as pain. It is to be noted that the gate-setting and the critical firing level are different facets of the pain mechanism even though both bear on the functioning of the gate control system.

Central Control Trigger

Another feature of the gate control theory has to do with the effect of the higher centers on both presetting and resetting the synaptic gate. The neurologic control of the gate-setting is by way of descending efferent fibers, which are activated by the brain.

The descending efferent circuits to the gate control system are influenced by past experience of the individual as well as by the noxious stimulus itself. Thus the total emotional level of the individual presets the gate before the noxious stimulus occurs. The gate is also reset by the effect of the noxious stimulus on the higher brain centers prior to being perceived or acted upon.

The presetting of the gate relates to such factors as past experience, conditioning, attention directed toward one's suffering, and the emotional state of the individual at any given time. The calm, placid, philosophic, emotionally adjusted person perceives pain and reacts to it differently from the distraught, anxious, frightened, emotionally unstable person. The difference is not one of emotional response but of actual organic perception of and physical reaction to the noxious stimulation. The intensity of suffering is not the same for the two. The emotionally unstable person feels more pain due to the setting of the synaptic gate. The person whose gate is opened not only suffers more from the same noxious stimulus but also may perceive as pain stimuli that normally should not be painful.

Still another feature relates to the action taken by the brain to reset the gate in direct response to the noxious stimulus itself prior to conscious recognition of it. When such stimulation occurs, certain fast-conducting large fibers bypass the substantia gelatinosa and carry the sensation directly to the brain by synapsing initially in the thalamus and thence to the somatosensory cortex. These nerve impulses reach the higher centers at extremely high conduction velocity, bypassing the gate and supplying precise information about the nature, intensity, and location of the noxious stimulation before such impulses reach the synaptic gate. This sensation is not perceived as pain, but, rather, is acted on by the higher centers in two ways. It sets the receptivity of cortical neurons for the subsequent afferent volley of impulses from the transmission cells fired from the gate control system. It also resets the gate itself by nerve impulses transmitted by descending efferent circuits from the higher centers to the gate control mechanism. *The signals received in the higher centers are identified and evaluated in terms of prior experience as well as by the contemporary meaning of the noxious stimulus itself and influence the setting of the gate.* All this occurs before the nerve impulses from the noxious stimulation have had time to arrive at the gate. Impulses initiated by the noxious stimulation are centrally inhibited before they are perceived, and not only the perception of pain but also its reaction are influenced through presetting and resetting the gate as a result of the total emotional state of the individual as well as by the contemporary meaning such noxious stimulation has for the individual at the very moment it occurs. The full emotional impact of the subject is therefore brought to bear on all painful sensations. The action of the higher centers constitutes not so much a part of the response to pain as an actual determinant in the passage of impulses through the synaptic gate where the transmission cells can be fired.

If the central inhibitory feedback control on the synaptic gate is total, no pain is felt regardless of how severe the noxious stimulation may be. If this central inhibitory system fails, all sensation—even that which is normally unconscious—may be perceived as pain. In effect, the first condition has a closed gate; the second, a wide-open gate. An essential part of the gate control theory is the functioning of the central control trigger that alters the presetting of the synaptic gate in the substantia gelatinosa. It provides the modulating effect of mentation as related to prior experience, conditioning, and current emotional state of the individual. This trigger is able to evaluate the noxious stimulus itself in terms of its intensity, location, and duration. It thus affects the receptivity of cortical neurons to the painful barrage to follow. It also resets the gate so as to influence the passage of the barrage through the initial synapse.

The modulating effect of this central control trigger on the gate control system is via descending efferent circuits from the higher centers to the synaptic gate in the substantia gelatinosa. It is a central inhibitory feedback system. Its effect occurs prior to conduction of the nervous impulses constituting the noxious stimulation to the gate control system and therefore acts prior to either the perception of that noxious stimulation or to any physical reaction to it.

Action System

The third major element in the gate control theory concerns reaction to painful nerve impulses transmitted to the higher centers by the firing of transmission cells, the second-order neurons. Depending on the setting of the synaptic gate and the critical firing level, the action system is triggered, causing a sequence of responses that includes both conscious perception and physical reaction. Until the action system is activated, pain is neither perceived nor acted on. Once the action system responds, both *pain perception and pain reaction become inseparable responses* recruiting vast numbers of neural circuits that involve action on the part of much of the brain. Many responses are set in motion. A sudden unexpected noxious stimulation excites a startle response, with flexion reflex and postural changes. There may be vocalization and visual and tactile inspection of the pained site. Autonomic responses occur. Memory of past similar or contrasting experiences flash by to color the emotional evaluation of the experience, and many patterns are set in motion to palliate the source of discomfort. To separate perception from reaction is impossible, and indeed impractical, because pain is more than a warning signal—it is a whole physiologic process.

The action system is the process of suffering and depends on the interaction of many factors that modulate the noxious impulses *prior to perception and response*. These factors include (1) the presetting of the gate due to mentation, emotions, and ongoing low-level small-fiber activity and the resetting of the gate by the noxious stimulus itself, both directly through the balance of large- and small-fiber activity and indirectly through central feedback mechanisms; (2) the critical firing level that must be attained before the action system is activated, this level being influenced by the balance between large- and small-fiber activity; and (3) central triggering of the gate control mechanism by efferent feedback inhibitory circuits, the effect being induced by cerebral evaluation of the threat at the moment of its inception, based on the quality and location of the threat against the whole background of past experience.

Summary

The gate control theory as initially presented has been subjected to further elaboration[5] (Fig 4–2). This combines the more obvious sen-

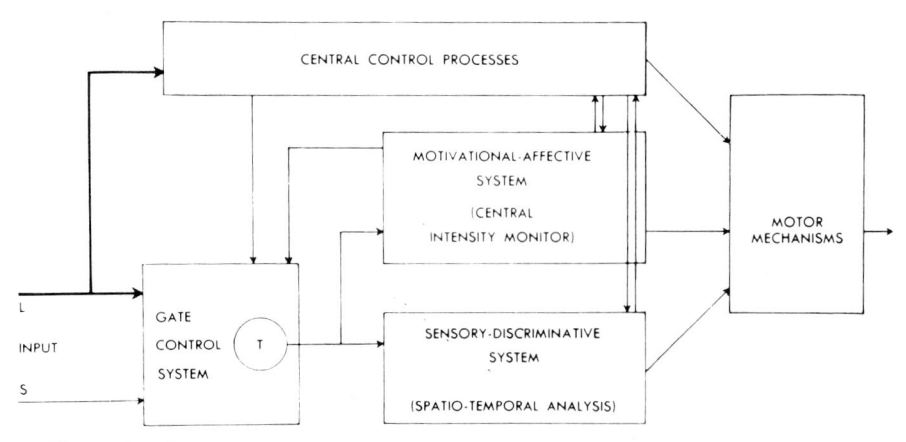

Fig 4-2.—Conceptual model of the sensory, motivational, and central control determinants of pain. The output of the *T* cells of the gate control system projects to the sensory-discriminative system (via neospinothalamic fibers) and the motivational-affective system (via the paramedial ascending system). The central control trigger (comprising the dorsal-column and dorsolateral projection systems) is represented by a line running from the large-fiber system to central control processes; these, in turn, project back to the gate control system, and to the sensory-discriminative and motivational-affective systems. All three systems interact with one another, and project to the motor system. (From Casey K.L., Melzack, R.: Neural mechanisms of pain: A conceptual model, in Way E.L. (ed.): *New Concepts in Pain and Its Clinical Management.* Philadelphia, F.A. Davis Co., 1967, pp. 13-31. Reproduced with permission.)

sory-discriminative component of pain with a motivational-affective dimension as an integral part of the pain experience on an anatomical and physiologic basis. The sensory-discriminative system, which renders spatio-temporal analysis of transmission cell activity, interacts with the central control processes that feed back to the gate control system. Likewise, the motivational-affective system, the central intensity monitor of transmission cell activity, feeds back inhibitory influence on the gate control system as well as interacting with central control processes, which in turn feed back controlling influence on the gate control system. The central control processes are activated directly by large-fiber activity from the periphery as well as by interacting influences from both the sensory-discriminative and motivational-affective systems, thus regulating the gate control system by both peripheral and central mechanisms. All these physiologic systems in turn influence the motor mechanisms responsible for the complex pattern of responses to pain. It appears that the rapid-conducting large-fiber activity that bypasses the gate control system and goes directly to the central control system acts as the afferent feed-forward peripheral input to the central control system. Further central input is received by interaction with both the sensory-discriminative and motivational-affective systems in response to monitoring of transmission cell activity. The gate control system in turn receives efferent feedback controlling impulses from both the motivational-affective monitor and the integrated central control system. All this influence affects directly and indirectly the motor mechanisms that finally make up the total response to painful stimulation.

Once the action system is activated, the suffering and physical response are nearly automatic since all cerebral effects have already had their bearing on the outcome prior to the conscious perception of the noxious threat. *If the stimulation continues,* if it changes in character and especially if the therapist fails to manage it well, *the suffering becomes experience upon which further cerebral evaluation rests, and marked changes in reaction may occur.*

It is believed that the interaction between the gate control system and the action system is not limited to the initial synapse in the substantia gelatinosa but that similar physiologic phenomena may occur at successive synapses at any level of the central nervous system. Thus, there may well be a filtering process involving sensory input that is more or less continuous and progressive. Central influence may take place at a series of levels also. The gate control system may therefore be set and reset a number of times as the temporal and spatial patterning of the input is analyzed and acted on by the brain.

In 1978, Wall[6] reexamined the gate control theory in the light of 13 years of additional neurophysiologic investigation. He confirmed that the substantia gelatinosa did play an important role in organizing the nociceptive input. However, he noted that all nociceptive neurons of the dorsal horn received inhibitory impulses from regions of the brain. He concluded that the theory in its original detail could no longer be sustained, but that the underlying concepts were still valid when restated in a more basic form.

TRANSCUTANEOUS ELECTRICAL NERVE STIMULATION

The chief product of the gate control theory has been the introduction of transcutaneous nerve stimulation as a therapeutic modality. The mechanisms involved give considerable insight into pain modulation. Kane and Taub[7] reviewed the history of local electrical analgesia from the time the early Egyptians used electric fish to minimize pain. They related that, in 1858, Francis used forceps charged with electricity to extract teeth with less pain. The use of electricity to reduce pain has been "discovered and rediscovered" many times down through the years. It lay dormant until resurrected by Wall and Sweet[8] in 1967. The Chinese have recently added electrical stimulation to their age-old acupuncture method of pain control. In 1975, Long and Hagfors[9] reviewed the resurgent use of electricity in various forms in treating some 3,000 patients.

The rationale of transcutaneous electrical nerve stimulation according to the gate control theory is based on the antinociceptive effect of stimulating cutaneous sensory nerves. An interrupted faradic current of very low intensity at a frequency of 50 to 100 Hz is used.[10] The stimulation is usually below what is required to activate A-delta and C nociceptive fibers.[11] No more than a tingling or vibratory sensation should be felt. Although the antinociceptive effect results from stimulation of the thick A-beta fibers,[12] stimulation of A-delta and C fibers also yields the same effect as long as it does not reach noxious levels.[13] The effect is immediate and usually disappears rapidly. Pain relief is localized to the segments stimulated.[10] The effect is not reversed by naloxone, indicating that it is not dependent upon the release of endorphins.[14-19]

It should be noted that transcutaneous electrical nerve stimulation and electroacupuncture are different procedures, mediated by different mechanisms, and should not be confused. The latter activates the endogenous antinociceptive system that releases endorphins and is reversed by naloxone. Since at a clinical level the two techniques somewhat overlap, there may be good reason for conflicting research reports relative to the release of endorphins by the two methods.[20-22]

MODULATING EFFECT OF NONNOXIOUS CUTANEOUS STIMULATION

The nonnoxious stimulation of cutaneous afferents activates neurons of the descending inhibitory system, particularly those of the nucleus raphe magnus in the brain stem and the periaqueductal gray (PAG) in the midbrain.[23] The stimulation of serotoninergic neurons in the raphe nucleus releases serotonin which reduces stimulation-evoked excitation of nociceptive dorsal horn neurons.[24] Stimulation of periaqueductal gray reduces the aversive reaction to pain.[13]

At a clinical level, the modulating effect of cutaneous stimulation has been known for ages. The almost instinctive act of grabbing, holding, pressing, or rubbing a painful site exemplifies this effect. Many useful pain-reducing remedies are of this category. Massage, analgesic balms, counterirritants, mustard plasters, hot and cold compresses, vibration, hydrotherapy, and vapocoolant therapy are examples.[25,26]

ENDOGENOUS ANTINOCICEPTIVE SYSTEM

The discovery of the endogenous antinociceptive system in 1975 opened a new avenue in pain research. This new knowledge brought considerable insight into the mechanisms of pain modulation. Endorphins were discovered in connection with research seeking an answer to why we have "morphine receptors" in the CNS. The term *endorphin* is a contraction of the words "endogenous morphine." There are five endorphins, namely, methionine-enkephalin, leucine-enkephalin, alpha-endorphin, beta-endorphin, and gamma-endorphin. The two enkephalins and beta-endorphin are particularly associated with antinociceptive mechanisms. No doubt these substances have other functions also.[27]

The endorphins are polypeptides, chains of amino acids. They are identical to portions of the pituitary hormone beta-lipotropin, which consists of 91 amino acids.[28-30] They behave like morphine, binding to morphine receptors to obtund pain. Like morphine, they are displaced from these receptors by the morphine antagonist naloxone. Repeated injections of enkephalin and beta-endorphin will cause tolerance and physical dependence.[27]

The short-chain enkephalins appear to act chiefly in the cerebrospinal fluid (CSF). They have short, rapid action and serve especially to limit the experience of excessive, sudden pain more than as an analgesic. The longer chain beta-endorphin appears to be closely related to pituitary function and may act somewhat like a hormone. It is longer lasting, requires the passage of a latent period before it becomes active, and has high antinociceptive potency.[27,31,32] Evidence exists that the endogenous opiates may act more as neuromodulators of postsynaptic activity than as classical neurotransmitters.[30] It has been shown that endorphins are important contributors to pain threshold and pain tolerance.[33] There is considerable interneurotransmitter action associated with the antinociceptive system in that endorphin is potentiated by serotonin that is released from serotoninergic neurons only in the presence of dopamine, while norepinephrine exerts a deterring effect.[34,35] It should be noted that Kosterlitz has remarked, "While it has been shown in many laboratories that the enkephalins and endorphins have antinociceptive effects, the underlying mechanisms have not been fully analyzed, and, in particular, the conditions controlling the release of opioid peptides are still not understood."[36]

It should be noted that beta-endorphin is appreciably released in long-distance runners.[37] It is also significant that placebo analgesia is endorphin mediated and naloxone reversible.[38,39] Analgesia produced by hypnosis, however, is not reversed by naloxone.[40,41] Hypnoanalgesia no doubt is based on other mechanisms, probably similar to that of psychological modulating effects.

ACUPUNCTURE AND ELECTROACUPUNCTURE

Although acupuncture has been in Chinese medicine for centuries, it came to public notice in the United States in 1972. Since then, much research has been directed toward this ancient modality of pain control. Needle acupuncture and electroacupuncture, which employs an electric current applied on the surface over acupoints, appear to work in the same general way. Both depend on noxious stimulation of specific sites. Both induce the release of beta-endorphin into the peripheral circulation.[42–46] Animal studies indicate a similar mechanism.[47] Some investigators believe, however, that acupuncture analgesia involves other mechanisms than the release of endorphin.[48]

Electroacupuncture differs from transcutaneous electrical nerve stimulation as described previously. This method requires a current of sufficient intensity to cause pain and phasic muscle contractions, but of very low frequency (2 Hz). The current must also be applied at specific sites where electrical impedance is lowest and where deeper nociceptors are available to be stimulated.[10]

Although unrelated to acupuncture, it should be noted that other deep noxious stimulation, such as strong visceral pain, may activate a similar antinociceptive effect.[49] Stimulation of the thalamus also exerts a powerful antinociceptive effect, presumably by way of activated raphe neurons.[50] Other antinociceptive amines such as gamma aminobutyric acid (GABA) and glycine act as inhibitory neurotransmitters and likely are involved in the mechanism of stimulation-produced analgesia.[51]

PSYCHOLOGICAL MODULATING EFFECTS

Although the mechanisms involved in the antinociceptive action of both nonnoxious and noxious electrical stimulation are important in understanding pain modulation, more important at a clinical level is an appreciation of the modulating effect of psychological factors. The mechanisms involved have yet to be elucidated. Several psychological conditions have marked modulating impact on the subject's pain experience. Some are excitatory; some are inhibitory.

Excitatory Modulating Factors

As a rule of thumb, egocentric psychological conditions that center the subject's attention toward himself have an excitatory effect on pain. This is borne out especially in the matter of attention. Wall determined that the level of pain due to injury related to the degree of attention directed toward the injury at the time.[52,53] So, too, with all pain; the more one is absorbed with his suffering, the more intense it becomes. Expectancy is another important factor.[54] Whether due to memory, anticipation, or prior conditioning, whatever one expects in the way of pain is likely to be what he experiences.[55,56]

The really potent excitatory modulators, however, are anxiety and fear, products of emotional reaction bearing on the consequences of the pain experience. Then, as maladaptive behavior ensues, depression and despair flourish, and chronicity associated with the depletion of endorphins sets in.[57] Problems of neuroticism[58] and the matter of secondary gains[56,59] that sometimes accompany suffering may further modulate the pain.

Inhibitory Modulating Factors

Generally, outgoing psychological conditions that direct one's attention and energies away from self have a favorable modulating effect on pain. A feeling of serenity born of confidence and assurance has marked inhibitory influence. Distraction is particularly inhibitory, as demonstrated by the effect of extraneous sounds,[60] suggestion and hypnosis,[61] mental absorption, and physical activities of different kinds.[62] Overcoming maladaptive behavior by constructively coping with the painful situation has very favorable modulating influence.

Not only does a knowledge of psychological modulation of nociceptive impulses help to understand pain better, it also gives important clues that can be useful in the treatment of people who suffer pain.

REFERENCES

1. Marshall H.R.: *Pain, Pleasure and Anesthesia*. London, Macmillan and Co. Ltd., 1894.
2. Strong C.A.: The psychology of pain. *Psychol. Rev.* 2:329, 1895.
3. Maurice C.G.: Differential diagnosis of dental pain. *J.A.D.A.* 50:316, 1955.

4. Melzack R., Wall P.D.: Pain mechanisms: A new theory. *Science* 150:971–979, 1965.
5. Casey K.L., Melzack R.: Neural mechanisms of pain: A conceptual model, in Way E.L. (ed.): *New Concepts in Pain.* Philadelphia, F.A. Davis Co., 1967, pp. 13–31.
6. Wall P.D.: The gate control theory of pain mechanisms: A reexamination and restatement. *Brain* 101:1–18, 1978.
7. Kane K., Taub A.: A history of local electrical analgesia. *Pain* 1:125–138, 1975.
8. Wall P.D., Sweet W.H.: Temporary abolition of pain in man. *Science* 155:108–109, 1967.
9. Long D.M., Hagfors N.: Electrical stimulation in the nervous system: The current status of electrical stimulation of the nervous system for relief of pain. *Pain* 1:109–123, 1975.
10. Andersson S.A.: Pain control by sensory stimulation, in Bonica J.J., Liebeskind J.C., Albe-Fessard D.G. (eds.): *Advances in Pain Research and Therapy.* New York, Raven Press, 1979, vol. 3, pp. 569–585.
11. Swett J.E., Law J.D.: Analgesia with peripheral nerve stimulation: Absence of a peripheral mechanism. *Pain* 15:55–70, 1983.
12. Zimmermann M.: Peripheral and central nervous mechanisms of nociception, pain, and pain therapy: Facts and hypotheses, in Bonica J.J., Liebeskind J.C., Albe-Fessard D.G. (eds.): *Advances in Pain Research and Therapy.* New York, Raven Press, 1979, vol. 3, pp. 3–32.
13. Bowsher D.: Role of the reticular formation in response to noxious stimulation. *Pain* 2:361–378, 1976.
14. Sjolund B.H., Eriksson M.B.E.: Endorphins and analgesia produced by peripheral conditioning stimulation, in Bonica J.J., Liebeskind J.C., Albe-Fessard D.G. (eds.): *Advances in Pain Research and Therapy.* New York, Raven Press, 1979, vol. 3, pp. 587–592.
15. Walker J.B., Katz R.L.: Nonopioid pathways produce prolonged pain suppression in humans. *Pain,* suppl. 1, 1981, p. S141.
16. Long D.M., Campbell J., Freeman T.: Failure of naloxone to affect chronic pain or stimulation-induced pain relief in man. *Pain,* suppl. 1, 1981, p. S111.
17. Pertovaara A., Kemppainen P., Johansson G., et al.: Dental analgesia produced by nonpainful, low-frequency stimulation is not influenced by stress or reversed by naloxone. *Pain* 13:379–384, 1982.
18. Willer J., Roby A., Boulu P., et al.: Comparative effects of electroacupuncture and transcutaneous nerve stimulation on the human blink reflex. *Pain* 14:267–278, 1982.
19. Freeman T.B., Campbell J.N., Long D.M.: Naloxone does not affect pain relief induced by electrical stimulation in man. *Pain* 17:189–195, 1983.
20. Boureau F., Luu M., Kisielnicki E.: Effects of transcutaneous nerve stimulation (TNS), electrotherapy (ET), and electroacupuncture (EA) on chronic pain: A comparative study. *Pain,* suppl. 1, 1981, p. S277.
21. Chapman C.R., Colpitts Y.M., Benedetti C., et al.: Evoked potential assessment of acupuncture analgesia: Attempted reversal with naloxone. *Pain* 9:183–197, 1980.
22. Peets J.M., Pomaranz B.: Intrathecal or systemic naloxone antagonizes TNS analgesia. *Pain,* suppl. 1, 1981, p. S179.
23. Basbaum A.T.: Brainstem control of nociception: The contribution of the monoamines. *Pain,* suppl. 1, 1981, p. S231.

24. Belcher G., Ryall R.W., Schaffner R.: The differential effects of 5–hydroxytryptamine, noradrenalin, and raphe stimulation on nociceptive and nonnociceptive dorsal horn interneurons in the cat. *Brain Res.* 151:307–321, 1978.
25. Ellis M.: The relief of pain by cooling of the skin. *Br. Med. J.* January 28, 1961, p. 250–252.
26. Steinman J.L., Komisaruk B.R., Yaksh T.L., et al. Spinal cord monoamines modulate the antinociceptive effects of vaginal stimulation in rats. *Pain* 16:155–166, 1983.
27. Synder S.H.: Opiate receptors and internal opiates. *Scientific American* 236:44–56, 1977.
28. Allen G.D.: *Dental Anesthesia and Analgesia*, ed. 2. Baltimore, Williams & Wilkins Co., 1979.
29. Kroening R., Donaldson D.: Proposed mechanism of acupuncture. *S.A.A.D. Digest* 4:28, 1979.
30. Watkins L.R., Mayer D.J.: Organization of endogenous opiate and non-opiate pain control systems. *Science* 216:1185–1192, 1982.
31. Kosterlitz H.W.: Interaction of endogenous opioid peptides and their analogs with opiate receptors, in Bonica J.J., Liebeskind J.C., Albe-Fessard D.G. (eds.): *Advances in Pain Research and Therapy.* New York, Raven Press, 1979, vol. 3, pp. 377–384.
32. Stacher G., Bauer P., Steinringer H., et al: Effects of the synthetic enkephalin analogue FK33–824 on pain threshold and pain tolerance in man. *Pain* 7:159–172, 1979.
33. Von Knorring L., Almay B.G.L., Johansson F., et al.: Pain perception and endorphin levels in cerebrospinal fluid. *Pain* 5:359–365, 1978.
34. Akil H., Liebeskind J.C.: Monoaminergic mechanisms of stimulation-produced analgesia. *Brain Res.* 94:279–296, 1975.
35. Mayer D.J., Price D.D.: Central nervous system mechanisms of analgesia. *Pain* 2:379–404, 1976.
36. Kosterlitz H.W.: Opioid peptides and pain: An update, in Bonica J.J., Lindblom U., Iggo A. (eds.): *Advances in Pain Research and Therapy.* New York, Raven Press, 1983, vol. 5, pp. 199–208.
37. Colt E.W.D., Wardlaw S.L., Frantz A.G.: The effect of running on plasma endorphin. *Life Sci.* 28:1637–1640, 1981.
38. Levine J.D., Gordon N.C., Fields H.L.: The role of endorphins in placebo analgesia, in Bonica J.J., Liebeskind J.C., Albe-Fessard D.G. (eds.): *Advances in Pain Research and Therapy.* New York, Raven Press, 1979, vol. 3, pp. 547–551.
39. Grevert P., Albert L.H., Goldstein A.: Partial antagonism of placebo analgesia by naloxone. *Pain* 16:129–143, 1983.
40. Barber J., Mayer D.: Evaluation of the efficacy and neural mechanism of a hypnotic analgesia procedure in experimental and clinical dental pain. *Pain* 4:41–48, 1977.
41. Mayer D.J.: Endogenous analgesia systems: Neural and behavioral mechanisms, in Bonica J.J., Liebeskind J.C., Albe-Fessard D.G. (eds.): *Advances in Pain Research and Therapy.* New York, Raven Press, 1979, vol. 3, pp. 385–410.
42. Sjolund B., Terenius L., Eriksson M.: Increased cerebrospinal fluid levels of endorphins after electroacupuncture. *Acta Physiol. Scand.* 100:382–384, 1977.

43. Pomeranz B., Cheng R.: Suppression of noxious responses in single neurons of cat spinal cord by electroacupuncture and its reversal by the opiate antagonist naloxone. *Exp. Neurol.* 64:327–341, 1979.
44. Cheng R.S.S., Pomeranz B.H.: Electroacupuncture analgesia is mediated by stereospecific opiate receptors and is reversed by antagonists of type 1 receptors. *Life Sci.* 26:631–638, 1980.
45. Salar G., Job I., Mingrino S., et al.: Effect of transcutaneous electrotherapy on CSF beta-endorphin content in patients without pain problems. *Pain* 10:169–172, 1981.
46. Stratton S.A.: Role of endorphins in pain modulation. *J. Orthoped. Sports Phy. Ther.* 3:200, 1982.
47. Han J., Zhou Z., Xuan Y.: Acupuncture has an analgesic effect in rabbits. *Pain* 15:83–91, 1983.
48. Chapman C.R., Benedetti C., Colpitts Y.H., et al.: Naloxone fails to reverse pain thresholds elevated by acupuncture: Acupuncture analgesia reconsidered. *Pain* 16:13–31, 1983.
49. Kraus E., LeBars L., Besson J.M.: Behavioral confirmation of 'diffuse noxious inhibitory controls' (DNIC) and evidence for a role of endogenous opiates. *Brain Res.* 206:495–499, 1981.
50. Dickenson A.: The inhibitory effects of thalamic stimulation on spinal transmission of nociceptive information in the cat. *Pain* 17:213–224, 1983.
51. Lovick T., Wolstencroft J.H.: Actions of GABA, glycine, methionine-enkephalin, and beta-endorphin compared with electrical stimulation of nucleus raphe magnus on responses evoked by tooth pulp stimulation in the medial reticular formation in the cat. *Pain* 15:131–144, 1983.
52. Wall P.D.: On the relation of injury to pain. *Pain* 6:253–264, 1979.
53. Melzack R., Wall P.D., Ty T.C.: Acute pain in an emergency clinic: Latency of onset and descriptor patterns related to different injuries. *Pain* 14:33–43, 1982.
54. Price D.D., Barrell J.J., Gracely R.H.: A psychophysical analysis of experimental factors that selectively influence the affective dimension of pain. *Pain* 8:137–149, 1980.
55. Dworkin S.F., Chen A.C.N., Schubert M.: Expectancy, nitrous oxide (N_2O) and modification of pain in a clinical setting. *Pain*, suppl. 1, 1981, p. S171.
56. Fordyce W.E.: Behavioral conditioning concepts in chronic pain, in Bonica J.J., Lindblom U., Iggo A. (eds.): *Advances in Pain Research and Therapy.* New York, Raven Press, 1983, vol. 5, pp. 781–788.
57. Lindblom U., Tegner R.: Are the endorphins active in clinical pain states? Narcotic antagonism in chronic pain patients. *Pain* 7:65–68, 1979.
58. Sternbach R.A., Timmermans G.: Personality changes associated with reduction of pain. *Pain* 1:177–181, 1975.
59. Sternbach R.A.: Varieties of pain games, in Bonica J.J. (ed.): *Advances in Neurology.* New York, Raven Press, 1974, vol. 4, pp. 423–430.
60. Gardner W.J., Licklider J.C.R.: Auditory analgesia in dental operations. *J.A.D.A.* 59:1144, 1959.
61. Orne M.T.: Hypnotic methods for managing pain, in Bonica J.J., Lindblom U., Iggo A. (eds.): *Advances in Pain Research and Therapy.* New York, Raven Press, 1983, vol. 5, pp. 847–856.
62. Szechtman H., Hershkowitz M., Simantov R.: Sexual behavior decreases pain sensitivity and stimulates endogenous opioids in male rats. *Europ. J. Pharmacol.* 70:279, 1981.

5

Secondary Effects of Deep Pain

IT IS WELL KNOWN that pain frequently is felt at a site other than where it originates—so-called referred pain. This and other phenomena associated with nociception need to be understood and appreciated if pain management is to be effective. Diagnostic differentiation between true primary pain and symptoms that occur as secondary effects of that pain is essential. Such manifestations are usually referred to as central excitatory effects on the presumption that they result from hyperexcitability of (CNS) interneurons.

CENTRAL EXCITATORY EFFECTS

The neurologic mechanisms involved in the secondary effects of pain have not been well investigated. Some researchers think that reflex activity is involved.[1] There seems to be little doubt that unusual convergence of impulses among CNS interneurons takes place.[2] However the factors that control the mechanisms involved have not been elucidated.

Clinically, secondary excitatory effects are induced by more or less continuous barrages of noxious sensation emanating from deep somatic structures. Intermittency of primary input limits their occurrence; intensity and duration favor them. In the absence of afferent synapses outside the CNS, the transfer of signals must involve interneuron activity. The neural pathways that mediate these effects, however, have not been identified. In effect, symptoms of central hyperexcitability are expected to complicate deep somatic pains that are continuous, and these effects tend to increase with the intensity and duration of the primary pain. Such symptoms occur in otherwise normal structures, and the cause of them must be sought elsewhere.

There is a close segmental relationship between the primary initiating pain and secondary effects. Most secondary symptoms occur in structures innervated by the same major nerve that mediates the primary pain. Familiarity with dermatome mapping helps one to understand these segmental relationships. A dermatome is a sensory root field on the skin where pain is felt when a particular neural segment mediates painful sensation. These have been well charted (Fig 5–1). Each nerve has a corresponding dermatome. There is considerable

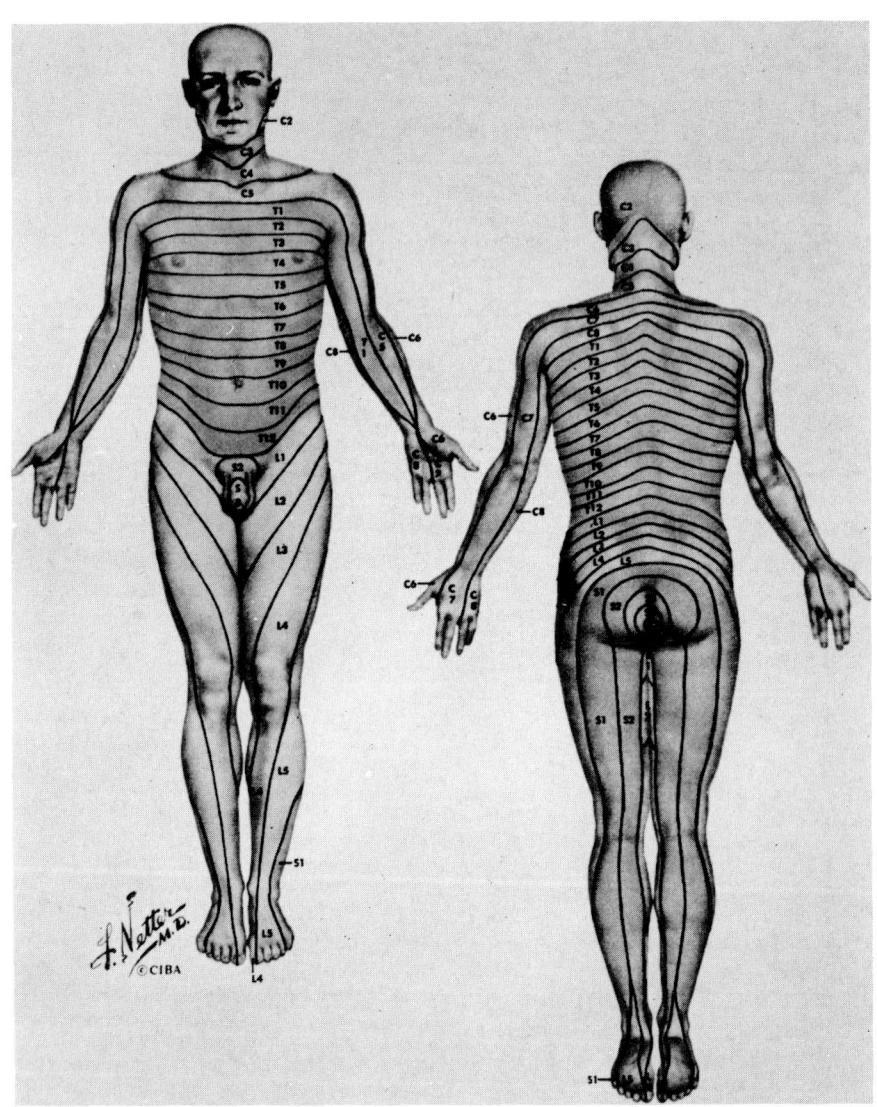

Fig 5–1.—Dermal segmentation as represented by Netter, based essentially on the work of Keegan. (Copyright 1953, 1972 CIBA Pharmaceutical Company, Division of CIBA-GEIGY Corporation. Reproduced with permission from *The CIBA Collection of Medical Illustrations* by Frank H. Netter, M.D. All rights reserved.)

SECONDARY EFFECTS OF DEEP PAIN 63

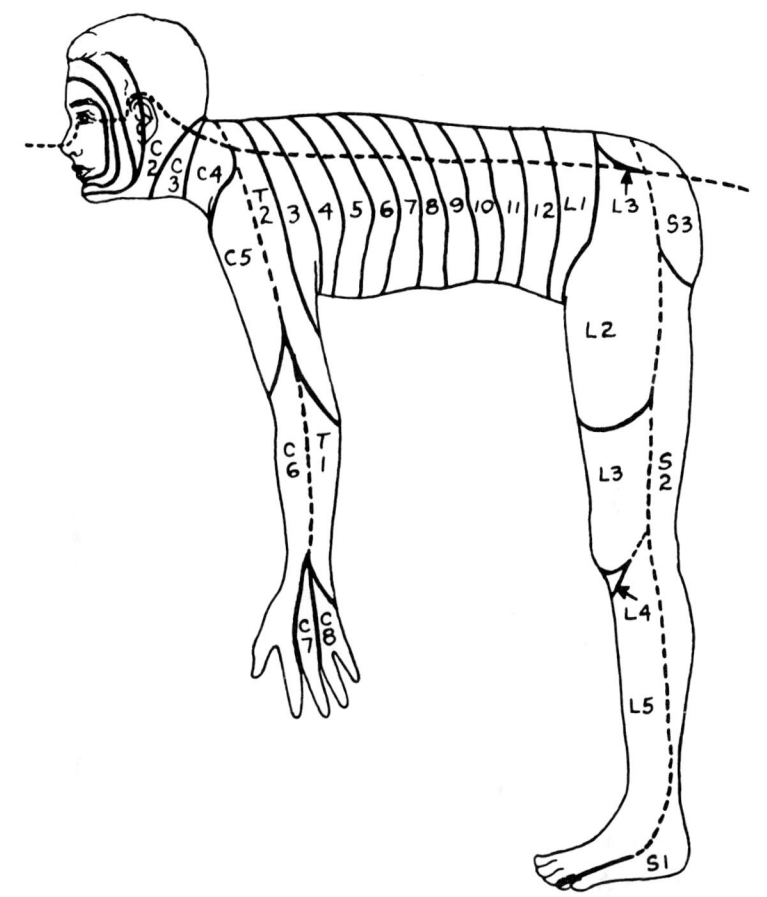

Fig 5–2.—The orderly metameric arrangement of dermatomes becomes apparent if we visualize man in the quadruped position. (From Finneson B.E.: *Diagnosis and Management of Pain Syndromes*, ed. 2. Philadelphia, W.B. Saunders Co., 1969. Reproduced with permission.)

overlapping, however. Man's upright posture causes some confusion in dermatome arrangement, especially in the extremities. They are better visualized with the subject in the quadruped position (Fig 5–2). This places them in a more logical metameric arrangement and helps considerably to identify the proper segmental relationships.[3] When intersegmental spreading of secondary effects takes place, it occurs predominantly in a cephalad direction. Only very intense primary pain causes excitatory effects in a segment caudal to the site of initiating input.[4]

The secondary effects of deep pain may be classified as (1) sensory, (2) autonomic, and (3) motor. The sensory effects include referred pains and secondary hyperalgesias; autonomic effects refer to vasomotor and

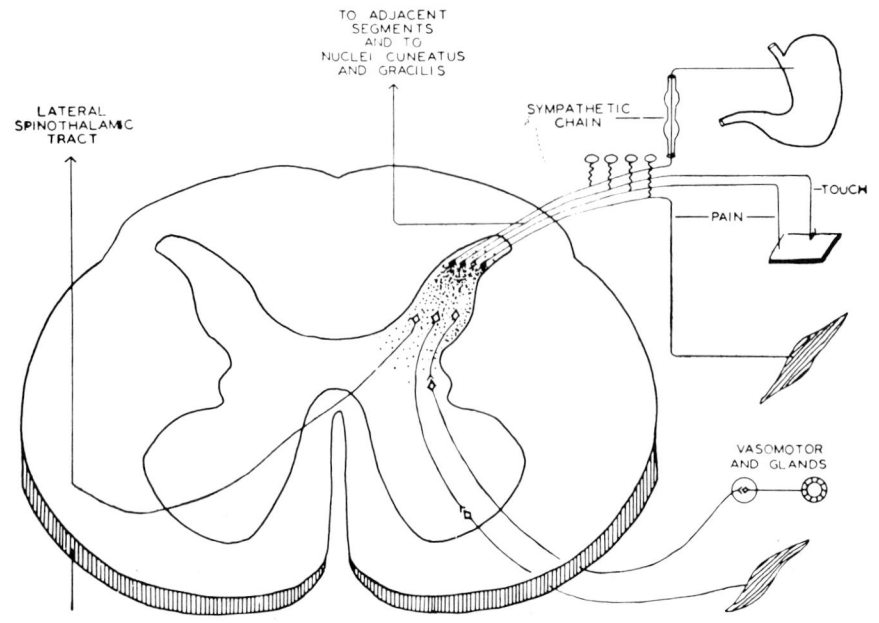

Fig 5-3.—Schematic representation of spinal segment showing various effects of noxious impulses from primary noxious stimulus in the stomach. The skin becomes hyperalgesic and hyperesthetic, and muscles become tender. Effector structures innervating blood vessels and glands (sweat and sebaceous) are involved as well as those innervating skeletal muscle causing contractions, which may in themselves become painful. (From Wolff H.G., Wolf S.: *Pain*, ed. 2. Springfield, Ill., Charles C Thomas, Publisher, 1958. Reproduced with permission.)

glandular symptoms; motor effects include trigger point and myospastic activity in segmentally related skeletal muscles. Wolff and Wolf[5] have schematically represented these effects involving a spinal segment (Fig 5-3). Wolff[4] and Bonica[6] have reviewed the clinical aspects of central excitatory effects in depth.

SENSORY EFFECTS OF DEEP PAIN

Heterotopic Pain

The term *heterotopic pain* refers to any pain that is felt in an area other than its true source. Such pain is broadly classified as allodynia—pain that occurs without noxious stimulation. Although the terms *referred* and *heterotopic* are frequently used interchangeably, a more restricted usage of the term *referred* is advocated. In this book, therefore, *referred pain* will be used to mean *spontaneous heterotopic pain that occurs as a central excitatory effect*. It should be distinguished from *secondary hyperalgesia*, another central excitatory effect, as well as from *projected pain*, a manifestation of neurogenous pain.

There are several types of heterotopic pain: (1) central pain, (2) projected pain, and (3) central excitation pain.

CENTRAL PAIN.—Pain that emanates from structures of the CNS is felt peripherally as heterotopic pain. Pain emanating from intracranial pain–sensitive structures on or above the tentorium cerebelli is felt in the peripheral distribution of the trigeminal nerve.

PROJECTED PAIN.—Projected pain is felt in the peripheral distribution of the *same nerve* that mediates the primary input. Pain due to noxious stimulation of a sensory root or a major nerve trunk is felt in the exact anatomical distribution of that nerve. An example is the radicular pain of posterior root compression. It has been assumed that compression due to herniation of an intervertebral disc produces prolonged firing in the injured sensory fibers. It should be noted, however, that acute peripheral nerve compression is usually painless and rarely lasts more than a few seconds. It is likely, therefore, that radicular pain is felt in the peripheral structures through activation of deeper interneurons.[7] The mechanism, however, seems to be different from that of central excitation in that projected pain follows a more precise anatomical pattern relative to the peripheral distribution, while central excitation pain is felt in a reference zone that is only segmentally related to the primary pain source. Projected sensory nerve pain is primarily neurogenous and follows dermatome mapping faithfully. Examples of projected pain include neuritic neuralgia, paroxysmal neuralgia, herpes zoster, and postherpetic neuralgia.

It has long been known that noxious stimulation of a motor root or major motor nerve also induces pain—but of a different type and felt in different areas. Rather than the bright, burning, neurogenous pain felt in the dermatome distribution, motor nerve pain is sensed as dull, deep somatic pain diffusely located in the muscles innervated by that nerve. Such pain is now explicable on the basis of recently identified afferent neurons that are present in the motor nerves. No doubt, such pain should be classified as projected pain, even though it displays a deep somatic rather than neurogenous quality and follows a motor nerve route rather than a dermatome field. Although the neural mechanisms have not been identified, it is likely that interneurons are involved in a manner similar to that for projected sensory nerve pain. It likewise differs from the heterotopic pain of central excitation.

It should be noted that heterotopic pain may be generated by stimulating certain sites within skeletal muscles or their fascial sheaths—so-called myofascial trigger points. It is interesting that some such heterotopic pain is felt peripherally at more distal sites in a manner similar to other projected motor pain. Most myofascially generated heterotopic pains, however, are felt in reference zones situated at segmentally related sites outside the involved muscle and innervated by different nerves. Such pains no doubt are true central excitatory effects as described below.

Projected pains may be accompanied by areas of secondary hyperalgesia that are hypersensitive to stimulation without appreciable reduction in local pain threshold. Whatever the mechanism responsible for this phenomenon, it is likely similar to that which induces the secondary hyperalgesia of central hyperexcitability as described below.

CENTRAL EXCITATION PAIN.—Heterotopic pain may be induced by deep somatic pain as a central excitatory effect. It differs from projected pain in that it remains dependent upon a primary pain input and is felt in a reference zone that is only segmentally related to the site of the primary pain. Although there is a neurologic relationship between the primary pain and the secondary effects, it follows a pattern that is unrelated to the peripheral distribution of the nerve that mediates the primary pain. The zone of reference may be some distance away and is innervated by a different sensory nerve. Thus, an aura of mystery is created that presents problems both diagnostic and therapeutic.

Other symptoms of central excitation may accompany the heterotopic pain. The primary deep pain may be modulated into complete silence, leaving only the secondary effects as the symptomatic complaint of the patient. When this occurs—which is commonplace—careful diagnostic differentiation is required to determine the correct location and cause of the initiating deep pain that is responsible for the symptoms.

Central excitation pain may be expressed in either or both of two ways: (1) *spontaneous* referred pain, and (2) *stimulation-evoked* secondary hyperalgesia.

Referred Pain

Referred pain due to central excitation is wholly spontaneous as far as the site of reference is concerned. It is not accentuated by provocation of the site where the pain is felt; it is accentuated only by manipulation of the primary pain source. It is dependent on continuance of the primary initiating pain; it ceases immediately if the primary pain is arrested or interrupted. Anesthesia of the structure where the referred pain is felt does not arrest the pain.[8] Only by anesthetizing the neural pathway that mediates the primary pain is the referred pain arrested.[9]

The diagnostic criteria for identifying referred pain are as follows:
1. It is not accentuated by provocation of the referred pain site.
2. It is not arrested by anesthesia of the referred pain site.
3. It is accentuated by exacerbation of the primary pain.
4. It is arrested by analgesic blocking of the primary pain.

It should be noted that although the primary initiating pain is of the deep somatic type, the secondary referred pain may be felt in either deep or superficial structures. This may present a bizarre clinical picture. When reference is felt superficially, it must be differentiated from superficial somatic pain and from projected neurogenous pain. When it is felt deeply, it must be differentiated from other deep somatic pains.

Secondary Hyperalgesia

Hyperalgesia is defined as increased sensitivity to pain *evoked by stimulation at the site of pain.* Primary hyperalgesia occurs as the result of lowered pain threshold due presumably to the presence of algogenic substances such as bradykinin, potassium, histamine, and serotonin. Secondary hyperalgesia is different. It is heterotopic pain, an increased response to stimulation at the site of pain, but without a lowered pain threshold and without the action of algogenic substances. It may occur with or without accompanying referred pain.

Secondary hyperalgesia is also different from referred pain in that it occurs in response to stimulation (provocation) at the site of pain, while referred pain is wholly spontaneous as far as the site of pain is concerned. Both referred pain and secondary hyperalgesia are initiated by deep pain input and remain dependent upon the continuance of such input. They differ, however, in that secondary hyperalgesia persists for a while after the primary pain ceases. Thus, analgesic blocking of the primary pain site does not immediately arrest the hyperalgesia as it does referred pain.

As with referred pain, secondary hyperalgesia may be felt in either superficial or deep structures. Superficial secondary hyperalgesia is felt as touchy or sensitive skin, scalp, hair, or gingiva. Deep secondary hyperalgesia is sensed as an area of palpable tenderness, discomfort due to functional manipulation, or hypersensitive or tender teeth.

At a clinical level, superficial secondary hyperalgesia usually presents no great problem because of the obvious lack of local cause. Deep secondary hyperalgesia, however, cannot be distinguished from primary hyperalgesia on the basis of manual palpation or functional manipulation. Special diagnostic effort is required to make this judgment—an important one therapeutically. It should be noted that palpable tenderness or deep discomfort from functional manipulation identifies only a *site of pain*, not a *source of pain*. Whether such an identified site of pain is primary hyperalgesia from local cause, such as inflammation or myospasm, or a heterotopic manifestation of deep pain input located elsewhere is a judgment that must precede definitive therapy.

Although secondary hyperalgesia occurs in otherwise normal structures, there usually is a small central area of hyperemia indicating some local tissue reaction. In this flare area of an axon reflex, the pain threshold is lowered, thus indicating that this portion of the hyperalgesic area is primary and reflects local tissue change. The entire area of sensitivity, however, extends far beyond the hyperemic zone. The wider area represents true secondary hyperalgesia that is dependent on continuance of primary deep pain impulses.[4] Analgesic blocking of such an area of secondary hyperalgesia does in fact decrease the total discomfort, due presumably to its effect on the component of primary hyperalgesia that is present.[5] It does not render the area entirely painless, however, as would be the case with primary hyperalgesia from local cause.

The diagnostic criteria for identifying secondary hyperalgesia are as follows:
1. It is accentuated by provocation of the hyperalgesic site.
2. It is not wholly arrested by anesthesia of the painful site.
3. It is accentuated by exacerbation of the primary pain.
4. It is not arrested by analgesic blocking of the primary pain.

Significance of Facial Lamination

According to Kunc,[10, 11] the location of trigeminal nociceptive terminals within the nucleus caudalis is as follows:
1. The fibers from parts near the sagittal midline of the face terminate *highest* in the nucleus (cephalad).
2. The fibers from parts located more laterally terminate *lowest* in the nucleus (caudad).
3. The intermediate fibers terminate *intermediately* in the nucleus (Fig 5–4). This laminated arrangement of facial innervation ap-

pears to coincide with Finneson's[3] metameric arrangement of the dermatomes in the quadruped position.

This grouping of the terminals of the primary trigeminal neurons should influence the location of clinical effects of central excitation, especially with regard to referred pain. It probably accounts for some effects not otherwise readily explained on the basis of what formerly

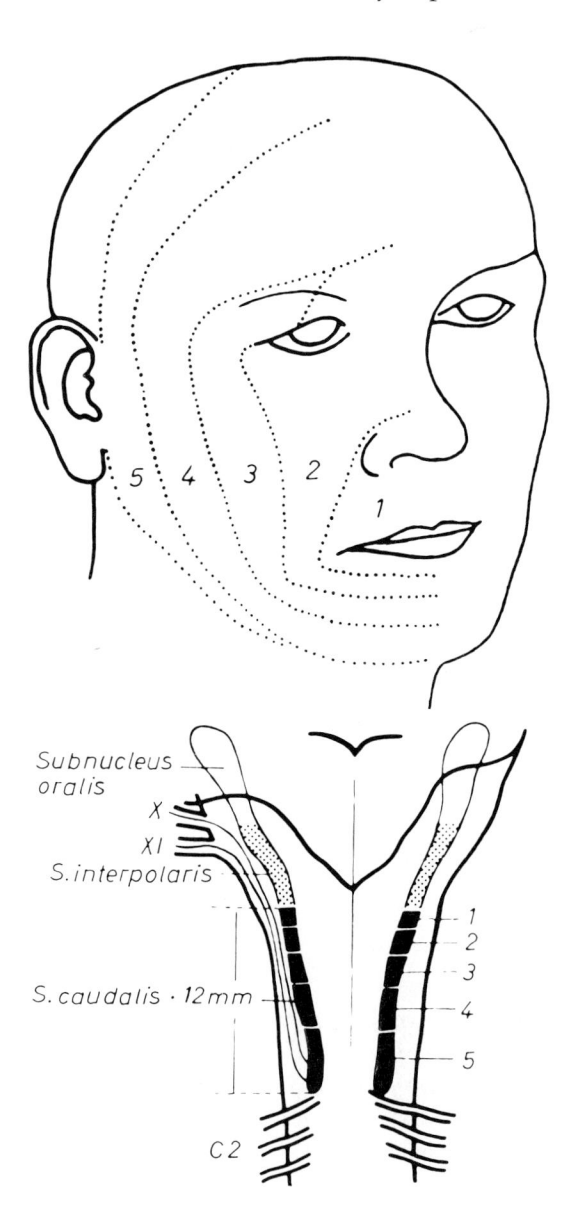

Fig 5–4.—Schema of spinal trigeminal nucleus. Only subnucleus caudalis serves for termination of fibers for pain. It has a segmentary arrangement. (From Kunc Z.: Significant factors pertaining to the results of trigeminal tractotomy, in Hassler R., Walker A.E. (eds.): *Trigeminal Neuralgia, Pathogenesis and Pathophysiology.* Stuttgart, Georg Thieme Verlag, 1970. Reproduced with permission.)

had been thought to be the grouping of the primary trigeminal synapses, i.e., terminals of mandibular, maxillary, and ophthalmic division fibers, respectively, are located in the trigeminal nucleus from above downward. Kawamura and Nishiyama[12] showed that a molar tooth projects dorsal to a canine, and a canine projects dorsal to an incisor, confirming the vertical lamination cited above.

The significance of an understanding of the lamination arrangement of the trigeminal afferent terminals has to do with the anatomical location of central excitatory effects in the trigeminal region. Although the most frequently encountered effects occur in structures innervated by fibers of the same neural division that mediates the primary pain impulses, when other divisions are involved, the location of such effects follows a vertical lamination pattern. Following this principle, referred pain is more likely to occur from maxillary molar to mandibular molar than from maxillary molar to mandibular incisor. Likewise, referred earache almost invariably arises from a molar tooth, and referred masseter muscle pain is characteristically felt in the temporomandibular joint or molar tooth.

AUTONOMIC EFFECTS OF DEEP PAIN

Deep somatic pain may induce autonomic effects in an area segmentally related to the site of primary pain. Vasomotor and glandular effects may occur. The symptoms include such things as temperature and color changes in the skin (flushing, blanching), puffy swelling of the eyelids and other loose cutaneous tissue, injection of the conjunctiva, lacrimation, nasal secretion, and nasal congestion. Such symptoms may simulate allergic rhinitis or maxillary sinusitis.

The autonomic changes induced by deep pain are thought to be central excitatory effects. Their behavior is similar to other such effects and remains dependent upon deep pain input. There is a recovery time lag, however, when the primary pain ceases; the autonomic symptoms may persist for a day or so.

MOTOR EFFECTS OF DEEP PAIN

Deep somatic pain may induce motor effects of two types: (1) myofascial trigger point pain mechanisms, and (2) spasm of skeletal muscles. The muscles that are affected are usually those innervated by the same major nerve that mediates the deep pain input, thus establishing a segmental relationship. If the primary pain is mediated by the trigeminal nerve, the muscles most likely to be affected are those innervated by the trigeminal nerve. They are eight in number: the masseter, the temporalis, the medial pterygoid, the lateral pterygoid, the mylohyoid, the anterior belly of the digastric, the tensor palati, and the tensor tympani muscles. It should be noted that if intersegmental spreading of such secondary effects occurs, it is predominantly in a cephalad direction. Thus, cervical deep pain input may induce myospasm activity in facial and masticatory muscles; the reverse, however, seldom if ever occurs.[4]

Trigger Point Mechanisms

A continuing deep pain input of some intensity may induce a myofascial trigger point mechanism involving a muscle(s) that is segmentally related to the site of primary pain. The masseter and temporalis are the masticatory muscles most frequently affected. The trigger point, in turn, refers pain that is frequently felt at or near the site of the initiating primary pain. The trigger itself, however, is usually silent unless manually palpated; then local muscle pain is felt. Although this mechanism may be initiated by pain, once trigger points become established, they remain active or latent until eliminated by therapeutic effort. Thus, pain at or near the initial site of primary pain may persist as a continuing or recurrent heterotopic manifestation long after the original pain has ceased. The complexity of such pain problems makes accurate diagnosis all the more necessary for effective management of the patient's complaint.

Muscle Spasm Activity

Another important secondary effect of deep pain is the development of myospastic activity in skeletal muscles innervated by the same neural segment that mediates the primary pain. Deep somatic pain may induce contraction of one or more segmentally related muscles. If this continues, a cycling myospasm may develop, and, once established, such spastic activity becomes wholly independent of the initiating cause. Cycling muscle spasms become self-perpetuating and may continue indefinitely. A myospasm constitutes a new and independent source of deep somatic pain that has the propensity to cause other central excitatory effects. Thus, a pattern of spreading pain and muscle spasm may develop.

Some muscular dysfunction accompanies myospasms. Isometric contraction leads to muscle rigidity and resistance to stretch. Isotonic contraction shortens the muscle and causes skeletal displacement.

As with other central excitatory effects, muscle spasm activity that follows intersegmental spreading occurs in the cephalad direction, not vice versa. It is commonplace, therefore, to encounter facial or masticatory muscle spasm induced by deep cervical pain, while the reverse seldom if ever occurs.[4] Since cycling muscle spasms become independent of initiating cause, such conditions may present difficult diagnostic problems when the initiating cause is no longer present.

REFERENCES

1. Procacci P., Zoppi M.: Pathophysiology and clinical aspects of visceral and referred pain, in Bonica J.J., Lindblom U., Iggo A. (eds.): *Advances in Pain Research and Therapy.* New York, Raven Press, 1983, vol. 5, pp. 643–658.
2. Milne R.J., Foreman R.D., Giesler G.J., et al.: Viscerosomatic convergence into primate spinothalamic neurons: An explanation for referral of pelvic visceral pain, in Bonica J.J., Lindblom U., Iggo A. (eds.): *Advances in Pain Research and Therapy.* New York, Raven Press, 1983, vol. 5, pp. 131–137.
3. Finneson B.E.: *Diagnosis and Management of Pain Syndromes*, ed. 2. Philadelphia, W.B. Saunders Co., 1969.
4. Dalessio D.J.: *Wolff's Headache and Other Head Pain*, ed. 3. New York, Oxford University Press, 1972.
5. Wolff H. G., Wolf S.: *Pain*, ed. 2. Springfield, Ill., Charles C Thomas, Publisher, 1958.
6. Bonica J.J.: *The Management of Pain.* Philadelphia, Lea & Febiger, 1953.
7. Howe J.F., Loeser J.D., Calvin W.H.: Mechanosensitivity of dorsal root ganglia and chronically injured axons: A physiological basis for the radicular pain of nerve root compression. *Pain* 3:25–41, 1977.
8. Wolff H.G., Hardy J.D.: On nature of pain. *Physiol. Rev.* 27:167, 1947.
9. Kunkle E.C., Kibler R.F., Armstead G.C., et al.: Central sensory excitation and inhibition in response to induced pain. *Trans. Am. Neurol. Assoc.* 74:64, 1949.
10. Kunc Z.: Significance of fresh anatomic data on spinal trigeminal tract for possibility of selective tractotomies, in Knighton R.S., Dumke P.R. (eds.): *Pain.* Boston, Little, Brown & Co., 1966, pp. 351–363.
11. Kunc Z.: Significant factors pertaining to the results of trigeminal tractotomy, in Hassler R., Walker A.E. (eds.): *Trigeminal Neuralgia.* Stuttgart, Georg Thieme Verlag, 1970, pp. 90–100.
12. Kawamura Y., Nishiyama T.: Projection of dental afferent impulses to the trigeminal nuclei. *Jpn. J. Physiol.* 16:584–597, 1966.

6

Genesis of Pain

THE GENESIS OF PAIN is poorly understood—if, indeed, it is understood at all. There was a time when it was generally thought that noxious stimulation, meaning tissue-damaging stimulation, was the chief basis for nociception. It was presumed that pain was some kind of gauge of tissue injury: the greater the pain, the greater the injury that had been sustained. Pain occurring without an initiating antecedent was presumed to be generated by psychic phenomena and therefore was not really pain at all.

As the concept of pain modulation evolved, the question of genesis lost much of its significance. It is now recognized that factors other than noxious stimulation are determinants of suffering. For example, Wall[1] has shown that pain at the time of injury relates to the *attention* given; pain later relates to the *consequences* of the injury and its treatment. Algogenic substances that accompany inflammation incidental to tissue injury require time to develop and therefore are not immediate determinants in the matter of pain from tissue damage per se. So, structural injury from mechanical, chemical, or electrical trauma, as it relates to the genesis of pain, abounds in uncertainty.

An understanding of the mechanisms underlying different types of pain inception may be helpful in the diagnosis and management of nociceptive problems in general.

PAIN INDUCED BY INFLAMMATION

The traditional concept of noxious stimulation as the initiating determinant of pain genesis may very well stem from that induced by inflammation. Tissue injury initiates an inflammatory reaction that characteristically induces pain. The symptoms relate to the conditions that prevail such as (1) the kind, extent, and location of injury, (2) the reactivity of the injured structures, (3) the degree of confinement of the inflammatory exudate, and (4) the phase of inflammation.

Inflammatory pain is due chiefly to the action of prostaglandins and bradykinin, substances released by the inflammatory process. They act in conjunction with each other to increase local vasodilatation and capillary permeability as well as to alter the sensitivity and receptivity of receptors in the area.[2-5] Thus, pain threshold is lowered so that nociceptors become more sensitive to stimulation, and higher threshold mechanoreceptors are sensitized to a wider variety of stimuli. As a result, spontaneous primary pain and stimulation-evoked primary hyperalgesia take place. Along with these local effects, there is a prostaglandinlike substance released in the central nervous system (CNS) that sensitizes nociceptive interneurons to mechanical and chemical stimuli and renders neural pathways related to inflammatory pain more sensitive to the action of opiates. This is called *prostaglandin hyperalgesia*.[6]

Pain of inflammatory origin may involve different kinds of tissue innervated by receptors with different reactive responses. For example, superficial pain may be inflammatory, such as that of dermatitis or gingivitis. Examples of musculoskeletal inflammatory pain are those of myositis and cellulitis. Visceral inflammatory pain may be expressed as that of lymphadenitis or arteritis. Inflammatory neurogenous pain may be manifested as neuritis. Many physical ailments are inflammatory, and pain of inflammatory type is part of the symptom complex.

MUSCULAR GENESIS OF PAIN

Noninflammatory pain of muscle origin is probably the most frequent cause of human suffering, yet it remains poorly understood. A great deal of mystery continues to shroud myogenous pain in general; this affects doctors and patients alike. Without a good understanding of disorders of this type, one cannot effectively manage many pain complaints.

Most myogenous pain is noninflammatory. It frequently occurs in relationship to systemic responses. Some are protective, such as muscle splinting. Some are reactive, such as myofascial trigger point activity. Some comprise a component of myospasm.

Muscle Splinting Pain

So-called muscle splinting is considered to be a temporary protective mechanism. It is thought to occur in response to altered proprioceptive and sensory input that is interpreted as a threat to some part of the musculoskeletal system. Such activity is considered to be normal physiologic behavior of skeletal muscles.

Muscle splinting is recognized as local tenderness of the muscle, especially when it is being contracted. Muscle splinting is usually accompanied by a feeling of muscle weakness. This occurs without appreciable clinical dysfunction or significant increase in electromyographic (EMG) activity of the resting muscle. The inhibitory influence of pain and feeling of weakness, however, satisfactorily accomplish the objective of arresting functional use of the muscle. If these signals go unheeded, and if the splinted muscle is abused by continued use, myospastic activity may ensue. If the inhibitory influence of muscle splinting is permitted to take the part out of function and set it at rest, the effect rapidly disappears as the threat resolves.[7]

Trigger Point Pain

A frequent source of myogenous pain is due to the presence of myofascial trigger points located in muscles or their facial sheaths, a condition sometimes referred to as *fibrositis*. These phenomena have been described and documented by Travell and Simons.[8] A myofascial trigger point is a hyperirritable locus within a taut band of skeletal muscle that is painful on compression and can evoke characteristic referred pain and autonomic symptoms. The severity of trigger point symptoms ranges from painless reduction of movement to agonizing, incapacitating pain.[8] Zones of reference to which pains are referred have been well charted.[9] Even temporomandibular pain referred from myofascial sources in muscles of the head and neck has been identified.[10]

An active myofascial trigger point may generate pain when the muscle is at rest as well as during functional movements. Such pain is usually felt at a secondary site outside the muscle while the primary initiating pain remains silent. Thus, the patient may be wholly unaware of the true source of pain, the complaint consisting entirely of referred pain and secondary hyperalgesia. Manual palpation of the trigger point, however, elicits local discomfort at the site. The secondary symptoms may or may not be accentuated by such manipulation.

The etiology of trigger points and the mechanisms involved in myofascial pain have not been elucidated. It is not accounted for by local structural change at the trigger site. Only minor tissue changes are evident unless the trigger has been present for long periods. The pain is not due to myospastic activity because no increased EMG activity is evident with the muscle at rest. It has been postulated that group

III or group IV nerve endings or both have been sensitized by some algogenic substance.[11, 12] Trigger points display a slightly higher temperature, indicating an area of increased metabolism, decreased circulation, or both. They do not seem to be related to myoneural junctions, muscle spindles, or Golgi tendon organs.[8]

Trigger points may develop in response to deep somatic or visceral pain as a central excitatory effect. They may occur sequential to viral infections, inflammatory conditions of various types, visceral disease, nutritional disorders, or emotional stress.[13] Some appear to complicate problems of disuse atrophy. Some seem to develop spontaneously. Active triggers may become latent, but they do not disappear without therapy. Trigger points are activated by overload, fatigue, trauma, or chilling.

Trigger points may induce minor dysfunction manifested as (1) muscle weakness without atrophic change, (2) resistance to stretch, (3) stiffness especially after periods of inactivity, and (4) palpable hardenings within the muscle. Autonomic and proprioceptive disturbance may also ensue. Trigger points cause symptoms attended by considerable mystery and uncertainty. This generates anxiety and fear out of proportion to the true significance. Marked modulating effects may therefore occur. Muscles involved in a myofascial syndrome may become spastic, thus adding complications to the problem both diagnostically and therapeutically.

Muscle Spasm Pain

The term *muscle spasm* is used clinically to describe CNS-induced tonic contraction of a skeletal muscle. It is thought to occur in response to increased excitability of alpha motor neurons. It is characterized by increased EMG activity in the muscle at rest.[14] Painful myospastic activity renders it independent of initiating cause and sets up a self-perpetuating local muscle condition that can cycle indefinitely. As such, it represents a new and independent source of deep somatic pain.[15]

The cause of muscle spasm pain has not been fully explained. Since continued contraction of skeletal muscle in prime movers induces fatigue and ischemia, and since algogenic substances including bradykinin are released during such ischemic episodes,[16] the pain of spastic activity in muscle may likely be due to the presence of such substances.

Travell[13] lists a number of causes of muscle spasm, namely, sudden trauma, unusual or excessive exercise, chilling, immobilization, acute visceral pain, rupture of a vertebral disc, and acute emotional stress. Clinically, it seems that none of these initiating causes induces muscle spasm directly. It appears that one of three conditions prevails prior to the development of the spasm, namely, (1) muscle splinting activity, (2) a continuing input of deep somatic pain, or (3) a preexistent myofascial trigger point mechanism. Muscle spasm activity occurs in response to one of these prior conditions.

Muscle spasm pain can be distinguished from that of muscle splinting and trigger point pain by the muscular dysfunction that accompanies the complaint. Spasm constitutes tonic contraction that causes muscle rigidity (if it is isometric contraction), muscle shortening (if it is isotonic contraction), or both. It may also be distinguished by the presence of EMG activity when the muscle is at rest.

VASCULAR GENESIS OF PAIN

Once considered to be the most common pain complaint known to man, [17] and still perhaps ranking second only to myogenous pain, so-called vascular pain continues to be poorly understood by health professionals. Gross[18] has shown that blood vessels are innervated by afferent neurons of both the somatic and visceral nervous systems. Nociceptive impulses arising from vascular structures therefore may be mediated by either or both of these pathways.

It has long been presumed that vascular pain is initiated chiefly by dilatation of small arteries, which distorts and noxiously stimulates afferent fibers in vascular and perivascular tissues. Vasoconstricting medications such as ergotamine tartrate, which reduce the dilatation and amplitude of pulsation of arteries, decrease the pain. Pressure applied to the carotid artery also diminishes the pain.[15] The presumption, however, that vasodilation is the primary cause of vascular pain is no longer tenable because spontaneous dilatation of cranial arteries does not cause pain in *normal* subjects. Rather, dilating drugs provide relaxation of arteries, but not pain. Only algogenic substances such as bradykinin and histamine can evoke vasodilation *and* pain.[19]

Systemic more than local factors seem to play the major role in the incidence of vascular pain. It occurs in "pain patients," so-called *hypernoceptors,* who have some deficiency in opioid peptides and neurotransmitters of the antinociceptive system.[19] Serotonin deficiency in the CNS has been identified with the incidence of vascular pain.[20-23] Histamine administered to known "migraine patients" consistently precipitates an attack of pain, while nonmigrainous persons do not react in this way.[24] Patients with vascular pain frequently display a characteristic emotional overlay with personality features of insecurity with tension. This may be manifested as inflexibility, conscientiousness, meticulousness, perfectionism, and resentment. Frustration, fatigue, and prostration seem to set the stage for an attack.[15] In the light of serotonin depletion, which also characterizes depressive states,[25] the emotional symptoms and the pain may simply represent different facets of a common problem.[26]

According to Wolff,[27] four conditions contribute to the discomfort of vascular pain: (1) dilatation of blood vessels, (2) local edema of the painful site, (3) edema of the vessel wall and perivascular tissue, and (4) associated muscle pain (especially in the occipital area). It has been shown that attacks of common migraine display accompanying increased EMG activity in pericranial muscles.[28, 29] It appears that so-called tension headache (muscle contraction headache) and vascular headache (classic and common migraine) have much in common.[19] The clinical complaint frequently comprises elements of both varieties of pain. Likely, the systemic factors in these conditions stem from common cause, and the peripheral symptoms may represent little more than different facets of a common problem. The psychological implications of both conditions therefore are of great importance.

NEURAL GENESIS OF PAIN

Quite a different source of pain is that which is generated within the nervous system itself. Neurogenous pain is from two causes: (1) neuropathy and (2) deafferentation. Neuropathy pain results from structural change in neural components; deafferentation pain results from interruption of the flow of afferent impulses through peripheral neurons.

Demyelination

Myelination of peripheral neurons helps to isolate the transmission of impulses in single neurons. Transfer of signals from one neuron to another normally takes place at synapses only. In the absence of neuropathologic change, the transfer of afferent impulses between neurons outside the CNS is unlikely. Kerr,[30] however, has observed demyelination changes in peripheral neurons that make ephaptic transmission of impulses possible. (An *ephapse* is a point of lateral contact, other than a synapse, between nerve fibers across which impulses are conducted directly through the nerve membranes from one fiber to the other.) Experimental demyelination leads to antidromically propagated extra-action potentials as well as some postdischarge activity, followed by refractory periods.[31] Short-term peripheral nerve compression is usually painless and rarely lasts more than a few seconds.[32] Continued compression causes local demyelination without loss of axonal continuity. Chronic nerve entrapment causes demyelination initially, followed by progressive axonal degeneration. In traumatic neuroma, ephaptic cross-excitation may be a factor in the generation of pain.[33]

Paroxysmal Neuralgia Pain

Paroxysmal trigeminal neuralgia is one of the most painful conditions known to man, yet it remains an enigma to many health professionals. The specific etiology of idiopathic tic douloureux remains unknown. The pathologic change most consistently identified is demyelination of axons in the gasserian ganglion, dorsal root, or both (Figs 6–1 and 6–2).[34-36] Kerr contended that, since it is unlikely that minor lesions would cause the demyelination seen, an underlying degenerative process aggravated by otherwise negligible mechanical factors probably accounted for the paroxysms of pain. Hypertension and arteriosclerosis appear to have little bearing. Ephaptic response due to progressive degenerative change may be periodically and episodically activated by mechanical vascular influences.[37] This general concept is shared by others.[38] It has been established that the pathogenesis of trigeminal neuralgia is not correlative to endogenous opioids.[39] There is sufficient evidence that the neuropathy responsible is of peripheral rather than central origin.[40]

Symptomatic trigeminal neuralgia can be related more specifically to known neuropathies such as multiple sclerosis,[15,35,41-48] vascular lesions,[46] and extramedullary neoplasms.[43] Destructive lesions of the nerve located within the brain from the entrance of the trigeminal nerve into the pons throughout the numerous sensory circuits to the cortex do not cause paroxysmal neuralgia.[49]

Neuritic Neuralgia

Neuritic neuralgia is a clinical category of neurogenous pain manifested as an ongoing, unremitting, burning sensation in the peripheral distribution of the affected nerve.[15,50] It is to be distinguished from paroxysmal neuralgia, which consists of intermittent, sudden volleys

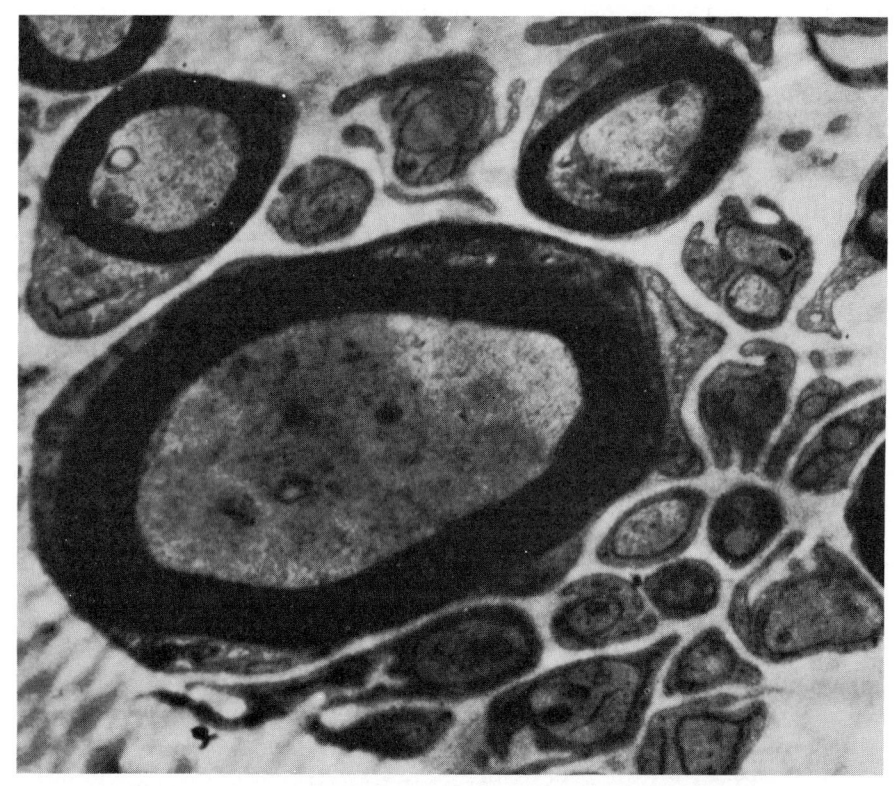

Fig 6–1.—Transverse section through posterior rootlet of trigeminal nerve in man, illustrating an area of unusually abundant unmyelinated fibers and several myelinated fibers, × 10,000. (From Kerr F.W.L.: Fine structure and functional characteristics of the primary trigeminal neuron, in Hassler R., Walker A.E. [eds.]: *Trigeminal Neuralgia, Pathogenesis and Pathophysiology.* Stuttgart, Georg Thieme Verlag, 1970. Reproduced with permission.)

of intense, burning pain. The distribution of neuritic pain closely follows dermatome geography. The symptom picture depends on the fiber population of the nerve at the site of neuropathy as well as on the kind and degree of involvement of each fiber type. Other sensory, motor, and autonomic symptoms may therefore accompany the complaint of pain.

Like many other clinical pain syndromes, the neural mechanisms are poorly understood. It is usually presumed that an inflammatory condition of the nerve is the generating cause of pain. The reason for such inflammation may be obscure. Metabolic and toxic disorders as well as neurovascular phenomena and viral infections are possible etiologic agents. Trauma, bacterial infection, and inflammation spreading from an adjacent site may be the cause. It is generally agreed that the pain of herpes zoster stems from a viral infection of the ganglion, dorsal root, or medullary tract of the involved nerve. The virus has been identified as similar to, if not identical with, that of varicella.[15, 36, 43]

It has been determined that in neuritic neuralgia the threshold of C-fibers is lowered, thus making them more sensitive to nociceptive stimuli. The reactivity of A-delta fibers, however, is partially or completely abolished.[51] As interpreted by the gate control theory, such altered ratio of large-small fiber activity would decrease the peripheral inhibitory mechanisms of pain modulation. This would permit the ongoing neural activity to be felt as pain.[52]

Traumatic Neuroma Pain

When a nerve trunk is sectioned, the regenerating axons may not find their proper neurilemma tubes. They may bundle into a disor-

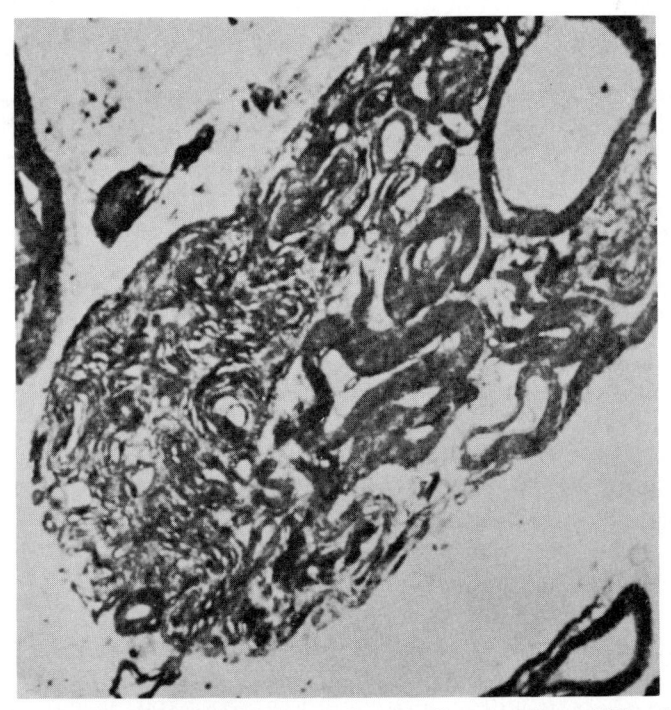

Fig 6–2.—Proliferative degenerative changes in a myelinated fiber in trigeminal neuralgia, × 10,700. (From Kerr F.W.L.: Pathology of trigeminal neuralgia, light and electron microscopic observations. *J. Neurosurg.* 26:151–156, 1967. Reproduced with permission.)

ganized, random overgrowth of intertwined extraneural and intraneural tissue and Schwann's cells. The neurogenous pain that results is thought to be largely due to ephaptic transfer of neural impulses generated by pressing or stretching the nerve tissue mass.[53]

Deafferentation Pain

Crushing or cutting a peripheral nerve induces anesthesia by interrupting the afferent impulses. Such deafferentation, however, may result in a variety of other symptoms, one of which is pain. Being part of a cell, a damaged peripheral sensory axon causes reactions in other peripheral and central cells that are in functional communication.[54] Deafferentation pains are initiated within the nervous system and are rarely altered significantly by the subject's activities or controlled by measures designed to reduce nociceptive stimulation.[55]

Experimental deafferentation utilizes capsaicin, the major pungent and irritating component of hot peppers. This substance selectively damages C-fibers, thus causing a depletion of substance P in the dorsal horn and expanding the sensory receptive field. These effects are quite similar to those of deafferentation due to sectioning a nerve.[56] Capsaicin affects unmyelinated fibers without inducing degeneration.[57] The enzyme, fluoride-resistant acid phosphatase (FRAP), disappears from central terminals within a few days, and substance P and cholecystokinin are depleted in the region of spinal cord terminals within two weeks.[58] It reduces nociceptive, heat, and nonnociceptive warm responses. However it does not alter touch, vibration, cold, or nonnociceptive pressure responses.[59] Fitzgerald[60] has reviewed the limitations of assumptions that should be drawn from the local and neonatal use of capsaicin to simulate the effects of mechanical deafferentation.

Deafferentation of peripheral nerves may induce various sensory symptoms, which include paresthesia, dysesthesia, hyperesthesia, hyperalgesia, and spontaneous pain. Symptoms may be felt, not only in the region of the initial anesthesia, but also in a considerably larger area. Anesthesia dolorosa, reflex sympathetic dystrophy (causalgia), and phantom pains are examples. Deafferentation effects have been identified following minor oral surgery[61] and tooth pulp extirpation.[62] Such symptoms are intimately related to efferent sympathetic activity and may often be alleviated by the interruption of sympathetic innervation to the area.[63] Some phantom pains are no doubt due to deafferentation[64]; some are not.[65]

The neural changes that take place as the result of peripheral deafferentation affect both the peripheral axons and the central terminals. Cutting the nerve peripheral to the dorsal ganglion arrests the afferent barrage of impulses and halts the movement of transport substances. Only limited anatomical degeneration takes place in the central terminals of the afferent fibers.[66] Some sprouts may find their proper neurilemma tubes, and relatively normal reinnervation may ensue. Axon-receptor mismatch and alien innervation due to misdirection or collateral sprouting may result in nonsense signals. Sprouts and axons peripheral to the site of damage become sensitive to norepinephrine, generated by activity in the sympathetic efferents. Retrograde shrinkage of axons proximal to the site of damage slows conduction velocity. Degenerative changes in the dorsal ganglion cells and central terminals yield abnormal, unbalanced input. Sprouting produces an increased number of small fibers proximal to the injury. The enzyme FRAP disappears at the terminals in the substantia gelatinosa, and there is depletion of substance P as well. In the dorsal horn, nearby intact afferents assume the ability to excite calls formerly dominated by the cut afferents, and spinal cord cells begin to respond to the nearest intact afferents. Thus, the sensory receptive field is enlarged.[54]

The peripheral effects of deafferentation chiefly may be attributed to alien innervation and mismatch and to sensitization of peripheral axons to sympathetic activity. The central effects relate primarily to the loss of C-fiber function, which normally is to maintain organization of the cord with respect to inhibitory mechanisms and the size of receptive fields. Deafferentation therefore markedly reduces normal inhibitory influences and enlarges the receptive fields.[66, 67]

The recent discovery by Wall and Devor[68] that dorsal ganglion cells normally initiate and maintain an ongoing, low-level background barrage of afferent signals may help to elucidate deafferentation phenomena. They observed that this ganglionic source of afferent input is increased considerably in response to peripheral nerve injury.

OTHER CAUSES OF OROFACIAL PAIN

Pain may result from numerous causes other than specific inflammatory conditions or other myogenous, vascular, or neurogenous phenomena. Pain may occur spontaneously with no identifiable cause of any kind. It may constitute an integral part of pathologic and pathophysiologic conditions of all types. Alterations in the endogenous antinociceptive mechanisms may occur. A degree or so of elevation in body temperature may induce pain in many structures. The general response to abnormal endocrine, metabolic, emotional, allergic, or toxic conditions may include a component of pain. Direct noxious stimulation by various mechanical, thermal, and chemical insults may induce pain. Cutaneous structures are sensitive to all such stimuli. Periosteum is especially reactive to compressive force; ligaments and fascia respond to distortion, strain, and traction; tendons and muscle tissue are particularly sensitive to torque and stretching. Glands react especially to pressure, while hollow viscera are sensitive to distension. Some structures are not pain sensitive at all, e.g., articular surfaces of joints and the parenchyma of the brain.

Headache and Intracranial Pain

Headache is perhaps the most frequent of all regional pain complaints. Most intermittent head pains are heterotopic manifestations. Being secondary in type, most such headaches are not as much a diagnostic concern for the pain itself as for the primary sources of deep somatic pain that initiate them. Primary intracranial head pain is rare. The parenchyma of the brain, including the vessels found within it, most of the dura and pia-arachnoid, the ependymal lining of the ventricles, and the choroid plexuses, are not sensitive to pain. The great venous sinuses and their tributaries from the surface of the brain, parts of the dura at the base, the dural arteries, and the cerebral arteries at the base of the brain are sensitive to pain. Stimulation of intracranial pain-sensitive structures on or above the superior surface of the tentorium cerebelli results in pain felt in the trigeminal distribution, whereas stimulation on or below the inferior surface of the tentorium cerebelli results in pain felt in the distribution of the glosso-pharyngeal and vagus cranial nerves and the upper cervical spinal nerves. Intracranial pain results from the following[15]:

1. Traction on veins that pass from the surface of the brain to the venous sinuses, on the middle meningeal arteries, and on the large arteries at the base of the brain and their main branches.
2. Displacement of the great venous sinuses.
3. Distension and dilatation of intracranial arteries.
4. Inflammation of pain-sensitive structures of the head.
5. Pressure by such lesions as tumors on nerves containing afferent pain fibers.

Pain From Tumors

Benign tumors may cause pain by encroachment onto pain-sensitive structures or by reason of pressure or weight. Malignant tumors cause pain also by direct involvement of neural structures.

The question of "brain tumors" may arise in the management of orofacial pains. Although the site of pain from brain tumors cannot accurately locate the tumor, the following guidelines are helpful[15]:
1. In the absence of papilledema (edema of the optic disc), lateral head pain is usually on the side of the tumor, and supratentorial tumors cause pain in the front of the head.
2. Posterior fossa tumors cause pain initially in the back of the head.
3. Frontal and occipital pain occurring simultaneously is without localizing value.

Pain from tumor involvement of the trigeminal root and ganglion may be divided into four groups[69]:
1. Cerebellopontine angle tumors rarely cause typical trigeminal neuralgia. Pain, if any, is usually a low-intensity, steady, dull ache. Hypoesthesia is considerably more common.
2. Middle fossa tumors may cause high-intensity paroxysms of 10 to 15 minutes' duration. Usually the pain, if any, is a sustained aching and burning sensation associated with areas of hypoesthesia.
3. Extracranial tumors that invade the ganglion from beneath may cause prolonged high-intensity paroxysms of burning pain. Anesthesia also may be the result.
4. Tumors arising from the envelopes of the ganglion cause a neuritic type of pain accompanied by other sensory and motor signs. Usually other nerves are simultaneously involved. Such pain is nonparoxysmal.

Psychogenic Pains

Psychogenic intensification of pain is a normal modulation phenomenon. If pain is intensified until it continues in the absence of significant peripheral input, a state of pain chronicity becomes evident. The psychogenic component of chronic pain syndromes of all types becomes a significant management problem. Pains due to conversion hysteria and the painful hallucinations of schizophrenia are manifestations of psychosis.

Iatrogenic Pains

Some pains result from therapeutic efforts. Although such phenomena may relate to the modulating effects of management, there are instances when dental or masticatory therapy directly initiates a pain problem. Treatment based on an incorrect or incomplete diagnosis may terminate this way. Therapy applied at the site of heterotopic pain rather than at the true source may cause injury. Injudicious occlusal grinding may increase the sensitivity of teeth. Alteration of the occlusal relationship may initiate pain involving muscles, the temporomandibular joints, or both as well as the teeth and peridontal structures. Any procedure (even corrective and otherwise beneficial measures) that alters the proprioceptive and sensory input may initiate protective muscle splinting pain, which, if not properly managed, can develop as myospasm or myositis. Overzealous therapy, rapid change in the functional relationship, or unwise selection of treatment may initiate a condition that has a component of pain. Many dental procedures, especially those that involve surgery, entail therapeutic hazards that can result in pain. Accidents happen; complications arise; unexpected results may follow therapy. Some procedures, such as the surgical interruption of nociceptive pathways, may generate irreversible sequelae that can offset the possible benefit.

The incidence of iatrogenic pain is sufficient to warrant a high degree of caution on the part of doctors of all types. The ancient maxim "At least do no harm!" should be heeded always.

REFERENCES
1. Wall P.D.: On the relation of injury to pain. *Pain* 6:253–264, 1979.
2. Burgess P.R. Perl E.R.: Cutaneous mechanoreceptors and nociception, in Iggo A. (ed.): *Handbook of Sensory Physiology*. Heidelberg, Springer-Verlag, 1973, Vol. 2, pp. 29–78.
3. Beitel R.E., Dubner R.: The response of unmyelinated (C) polymodal nociceptors to thermal stimuli applied to monkey's face. *J. Neurophysiol.* 35:1160, 1976.
4. Lim R.J.S.: Pain. *Ann. Rev. Physiol.* 32:269, 1970.
5. Handwerker H.O.: Influences of algogenic substances and prostaglandins on the discharges of unmyelinated cutaneous nerve fibers identified as nociceptors, in Bonica J.J., Albe-Fessard D.G (eds.): *Advances in Pain Research and Therapy*. New York, Raven Press, 1976, vol. 1, pp. 41–45.
6. Ferreira S.H.: Prostaglandins: Peripheral and central analgesia, in Bonica J.J., Lindblom U., Iggo A. (eds.): *Advances in Pain Research and Therapy*. New York, Raven Press, 1983, vol. 5, pp. 627–634.
7. Frost H.M.: Musculoskeletal pain, in Alling C.C., Mahan P.E. (eds.): *Facial Pain*, ed. 2. Philadelphia, Lea & Febiger, 1977, pp. 135–154.

8. Travell J.G., Simons D.G.: *Myofascial Pain and Dysfunction.* Baltimore, Williams & Wilkins Co., 1983.
9. Travell J., Rinzler S.H.: The myofascial genesis of pain. *Postgrad. Med.* 11:425, 1952.
10. Travell J.: Temporomandibular joint pain referred from muscles of the head and neck. *J. Prosthet. Dent.* 10:745, 1960.
11. Simons D.G., Travell J.: Letter to the editor. *Pain* 10:106–109, 1981.
12. Mense S., Meyer H.: Bradykinin-induced sensitization of high-threshhold muscle receptors with slowly conducting afferent fibers. *Pain,* suppl. 1, 1981, p. S204.
13. Travell J.: Referred pain from skeletal muscle. *N.Y. State J. Med.* 55:331, 1955.
14. Weisengreen H., Elliott H.W.: Electromyography in patients with orofacial pain. *J.A.D.A.* 67:798, 1963.
15. Dalessio D.J.: *Wolff's Headache and Other Head Pain.* New York, Oxford University Press, 1972.
16. Foreman R.D., Blair R.W., Weber R.N.: Effects on T3 to T5 primate spinothalamic tract cells of injecting bradykinin into the heart. *Pain,* suppl. 1, 1981, p. S212.
17. Bassoe P.: Migraine. *J.A.M.A.* 101:599, 1933.
18. Gross D.: Pain and autonomic nervous system, in Bonica J.J. (ed): *Advances in Neurology.* New York, Raven Press 1974, vol. 4, pp. 93–103.
19. Sicuteri F.: Headache as the most common disease of the antinociceptive system: Analogies with morphine abstinence, in Bonica J.J., Liebeskind J.C., Albe-Fessard D.G. (eds.): *Advances in Pain Research and Therapy* New York, Raven Press, 1979, vol. 3, pp. 359–365.
20. Appenzeller O.: Headache: Clinical and pathogenetic aspects, in Bonica J.J., Liebeskind J.C., Albe-Fessard D.G. (eds.): *Advances in Pain Research and Therapy.* New York, Raven Press, 1979, vol. 3, pp. 345–358.
21. Dvilansky A., Rishpon S., Nathan I., et al.: Release of platelet 5–hydroxytryptamine by plasma taken from patients during and between migraine attacks. *Pain* 2:315–318, 1976.
22. Anthony M., Hinterberger H., Lance J.W.: Plasma serotonin in migraine and stress. *Arch. Neurol.* 16:544–552, 1967.
23. Anthony M., Hinterberger H., Lance J.W.: The possible relationship of serotonin to the migraine syndrome. *Res. Clin. Stud. Headache* 2:29, 1969.
24. Krabbe A.A., Olesen J.: Headache provocation by continuous intravenous infusion of histamine: Clinical results and receptor mechanisms. *Pain* 8:253–259, 1980.
25. Seltzer S., Marcus R., Stoch R.: Perspectives in the control of chronic pain by nutritional manipulation. *Pain* 11:141–148, 1981.
26. Johansson F., Von Knorring L.: A double-blind controlled study of a serotonin uptake inhibitor (Zimelidine) versus placebo in chronic pain patients. *Pain* 7:69–78, 1979.
27. Wolff H.G.: *Headache and Other Head Pain,* ed. 2. New York, Oxford University Press, 1963.
28. Clifford T., Lauritsen M., Bakke M., et al.: Electromyography of pericranial muscles during treatment of spontaneous common migraine attacks. *Pain* 14: 137–147, 1982.
29. Bakke M., Tfelt-Hansen P., Olesen J., et al.: Action of some pericoronal muscles during provoked attacks of common migraine. *Pain* 14:121–135, 1982.

30. Kerr F.W.L.: Correlated light and electron microscopic observations on the normal trigeminal ganglion and sensory root in man. *J. Neurosurg.* 26:132, 1967.
31. Burchiel K.J.: Abnormal impulse generation in focally demyelinated trigeminal roots. *J. Neurosurg.* 53:674, 1980.
32. Howe J.F., Loeser J.D., Calvin W.H.: Mechanosensitivity of dorsal root ganglia and chronically injured axons: A physiological basis for the radicular pain of nerve root compression. *Pain* 3:25–41, 1977.
33. Ochea J., Noorrdenbes W.: Pathology and disordered sensation in local nerve lesions: An attempt at correlation, in Bonica J.J., Liebeskind, J.C., Albe-Fessard D.G. (eds.): *Advances in Pain Research and Therapy.* New York, Raven Press, 1979, vol. 3, 67–90.
34. Kerr F.W.L., Miller R.H.: The pathology of trigeminal neuralgia: Electron microscopic studies. *Arch. Neurol.* 15:308–309, 1966.
35. Kerr F.W.L.: Fine structure and functional characteristics of the primary trigeminal neuron, in Hassler R., Walker A.E. (eds.): *Trigeminal Neuralgia.* Stuttgart, Georg Thieme Verlag, 1970, pp. 11–21.
36. Sweet W.H.: Trigeminal neuralgia, in Alling C.C., Mahan P.E. (eds.): *Facial Pain,* ed. 2. Philadelphia, Lea & Febiger, 1977, pp. 71–93.
37. Kerr F.W.L.: Evidence for a peripheral etiology of trigeminal neuralgia. *J. Neurosurg.* 26:168–174, 1967.
38. Calvin, W.H., Loeser J.D., Howe J.F.: A neurophysiological theory for the pain mechanism of tic douloureux. *Pain* 3:147–154, 1977.
39. Salar G., Mangrino S.: Trigeminal neuralgia and endorphins. *Pain,* suppl. 1, 1981, p. S259.
40. Kerr F.W.L.: Peripheral versus central factors in trigeminal neuralgia, in Hassler R., Walker A.E. (eds.): *Trigeminal Neuralgia.* Stuttgart, Georg Thieme Verlag, 1970, pp. 180–190.
41. Parker H.L.: Trigeminal neuralgia associated with multiple sclerosis. *Brain* 51:46, 1928.
42. Harris W.: Rare forms of paroxysmal trigeminal neuralgia and their relationship to disseminated sclerosis. *Br. Med. J.* 2:1015, 1950.
43. Stookey B., Rausohoft J.: *Trigeminal Neuralgia.* Springfield, Ill., Charles C Thomas, Publisher, 1959.
44. Rushton J.G., Olafson R.A.: Trigeminal neuralgia associated with multiple sclerosis: A case report. *Arch. Neurol.* 13:383, 1965.
45. Olafson R.A., Rushton J.G., Sayre G.R.: Trigeminal neuralgia in a patient with multiple sclerosis: An autopsy report. *J. Neurosurg.* 24:755, 1966.
46. Gardner W. J.: Trigeminal neuralgia, in Hassler R., Walker A.E. (eds.): *Trigeminal Neuralgia.* Stuttgart, Georg Thieme Verlag, 1970, pp. 162–165.
47. Friedlander A.H., Zeff S.: Atypical trigeminal neuralgia in patients with multiple sclerosis. *J. Oral. Surg.* 32:301–303, 1974.
48. Lazar M.L., Greenlee R.G. Jr., Naarden A.L.: Facial pain of neuralgic origin mimicking oral pathologic conditions: Some current concepts and treatments. *J.A.D.A.* 100:884–888, 1980.
49. Kaemmerer E.F.: A review of the etiologic factors in trigeminal neuralgia, in Hassler R., Walker A.E. (eds.): *Trigeminal Neuralgia.* Stuttgart, Georg Thieme Verlag, 1970, pp. 175–179.
50. Wolff H.G., Wolf S.: *Pain,* ed. 2. Springfield, Ill., Charles C Thomas, Publisher, 1958.

51. Bigelow N., Harrison I., Goodell H., et al.: Studies on pain: Quantitative measurements of two pain sensations of the skin with reference to the nature of the 'hyperalgesia of peripheral neuritis.' *J. Clin. Invest.* 23:503, 1945.
52. Melzack R., Wall P.D.: Pain mechanisms: A new theory. *Science* 150:971, 1965.
53. Gregg J.M., Walter J.R., Driscoll R.: Neurosensory studies of trigeminal dysesthesia following peripheral nerve injury, in Bonica J.J., Liebeskind J.C., Albe-Fessard D.G. (eds.): *Advances in Pain Research and Therapy.* New York, Raven Press, 1979, vol.3, pp. 311–315.
54. Wall P.D.: Changes in damaged nerve and their sensory consequences, in Bonica J.J., Liebeskind J.C., and Albe-Fessard D.G. (eds.): *Advances in Pain Research and Therapy.* New York, Raven Press, 1979, vol. 3, pp. 39–52.
55. Loeser J. D.: Definition, etiology, and neurological assessment of pain originating in the nervous system following deafferentation, in Bonica J.J., Lindblom U., Iggo A. (eds.): *Advances in Pain Research and Therapy.* New York, Raven Press, 1983, vol. 5, pp. 701–711.
56. Wall P.D., Fitzgerald M., Gibson S.J.: The effect of local sciatic nerve capsaicin and sciatic nerve section on neurophysiological responses and peptide levels in rat lumbar dorsal horn. *Pain*, suppl. 1, 1981, p. S202.
57. Nagy J.I., Hunt S.P., Iversen L.L., et al.: Effects of capsaicin on dorsal root afferents, in Bonica J.J., Lindblom U., Iggo A. (eds,): *Advances in Pain Research and Therapy.* New York, Raven Press, 1983, vol. 5, pp. 77–82.
58. Ainsworth A., Hall P., Wall P.D., et al.: Effects of capsaicin applied locally to adult peripheral nerves: II. Anatomy and enzyme and peptide chemistry of peripheral nerve and spinal cord. *Pain* 11:379–388, 1981.
59. Buck S.H., Miller M.S., Burks T.F.: Specific sensory deficits in adult guinea pigs induced by the putative substance P neurotoxin, capsaicin, and its active analogs. *Pain*, suppl. 1, 1981, p. S134.
60. Fitzgerald M.: Capsaicin and sensory neurons: A review. *Pain* 15:109–130, 1983.
61. Gregg J.M.: Post-traumatic pain: Experimental trigeminal neuropathy. *J. Oral Surg.* 29:260–267, 1971.
62. Gobel S., Binck J.M.: Degenerative changes in primary trigeminal axons and in neurons in nucleus caudalis following tooth pulp extirpation in the cat. *Brain Res.* 132:347–354, 1977.
63. Bonica J.J.: Causalgia and other reflex sympathetic dystrophies, in Bonica J.J., Liebeskind J.C., Albe-Fessard D.G. (eds.): *Advances in Pain Research and Therapy.* New York, Raven Press, 1979, vol. 3, pp. 141–166.
64. Howe J. F.: Phantom limb pain: A re-afferentation syndrome. *Pain* 15:101–107, 1983.
65. Melzack R., Loeser J.D.: Phantom body pain in paraplegics: Evidence for a central 'pattern generating mechanism' for pain. *Pain* 4:195–210, 1978.
66. Wall P.D.: Alterations in the central nervous system after deafferentation: Connectivity control, in Bonica J.J., Lindblom U., Iggo A. (eds.): *Advances in Pain Research and Therapy.* New York, Raven Press, 1983, vol. 5, pp. 677–689.

67. Wall P.D.: Mechanisms of acute and chronic pain, in Kruger L., Liebeskind J.C. (eds.); *Advances in Pain Research and Therapy.* New York, Raven Press, 1984, vol. 6, pp. 95–104.
68. Wall P.D., Devor M.: Sensory afferent impulses originate from dorsal root ganglia as well as from the periphery in normal and nerve injured rats. *Pain* 17:321–339, 1983.
69. Cushing H.: The major trigeminal neuralgias and their surgical treatment. *Am. J. Med. Sci.* 160:157, 1920.

7

Classification of Orofacial Pain Syndromes

PAIN DIAGNOSIS IS MUCH TOO COMPLEX to be undertaken without reasonable guidance or some sense of direction. Serving as a sort of diagnostic roadmap to lead the examiner toward an accurate conclusion, a satisfactory classification of pain syndromes can become a valuable diagnostic tool. The more sophisticated the classification, however, the greater the requirement for a good understanding of pain mechanisms and examining techniques.

The first prerequisite in classifying pain is a common language with which to communicate intelligibly. Considerable improvement in the meaning of terms used to describe pain has been made in recent years. Some definitions as listed in a standard medical dictionary[1] are not sufficiently precise to prevent ambiguity and misunderstandings. The International Association for the Study of Pain has taken the lead in defining such terms more precisely.[2,3] A list of definitions as used in this monograph may be found at the front of the book. The reader is encouraged to become familiar with them.

CLASSIFICATIONS OF PAIN

The most elementary classification of pain is that which lists the anatomical locations where pain is felt. An example of such a classification follows:
1. Head and neck pain
2. Thoracic pain
3. Abdominal pain
4. Extremity pain

Subdivisions of head and neck pain would include (1) headache, (2) orofacial pains, and (3) cervical pains. The title of this book reflects this type of classification.

Such simple classification is useful to record the patient's subjective complaint. For example, it might list the complaint as headache, toothache, chest pain, backache, or leg pain. It should be understood, however, that it identifies only the *site* where pain is felt, not the location of its true *source*. A pain listed as "toothache" could be of dental origin and require dental therapy. But it could also be a heterotopic manifestation of some myogenous, vascular, or neurogenous condition that would require treatment on quite a different level. Therefore, such a classification has very little diagnostic value.

More refined pain classifications require additional knowledge of pain behavior and the expending of some diagnostic effort. To classify pain by the location of its source requires an understanding of heterotopic pains and entails the need for diagnostic differentiation between primary pain and its secondary effects. Thus, "toothache" in such a classification might become pulpal pain, periodontal pain, or heterotopic pain when its true site of origin is determined. It should be obvious that this more accurate classification of the patient's complaint implies important therapeutic considerations.

An understanding of the genesis of pain can add more refinement to pain classification. This brings into the picture considerations relative to the type of tissue from which the pain emanates. Utilizing this information, orofacial pains may be classified regionally as follows:
1. Cutaneous and mucogingival pains
2. Mucosal pains of the pharynx, nose, and paranasal sinuses
3. Pains of dental origin
4. Pains of the musculoskeletal structures of the mouth and face
5. Pains of the visceral structures of the mouth and face
6. Pains of the neural structures of the mouth and face
7. Chronic face pain syndromes

This type classification is utilized as headings for the chapters that follow.

The ultimate in pain classification, however, is that based also on the symptomatology. This requires an understanding of the clinical characteristics displayed by the different categories of pain. It is on the basis of the subjective and objective symptoms of the nociceptive condition under examination that proper identification is made. If one fully appreciates the concept of pain modulation, understands and can differentiate primary from secondary pain, has some knowledge of pain genesis, and can identify the categories of pain by their clinical characteristics, a truly sophisticated and useful classification of orofacial pains is possible. As concepts have evolved in recent years, this pain classification has undergone considerable metamorphosis. It now conforms quite well to current knowledge of nociceptive mechanisms.

CATEGORIES OF OROFACIAL PAIN

Pain syndromes about the mouth and face may be divided by their clinical characteristics into three categories, namely, (1) somatic pain, (2) neurogenous pain, and (3) psychogenic pain. *Somatic pain* results from the noxious stimulation of normal neural structures that innervate body tissues. *Neurogenous pain* is generated within the nervous system itself and is caused by abnormality of the neural structures that innervate body tissues. *Psychogenic pain* results neither from noxious stimulation nor from neural abnormality, but from psychic causes.

Somatic Pain

Somatic pains occur in response to the stimulation of neural receptors or peripheral nerve fibers. Local conditions including inflammation and sustained hyperemia increase the receptivity of the neural structures so that less intense stimulation becomes more noxious. Reduced central inhibitory control of the passage of peripheral impulses to the higher centers also causes less intense peripheral stimulation to become more noxious. The degree of pain therefore does not necessarily relate to the intensity of the stimulus.

The neural structures involved in such pain reception and transmission are presumed to be normal, and the sensation serves to warn, alert, or inform the patient about such noxious stimulation. The conscious sensation of pain under such conditions is an added component to the voluminous sensory input the brain receives constantly, and it serves the purpose of preparing the patient for appropriate response. Afferent neurons of both the somatic and visceral nervous systems participate in this mechanism. The clinical characteristics of pain that originates in superficial structures are distinctly different from those of deep origin. It is by these differences that the two types of somatic pain are distinguished.

Superficial Somatic Pain

The external surface of the body is richly innervated with receptors and sensory fibers of different types. These constantly feed information to the somatosensory cortex concerning the organism's environment. Not only does such sensation establish full conscious contact between the organism and its surroundings, but it furnishes the impetus for involuntary reflex activity. Superficial sensation serves a protective function so the organism may react appropriately to the constant and varied environmental threat to its well-being, comfort, and survival.

The sensory system provides input on conscious levels that allow precise definition of the physical characteristics of the stimulus including its modality, location, duration, and intensity. Pain emanating from these superficial structures presents characteristics *on a conscious level* of the definition of the physical properties of the noxious stimulus. These qualities are inherent in superficial somatic pain and furnish the examiner a means of identifying it.

Superficial pains have a bright, *stimulating* quality.[4–6] This probably results from the alarm reaction that such discomfort tends to create. As part of the environmental threat, superficial pain causes the patient to react in such a way as to escape such threat—fight or flight. The more severe the superficial pain, the more pronounced this stimulating quality becomes.

Superficial pains can be correctly located by the patient so that he is aware precisely of where he hurts. He is able to describe the location of the pain with anatomical accuracy.

Since the source of superficial pain is noxious stimulation of the very structures that hurt, the location of the pain clearly identifies where to look for its cause: the site of pain and site of origin are identical. In fact, if the cause of the pain is not immediately evident or reasonably explicable, the diagnosis of superficial pain should be questioned.

Since superficial somatic pain is due to lowered pain threshold, and since the site of pain and the location of its true source are the same, the discomfort that results from provocation at the site of pain relates *faithfully* to the stimulus. By this is meant that the reaction is immediate, it is proportional to the intensity of the stimulus, it lasts as long as the stimulus, and there is no reference of pain to other normal structures. Superficial pain responds faithfully to provocation. Effects of central hyperexcitability such as referred pain, secondary hyperalgesia, local autonomic effects, and secondary myospasm activity are not observed.

Since superficial pain emanates from the surface tissue, application of a topical anesthetic interrupts the pain. It should be noted that neither neuritic pain felt in superficial tissues nor pain referred from deeper structures to the surface is arrested by the application of topical local anesthesia.

Two types of superficial orofacial pain are recognized, namely, cutaneous pain and mucogingival pain.

To summarize, the clinical characteristics displayed by superficial somatic pain are as follows:
1. The pain has a bright, stimulating quality.
2. Subjective localization of the pain is excellent and anatomically accurate.
3. The site of pain identifies the correct location of its source.
4. Response to provocation at the site of pain is faithful in incidence, intensity, and location.
5. The application of a topical anesthetic at the site of pain temporarily arrests it.

Deep Somatic Pain

Sensory innervation of the deeper structures of the body supplies the somatosensory cortex with a constant inflow of information monitoring all the internal functioning of the body. No doubt the information has a certain precision of definition as to the physical characteristics of the stimulus including its modality, location, duration, and intensity, but this information is normally *below conscious levels* unless volition brings it to the attention of the subject. Functions that require precise definition of the physical characteristics of the stimulus, such as the action of skeletal muscles, are attended by some conscious sensation that is fairly precise for location. Functions that operate on an involuntary level, such as the action of smooth muscle, are attended by sensations that remain below conscious levels unless unusual conditions prevail such as distension, pressure, sustained hyperemia, or inflammation.[7] In such cases the conscious sensation usually is that of diffusely located and poorly defined discomfort or pain.

Deep pain has a dull, *depressing* quality,[4-6] sometimes causing a sickening sensation of nausea. The background sensation may be punctuated by momentary lancinating pains that the patient describes as stimulating and exciting. Such lancinating pain is usually initiated by sudden traction, distension, or distortion of deep tissues.

The depressing effect of pain arising in deeper body structures and mediated by either deep somatic or visceral afferent fibers is likely to be a manifestation of withdrawal reaction. In contrast to the alarm effect from environmental threat as witnessed in superficial pain syndromes, the usual reaction to discomfort emanating from deeper structures is to prepare the subject for conservation and recovery—a decrease in somatic skeletal activity in favor of increased visceral function. The characteristic quality of deep pain is that the discomfort induces a depressing effect leading to inactivity and withdrawal, sometimes accompanied by lassitude, depression, weakness, or nausea.

Deep pain is less accurately localizable by the patient. Some pains of deep origin, such as those from skeletal muscle or from the peridontal ligament, are fairly localizable. However, such localizing sensation is considerably less accurate, and the ability of the patient to describe the painful site anatomically less certain, than with superficial pain. The area where pain is sensed is usually greater than the site from which it arises. Many deep pains such as those emanating from the dental pulp or from blood vessels are hardly localizable and the patient's anatomical description of where he feels the pain may be diffuse indeed. Some deep pains manifest effects of central hyperexcitability so that the pain is felt in otherwise normal structures, and the descriptive location of the pain in nonanatomical.

Because of the variable and inconsistent localizability of deep pain syndromes generally, the site of pain may not indicate the true origin. This applies especially to pains that occur spontaneously or in response to normal function. *Pain provoked by manual palpation and manipulation more accurately identifies its true location, and this diagnostic maneuver often can be useful to isolate otherwise vague and diffusely located pain sites.* Muscle and organ pains especially show this trait. It is true that the site of some deep pains may clearly identify the origin, but even then it is considerably less precise and dependable than with superficial pain syndromes. Although some deep pains are felt in sites much larger than the true source of pain, others may be felt in entirely normal structures. Since these variabilities are characteristic of deep pain syndromes, it behooves the examiner to take measures that prove the location of the pain source and not to depend entirely on the site of pain for this information.

Deep pain may not be proportional to the stimulus. Although some deep pains (usually those with better localization behavior) respond rather faithfully to a stimulus, the response is not as faithful as with superficial pain. In contrast, some deep pains manifest little relationship between stimulus and response, and others cannot be provoked by manual palpation or the demands of function. Although the lack of faithful response to provocation is characteristic of deep pain—sometimes greater, sometimes less than the intensity of provocation would suggest—true summation effects are not seen. Therefore, triggering of intense pain by light touch or superficial movement is not characteristic of deep pain syndromes.

One of the most important identifying clinical characteristics of deep pain is its tendency to display effects caused by central hyperexcitability.[4,5] Deep pain input tends to provoke referred pains, secondary hyperalgesias, localized autonomic effects and secondary myospasm activity. This tendency relates to continuity, severity and duration of the deep pain input. When diagnostic evidence of such central excitatory effects is observed, a deep pain syndrome must be suspected, and a serious diagnostic search made for the primary pain source. Great care must be exercised not to confuse secondary pain effects, which may actually comprise the patient's clinical complaint, with the primary pain syndrome, which may be silent and therefore nonsymptomatic to the patient. It is the manifestation of such secondary effects that creates much of the diffuse variableness and spreading effect of some deep pains. Certainly, these effects are largely responsible for the confusion that surrounds many deep pain syndromes and the therapeutic failures that sometimes occur.

Deep pain usually is not arrested by application of a topical anesthetic except when it arises from visceral mucosa such as the nasal mucosa in so-called sinus headache. Analgesic blocking of the nerve that mediates the primary painful impulses usually arrests deep pain, and this technique is useful diagnostically in localizing the source of such pains. Vascular pains may not respond well to ordinary analgesic blocking.

To summarize, the clinical characteristics displayed by deep somatic pain are as follows:
1. The pain has a dull, depressing quality.
2. Subjective localization of the pain is variable and somewhat diffuse.
3. The site of pain may or may not identify the correct location of its true source.
4. Response to provocation at the site of pain is fairly faithful in incidence and intensity, but not in location.
5. Accompanying secondary central excitatory effects are frequently displayed.

There are two distinct types of deep somatic pain, namely, musculoskeletal pain and visceral pain. *Musculoskeletal pain* involves the action of receptors that respond to varying degrees of stimulation. Such pain therefore yields a graduated response to stimulation. Musculoskeletal pain relates intimately to function. It can be localized to the degree that such a sense of localization is required in the course of normal functioning. Musculoskeletal pain is further subdivided into: (1) muscle pain; (2) temporomandibular joint pain; (3) osseous and periosteal pain; (4) soft connective tissue pain, and (5) dental pain of periodontal origin. Muscle pains include protective muscle splinting, myofascial trigger point pain, muscle spasm pain; and muscle inflammation pain. Temporomandibular joint pain includes disc attachment pain, retrodiscal pain, capsular pain, and arthritic pain.

Visceral pain involves the action of high-threshold receptors of interoceptive type. Such pain usually is not felt at all until threshold is reached. It does not present a graduated response to stimulation. It has little or no relationship to biomechanical function and is nearly nonlocalizable by the subject. Visceral pain is further subdivided into (1) dental pain of pulpal origin, (2) vascular pains, (3) visceral mucosa pains, and (4) glandular, ocular, and auricular pains. Vascular pains include migrainous neuralgia, atypical odontalgia, common migraine, classic migraine, and vascular inflammation pain.

Neurogenous Pain

Neurogenous pains are those that are generated within the nervous system itself. Stimulation of receptors and nerve fibers is therefore unnecessary. Stimulation may cause summation effects so that the evoked response may be wholly disproportionate to the stimulus. Spontaneous, triggered, and unremitting types of pain are characteristic.

Neurogenous pain has a bright, stimulating, burning quality similar to superficial somatic pain, from which it must be differentiated. Usually, the subject is able to localize the pain quite well. Except for traumatic neuroma pain, the site of pain does not identify the correct location of its source. To a knowledgeable examiner, however, the site of pain bears an anatomical relationship to the location of the neuropathy or deafferentation that generates it. Response to provocation at the site of pain is unfaithful in all respects except perhaps with traumatic neuromas. Since central excitatory effects usually are not seen, neurogenous pain has a sameness, a clean-cut quality without reference or other secondary symptoms. Neuritic neuralgia and some deafferentation syndromes may be accompanied by other sensory, motor, and/or autonomic symptoms. Herpes zoster is characterized by the presence of herpetic lesions in the exact peripheral distribution where pain is felt. Deafferentation pain displays enlarged receptive fields and responds to efferent sympathetic activity.

To summarize, the clinical characteristics displayed by neurogenous pain are as follows:
1. The pain has a bright, stimulating, burning quality.
2. Subjective localization of the pain is good.

3. The site of pain (except traumatic neuroma) does not identify the correct location of its source.
4. Response to provocation at the site of pain is wholly unfaithful in incidence, intensity, and location. Summation effects may be displayed.
5. Other sensory, motor, and/or autonomic symptoms may accompany some neurogenous pain syndromes. Central excitatory effects usually are not displayed.

Neurogenous pain may be classified as neuropathic pain or deafferentation pain. Neuropathic pain may be divided into traumatic neuroma pain, paroxysmal neuralgia, and neuritic neuralgia. Paroxysmal neuralgia is further subdivided into idiopathic neuralgia and symptomatic neuralgia. Neuritic neuralgia, in turn, may be divided into peripheral neuritis, herpes zoster and postherpetic neuralgia. Deafferentation pain may be expressed as reflex sympathetic dystrophy, anesthesia dolorosa, and some forms of phantom pain.

Psychogenic Pain

Psychogenic pain is expressed as psychogenic intensification of somatic or neurogenous pain or as a manifestation of psychoneurosis. Psychogenic intensification of pain may proceed until the suffering is wholly disproportionate to the peripheral nociceptive input. Although the original pain complaint may have displayed the usual clinical characteristics of somatic or neurogenous pain, as psychogenic intensification converts it into a chronic face pain syndrome, the clinical symptoms take on features that identify it as psychogenic. Such pain lacks an adequate source of input that is anatomically related to the site of pain. It may be felt in multiple, and sometimes changeable, locations. Pain bilaterality may become evident in the absence of bilateral sources of noxious input. The complaint may display unusual or unexpected responses to therapy. It may respond too quickly or too slowly. It may respond in an exaggerated way or with unusual side effects or complications. The response may be followed by relapse without organic justification, or the condition may remain refractory in spite of otherwise effective therapy. Psychogenic pain may display changeableness in location, intensity, or temporal behavior without reasonable, identifiable organic cause. Occasionally, psychogenic intensification may be expressed in the form of phantom pain.

Psychoneurotic pain is further subdivided into conversion hysteria pain and delusional pain.

To summarize, the clinical characteristics displayed by psychogenic pain are as follows:
1. The site of pain lacks an adequate, anatomically related source of nociceptive input.
2. Its clinical behavior and responsiveness to reasonable therapy is unusual, unexpected, and nonphysiologic.

CLASSIFICATION OF OROFACIAL PAINS

I. Somatic pain
   A. Superficial somatic pain
      1. Cutaneous pain
      2. Mucogingival pain
   B. Deep somatic pain
      1. Musculoskeletal pain
         a) Muscle pain
            (1) Protective splinting pain
            (2) Myofascial trigger point pain
            (3) Muscle spasm pain
            (4) Muscle inflammation pain
         b) Temporomandibular joint pain
            (1) Disc attachment pain
            (2) Retrodiscal pain
            (3) Capsular pain
            (4) Arthritic pain
         c) Osseous and periosteal pain
         d) Soft connective tissue pain
         e) Periodontal dental pain
      2. Visceral pain
         a) Pulpal dental pain
         b) Vascular pain
            (1) Migrainous neuralgia
            (2) Atypical odontalgia
            (3) Common migraine
            (4) Classic migraine
            (5) Vascular inflammation pain
         c) Visceral mucosa pain
         d) Glandular, ocular, and auricular pain
II. Neurogenous pain
   A. Neuropathic pain
      1. Traumatic neuroma pain
      2. Paroxysmal neuralgia

a) Idiopathic neuralgia
   b) Symptomatic neuralgia
  3. Neuritic neuralgia
   a) Peripheral neuritis
   b) Herpes zoster
   c) Postherpetic neuralgia
 B. Deafferentation pain
  1. Reflex sympathetic dystrophy (causalgia)
  2. Anesthesia dolorosa
  3. Phantom pain
III. Psychogenic pain
 A. Chronic face pain
 B. Psychoneurotic pain
  1. Conversion hysteria pain
  2. Delusional pain

REFERENCES

1. *Dorland's Illustrated Medical Dictionary*, ed. 26. Philadelphia, W.B. Saunders Co., 1981.
2. Merskey H.: Pain terms: A list with definitions and notes on usage. *Pain* 6:249–252, 1979.
3. Merskey H.: Pain terms: A supplementary note. *Pain* 14:205–206, 1982.
4. Bonica J.J.: *The Management of Pain.* Philadelphia, Lea & Febiger, 1953.
5. Wolff H.G., Wolf S.: *Pain*, ed. 2. Springfield, Ill., Charles C Thomas, Publisher, 1958.
6. Procacci P., Zoppi M., Maresea M.: Experimental pain in man. *Pain* 6:123–140, 1979.
7. Dalessio D.J.: *Wolff's Headache and Other Head Pain*, ed. 3. New York, Oxford University Press, 1972.

8

Cutaneous and Mucogingival Pains

SUPERFICIAL SOMATIC PAIN in the orofacial region emanates from either the skin of the lips and face or the mucogingival tissues of the mouth (Fig 8–1). Cutaneous and mucogingival pains display identifying clinical characteristics that distinguish them from other structural and neurogenous pains and from heterotropic sensations that may be felt in the superficial structures. These symptoms are as follows:
1. The pain has a bright, stimulating quality.
2. Subjective localization of the pain is excellent and anatomically accurate.
3. The site of pain identifies the correct location of its source.
4. Response to provocation at the site of pain is faithful in incidence, intensity, and location.
5. The application of a topical anesthetic at the site of pain temporarily arrests it.

CUTANEOUS PAINS OF THE FACE

Cutaneous pain is usually described as an itching, pricking, raw, stinging, burning sensation depending chiefly on the intensity of the complaint. Stimulation-evoked pain is initially felt as a fast, sharp, pricking pain. Since this is prevented by A-fiber blocking, it is presumed that the initial sensation is mediated by A-delta nociceptive neurons.[1] The initial pricking sensation is followed by a slightly delayed, less sharp, less precisely localized, burning pain that quite assuredly is mediated by C-fiber nociceptive units.

Since the pain is felt precisely at the location of the initiating cause, usually no diagnostic effort is needed to determine its origin. When the cause of cutaneous pain is not immediately evident, the examiner should question whether the complaint might be heterotopic, such as referred pain from other deep pain input or as projected pain of neurogenous etiology.[2-4] A topical anesthetic applied at the site of pain

CUTANEOUS AND MUCOGINGIVAL PAINS 103

OROFACIAL PAIN SYNDROMES

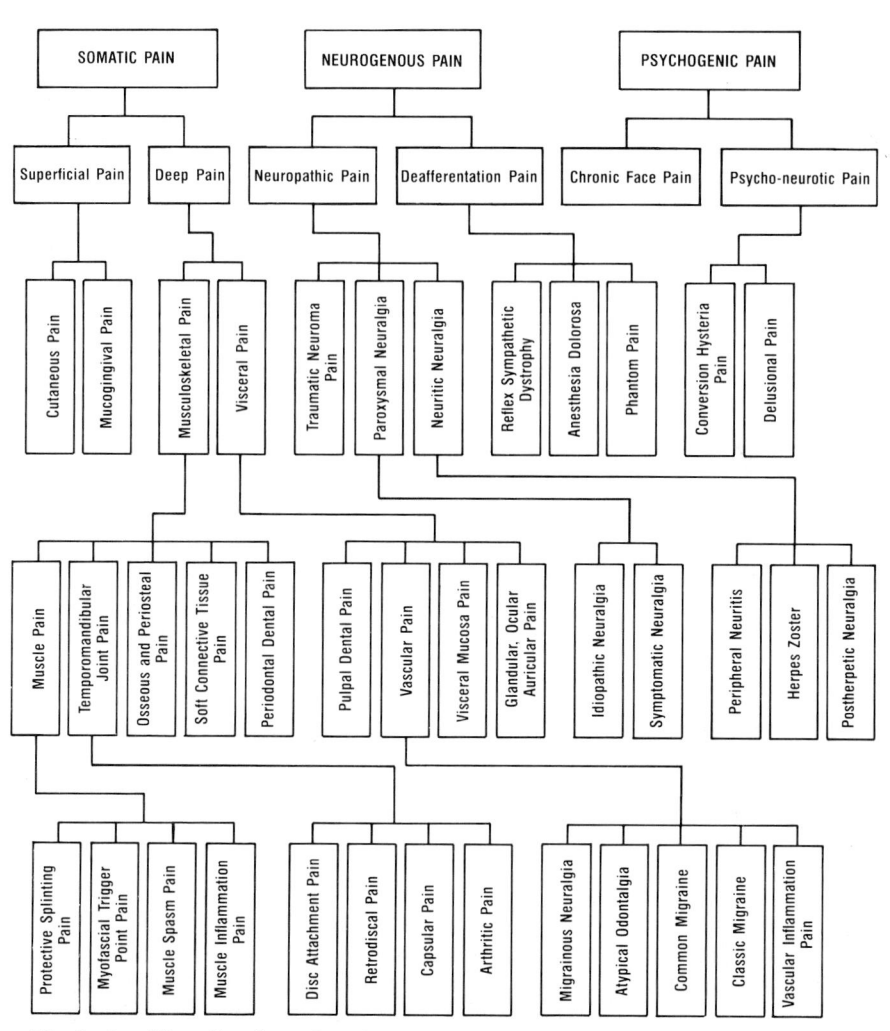

Fig 8–1.—Classification of orofacial pain syndromes.

temporarily arrests superficial somatic pain. It should be noted, however, that the irritating effect of the medication, when first applied, may initially increase the discomfort.

Caution should be exercised in assuming that a visible lesion at or near the site of pain necessarily represents the primary initiating cause. It may or may not be so. For example, the lesions of herpes zoster stem from a much more deeply located neural disorder and are not the *cause* of the peripheral pain. Again, one should not assume that the complaint does not emanate from cutaneous structures simply because the etiology is obscure. Subtle forms of noxious stimulation that cause itching and stinging may be encountered. When such confusing situations arise, the use of topical anesthesia to confirm the diagnosis is indicated.

MUCOGINGIVAL PAINS OF THE MOUTH

There may be some questions about classifying mucogingival pain in the same general category with pains of cutaneous origin. They are not identical in behavior. For example, mucogingival discrimination of painful sensation does not include the familiar pricking-burning pattern of cutaneous pain. Also, the number of thick fibers innervating the oral mucosa is negligible compared with that of the skin. However, palatal mucosa senses both itch and tickle, and all oral tissues feel stinging and burning sensations. The pains have a bright, *stimulating* quality; are easily localized and identify adequate local cause; respond faithfully to provocation at the site of pain; do not present central excitatory effects; and are arrested by application of a topical anesthetic at the site of pain. They therefore present the characteristics of superficial somatic pain by which identification can be made. The true site of origin of such pain is less evident than for cutaneous pain only because of the added difficulty of intraoral examination and failure on the part of the examiner to fully appreciate the implications of oral functioning.

The oral tissues are fragile and easily injured by rubbing against the teeth, tongue, and cheeks and each other during normal use. They are subject to countless insults from foods, beverages, burns, tobacco, alcohol, toothpastes, mouthwashes, medications, dental defects, dental restorations and appliances of all types, objects held in the mouth, habits of clenching the teeth, and unusual functional demands ad infinitum. The oral tissues are reactive to systemic disorders and diseases. The saliva, which normally acts as the oral lubricant, is especially responsive to the effects of emotional stress, physical disorders, and diseases as well as many medications now in common use. The identification of the cause of pain from these tissues is obviously more difficult than for cutaneous pains, but it should be within the capability of the knowledgeable dental examiner. As with cutaneous pain, when the cause of pain felt in the mucogingival tissues is not immediately evident, the examiner must differentiate between pain of true mucogingival origin and pain that stems from neurogenous or secondary deep pain sources.

Mucogingival pains are usually described as distinct raw, stinging, or burning sensations. Pains arising from the lining tissues of the oral cavity can be precisely located by the patient. Such pain may be generalized throughout the mouth when the cause widely affects the mucogingival tissues, or it may be isolated if the hyperalgesic area is small. In either case the patient can precisely locate the discomfort on an accurate anatomical basis, and the location changes only as the underlying cause varies. This precision of localization may become less accurate in the deeper recesses of the oral cavity.

The location of the pain accurately identifies its source. The pain arises from primary hyperalgesia due to *local* cause such as the irritating effect of foods, liquids, mouthwashes, dentrifices, and medications. It may be due to the abrasive effect of excessive rubbing of the tongue and cheeks, and this effect may be compounded when the quality and quantity of saliva do not afford adequate lubricative protection to the moving tissues. When the salivary deficit is great, normal functioning may become traumatic to the oral tissues. Localized hyperalgesia may occur from numerous causes such as trauma; infection by bacterial, fungoid, or viral agents; allergy; and neoplasia. Frequently one may identify objective signs of hyperemia, inflammation, vesiculation, ulceration, or some other pathosis at the site of pain. However primary hyperalgesia of the oral lining tissues may show no objective signs, and mucogingival tissues may appear entirely normal. Hyperalgesia may occur with no clinical signs of other tissue change. It is in such instances that the examiner should carefully consider a salivary deficit as the possible etiologic factor.

There is a precise, accurate, and proportional relationship between the noxious stimulation and the resulting discomfort. When no stimulus is applied, little or no discomfort occurs. When the stimulus is increased, the discomfort increases accordingly without summation effects. The suffering faithfully reflects the degree of hyperalgesia and the intensity of the stimulus.

Ordinarily, central excitatory effects are not seen as a result of mucogingival pains even when severe and continuous. Referred pains, secondary hyperalgesias, and the development of secondary painful muscle spasms do not occur. This gives the pain a constancy and sameness that is characteristic.

Since pain of mucogingival origin is an expression of primary hyperalgesia of the tissues that hurt, application of a topical anesthetic to those tissues arrests the pain due to action of the medication on the receptors and pain fibers in the mucogingival tissues. This is an important point of differentation from referred pain of superficial type and neuritic pain, neither of which is arrested by the application of topical anesthesia.

GLOSSODYNIA, "BURNING MOUTH," AND "BURNING TONGUE."—These common oral complaints are described as steady, continuous, typical superficial somatic pain. Very frequently, the oral examination reveals a clean hygienic mouth with little objective evidence of pathosis of any kind. A distinguishing characteristic of this condition is the fact that the *location of the pain corresponds to areas of greatest movement*, thus revealing the cause as the abrasive effect of the tissues rubbing against themselves and the teeth. Pain location depends on which tissues are being rubbed and where. At times, hyperemia may be observed as well as actual inflammation and ulceration. Secondary infection of the irritated tissues may complicate the symptom picture. There is a tendency for the complaint to be better and worse in a cyclic pattern presumably because of the inhibitory effect of pain on functional movements, permitting some regression of the complaint, only to be followed by an exacerbation from increased rubbing when the discomfort ceases.

The tip of the tongue or one side of the tongue may be involved. The inner surface of the lips is also a common site. Although the gingiva proper is more resistant to such irritation, localized burning gingival pain may occur, especially from rubbing with the tongue.

All oral irritants increase the patient's discomfort. This includes especially highly spiced foods, hot liquids, carbonated drinks, strong coffee and tea, certain juices, dentrifices, mouthwashes and medications. Sometimes mastication becomes so painful that nutritional difficulties arise.

A common cause of this condition is *xerostomia*. Inadequate quantity of saliva as well as low mucinous content contributes to the condition. Many modern medicines have an anticholinergic action that alters and depresses salivation. Certain emotional states cause the same effect. This includes especially such conditions as anxiety, insecurity, and resentment sustained over a period of time. Functional failure due to the aging process and radiation also may be etiologic factors. Sjögren's syndrome has been implicated. This is described as keratoconjunctivitis sicca associated with pharyngitis sicca, enlargement of the parotid glands, and chronic polyarthritis.

Other causes of burning mouth and burning tongue are emotional tension, oral consciousness, dental appliances of all types, and habits. Quinn found that tongue-thrusting predominated in patients with glossodynia.[5] Bruxism no doubt is a contributing factor. Dietary influence and systemic conditions affect salivary functioning also.

The condition of glossodynia and burning mouth seems to be poorly understood. Much of it is iatrogenic from medications such as the antihistamines, belladonna, and other anticholinergic agents; some tranquilizers and muscle relaxants; diuretics; and some antihypertensive drugs. Anxiety and emotional tension frequently induce or aggravate the condition. It is especially common in women of menopause age. The condition is frequently iatrogenic from increased tongue and mouth movements due to oral consciousness following dental treatment. Although dentures normally require more lubrication from saliva than natural teeth, they may at times depress salivary flow due to apprehension and resentment that their presence induces in some individuals. Thus, a normally difficult situation becomes compounded by the emotional problems that accompany it.

The diagnostic key to this problem is a simple one—use of a topical anesthetic applied to the painful site. Its penetration is too limited to appreciably affect pain sources situated more deeply in the tissues. Referred pains are not affected. Therefore, if application of a topical anesthetic promptly and effectively arrests the pain and induces numbness, the condition truly represents primary hyperalgesia, and the diagnosis is confirmed. It should be noted that some neuralgias are triggered by stimulation of the oral and pharyngeal mucosa, and such triggering may be temporarily arrested by application of a topical anesthetic. This phenomenon should never be confused with the problem under consideration, due to the clinical difference in the two complaints.

MASSIVE SUPERFICIAL INJURY.—Generalized surface injuries cause mucogingival pains, but the cause is usually so evident that no diagnostic problem is presented. Other signs are present—or promptly become so—namely, hyperemia, inflammation, vesiculation, or ulceration. Such traumatic effects may have mechanical, thermal, or chemical causes such as scalding with hot foods or liquids, excessive smoking or other use of tobacco, abrasions from tooth brushes and other objects, chemical burns, accidents as a result of dental treatment, or use of harmful medications by the patient. Examples of the latter are aspirin burns and injuries produced by toothache remedies.

ALLERGIC RESPONSES.—Various allergic responses, including stomatitis medicamentosa and stomatitis venenata, may produce rather generalized mucogingival pain, the cause of which may at times be obscure. These conditions are usually accompanied by objective signs of tissue change, and the cause may be established by careful history-taking. Stomatitis venenata presents lesions of the oral mucosa resulting from contact with ordinarily innocuous substances such as denture materials, dentifrices, mouthwashes, lozenges, lipsticks, topical medications, foods, and flavoring materials (Figs 8–2 and 8–3). Sometimes desquamation of the protective surface layers of epithelium occurs, revealing the deeper vascular bed. When the shedding is extensive, the term *desquamative stomatitis* may be applicable.

Stomatitis medicamentosa is an allergic reaction to systemic medications such as antibiotics, sulfonamides, aminopyrine, quinine, arsphenamine, phenolphthalein, barbiturates, mercurials, and salicylates. Some cases of erythema multiforme (Fig 8–4) as well as variants described as Stevens-Johnson syndrome, Behçet's syndrome and ectodermosis erosiva pluriorificialis may represent allergic reponses of this type.

Other allergens may cause oral manifestations accompanied by superficial mucogingival pain. At times, such manifestations may require consultation with an allergist. From the standpoint of pain diagnosis, such conditions should be distinguished from localized autonomic effects that result from central excitation. The key to diagnosis relates to one's knowledge of the neuroanatomy of the visceral nervous sys-

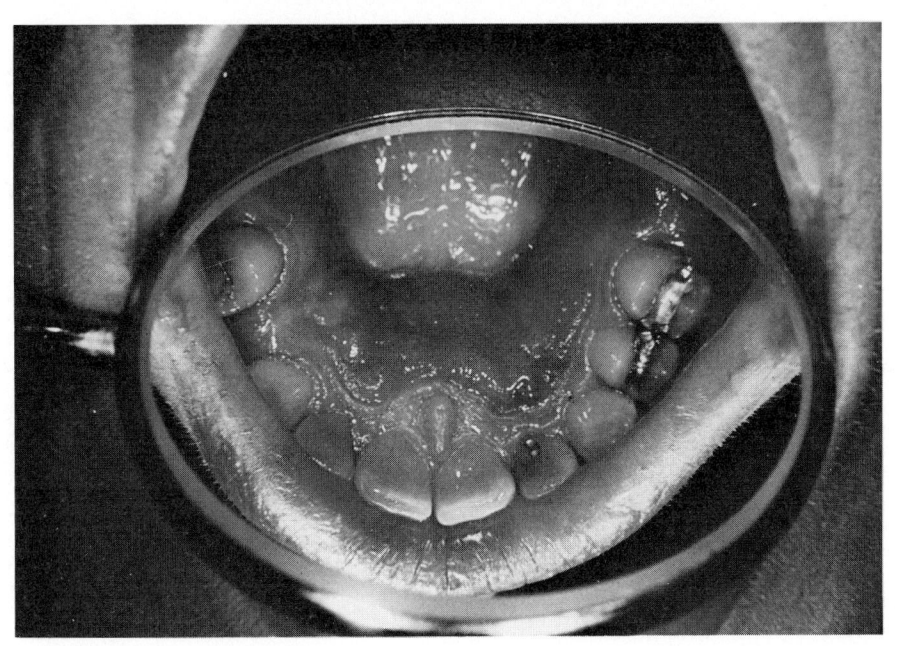

Fig 8–2.—Stomatitis venenata due to contact with denture base material. Note that tissue reaction conforms to shape of denture base.

Cutaneous and Mucogingival Pains 109

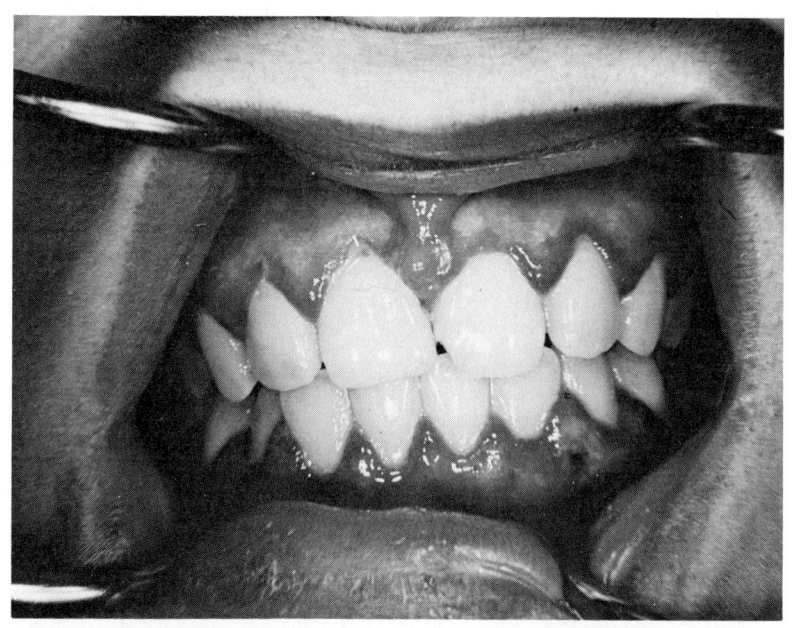

Fig 8-3.—Stomatitis venenata due to contact with dentifrice to which patient was sensitive.

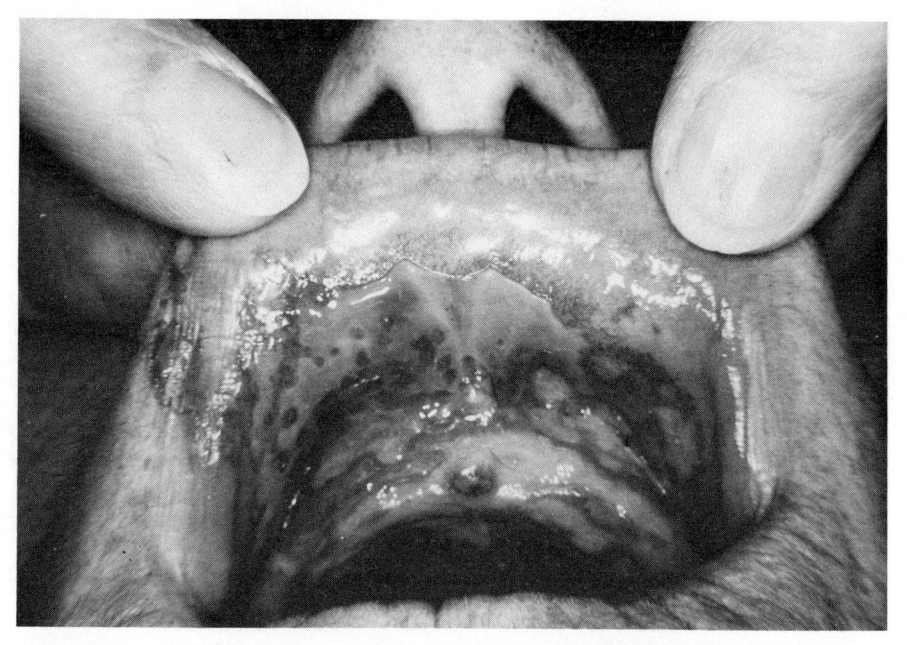

Fig 8-4.—Stomatitis medicamentosa expressed clinically as erythema multiforme due to ingestion of a laxative medicine that contained phenolphthalein.

tem. Systemic allergic responses do not follow neuroanatomical patterns and therefore are observed *bilaterally* and *diffusely,* whereas localized autonomic effects relate to the anatomical distribution of the neurons involved and are predominantly *unilateral.*

PREGNANCY.—Pregnancy and perhaps also the ingestion of oral contraceptive drugs may cause oral manifestations that become painful (Fig 8–5). Usually only the mucogingival tissues are involved, and the pain is characteristically superficial somatic in type. These conditions exhibit objective signs of congestion so that discoloration and swelling are evident. Such effects frequently occur at sites where other local irritation is present such as trauma, malocclusion, gingivitis, and periodontal involvement.

SYSTEMIC DISEASE.—Systemic disease may cause oral manifestations that affect the mucogingival tissues, inducing generalized superficial somatic pain. Included are nutritional deficiencies, intoxications, exanthematous diseases, anemia and other blood dyscrasias, pellagra, diabetes, pemphigus, infections, and general debilitation.

LOCAL INFECTIONS.—Widespread local infections of the mucogingival tissues cause generalized superficial somatic pain. Usually the

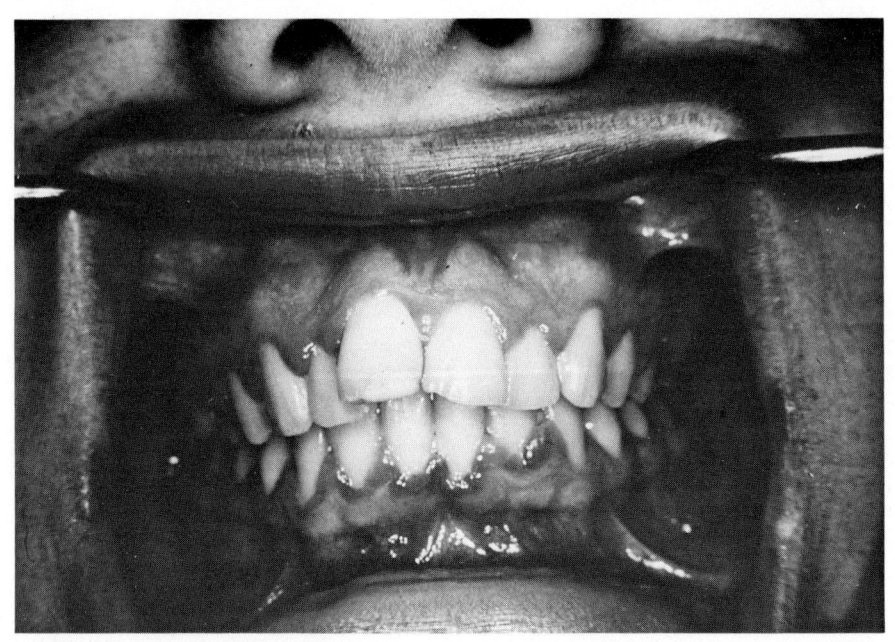

Fig 8–5.—Gingivitis that became acute during the third month of pregnancy and persisted five weeks post partum.

accompanying local signs of inflammation and ulceration make the cause of pain obvious. Examples of this are fulminating Vincent's infection and fungoid infections (Figs 8–6 and 8–7).

Isolated Pains

Most isolated pains emanating from the oral mucogingival tissues present no diagnostic problem because they are usually associated with local lesions clinically evident subjectively and objectively. Among such painful lesions may be listed the lip lesions of herpes simplex and the oral ulcerative lesions of aphthous stomatitis. Traumatic abrasions and ulcerations are common due to local tissue injury. Decubital ulcers from dental appliances may be identified (Fig 8–8).

Exostoses and bony prominences are especially vulnerable to injury, and, when severely traumatized, full-thickness mucogingival ulcers may develop, causing exposure and surface devitalization of the underlying cortical bone. Such lesions are slow to heal and cause pain with deep somatic characteristics in addition to the expected superficial somatic variety. Whenever the periosteal and osseous structures become involved, pains of mixed quality should be expected. This is

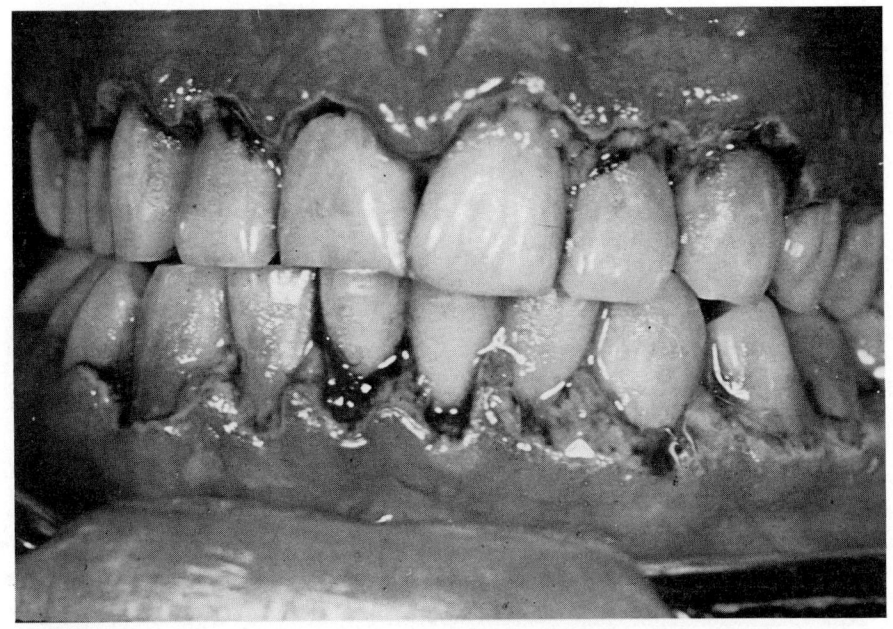

Fig 8–6.—Acute necrotizing ulcerative gingivitis (Vincent's infection).

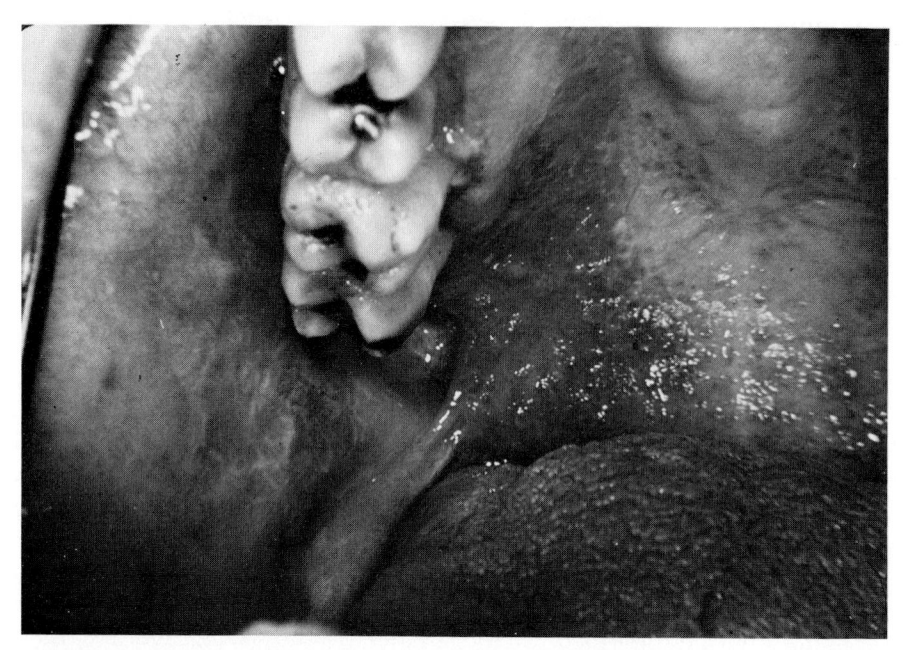

Fig 8-7.—Fungoid infection of oral mucosa.

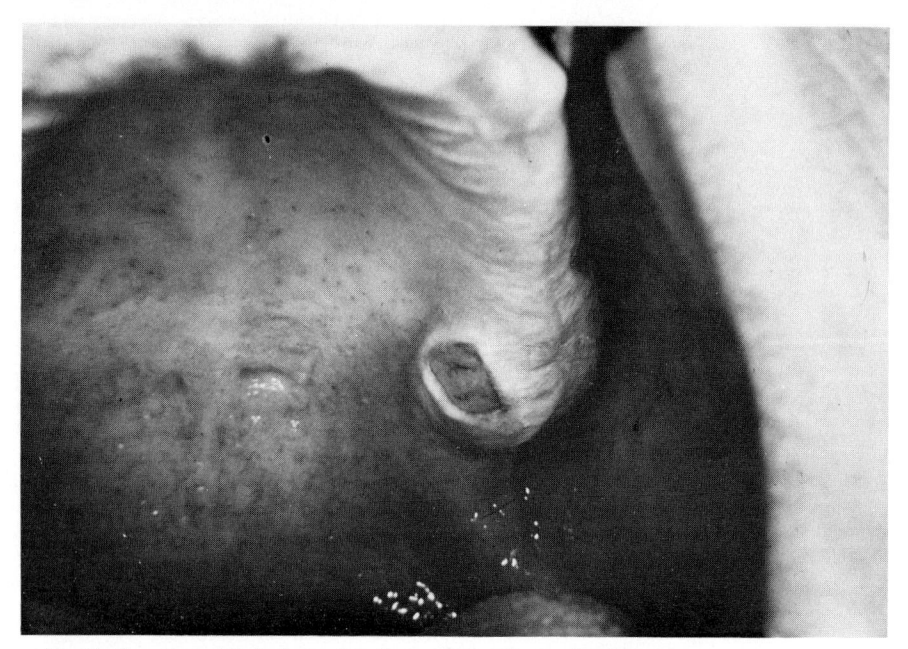

Fig 8-8.—Decubital ulcer due to pressure from denture.

true not only of the full-thickness ulcers but also of gingival lesions that involve the deeper periodontal structures. Examples of such lesions are acutely inflamed periodontal pockets and superficial infections that spread as cellulitis. *Pains of mixed quality are less likely to be arrested by application of a topical anesthetic.* They frequently present symptoms of central excitation.

Mucogingival Pain Without Local Cause

There are occasions when superficial somatic pain from mucogingival tissues arises without local cause of any kind. Such complaints usually are described as excessive sensitivity of the lining mucosa of the mouth. It goes without saying that in all such conditions one should thoroughly investigate the possibility of glossodynia and burning mouth, as previously described. The lowered local pain threshold, however, may be due to a deficiency in the endogenous antinociceptive system. It is thought that elevated emotional tension, stress, or anxiety may account for such effects. Nutritional and endocrine dysfunction as well as illnesses and various toxic conditions may also be contributing factors.

DIFFERENTIAL DIAGNOSIS

Pain felt in the cutaneous or mucogingival tissues may be heterotopic. The decisive diagnostic evidence that the complaint is heterotopic is failure of an effective topical anesthetic to arrest the pain even though surface anesthesia is attained. Therapeutic considerations require that the type and source of such heterotopic pain be identified.

Referred Pain and Secondary Hyperalgesia

Referred pain and/or secondary hyperalgesia induced as a central excitatory effect of deep somatic pain may involve the skin or the oral mucogingival structures. Spontaneous referred pain usually is readily recognized. Stimulus-evoked secondary hyperalgesia, however, can be difficult to identify. The clue to differential diagnosis in either case is to become suspicious that the problem is that of a secondary effect of deep pain input located elsewhere.

The diagnostic criteria of this phenomenon relate to identifying the primary pain source. Analgesic blocking or application of a topical anesthetic at the site where heterotopic pain is felt does not arrest the pain even though some altered sensation due to the local anesthesia may be felt.

Referred pains and areas of hypersensitivity in the mucogingival tissues may occur as a direct result of other deep pain sources such as toothache, earache, sinusitis, temporomandibular arthralgia, myogenous pains, and vascular pains. Frequently, other central excitatory effects such as local autonomic signs and secondary painful muscle spasms may be identified as well.

Neurogenous Pains

Neurogenous pains present clinical characteristics that in some respects simulate those of superficial somatic pain, and differentiation between the two categories of pain is necessary.

Traumatic neuroma is characterized by its location relative to prior injury or surgery and by the specific induction of pain due to compressing or stretching the tissue involved. Topical anesthesia does nothing. Injection, however, of a drop or so of local anesthetic into the site of pain completely arrests it.

Paroxysmal neuralgia may be triggered by stimulation of the receptors in the peripheral distribution. In trigeminal neuralgia the sites of such triggering are predominantly cutaneous, being located especially in the lips. Mucogingival triggering, however, sometimes occurs, the tongue being a frequent site. Glossopharyngeal trigger sites are located in the pharyngeal mucosa, and pain is induced by swallowing, talking, and chewing. The clinical criterion for identifying mucosal triggering of paroxysmal neuralgia has to do with the summation effects displayed: the triggering provokes pain that is wholly disproportionate to the stimulus. Analgesic blocking of the peripheral receptors of the affected nerve prevents the triggering effect of superficial stimulation. Topical anesthesia of mucosal trigger sites such as those of glossopharyngeal neuralgia also prevents the paroxysms of pain.

Neuritic neuralgia that involves cutaneous and mucogingival structures may be more difficult to recognize because of the similarity to superficial somatic pain. One clinical criterion for identifying this neurogenous pain is its ongoing, persistent, unremitting character. It is not dependent on superficial stimulation even though such stimulation accentuates the discomfort. A more important criterion, however, is the presence of other neural effects (such as paresthesia, hypoesthesia, anesthesia, and paralysis) that may accompany the neuritic pain. Neuritic neuralgia of the facial nerve is characterized by widespread paralysis of facial muscles. Analgesic blocking central to the site of neuropathy arrests the pain.

Herpes zoster can be particularly difficult to distinguish from superficial somatic pain unless the typical lesions are present also. Cutaneous herpetic lesions are usually recognized because they occur in the neuroanatomical peripheral distribution of the affected nerve—exactly where the pain is felt. The intraoral mucosal lesions of trigeminal and geniculate herpes zoster, however, may be confused with aphthous ulcers. As such, the lesions may be thought to cause the pain. When herpetic lesions are absent, go unnoticed, or are misdiagnosed, leaving only the persistent neuritic pain, diagnosis may be extremely difficult. Perhaps the best criterion is that analgesic blocking of any type does not arrest the pain. If the condition persists more than a few weeks, a diagnosis of postherpetic neuralgia is indicated.

Deafferentation pain may become a complication sequential to trauma, surgery, tooth extraction, or tooth-pulp extirpation. The best differential criterion is a history of prior deafferentation. The pain complaint may be accompanied by paresthesia, dysesthesia, anesthesia, hyperesthesia, or hyperalgesia in an area considerably larger than that innervated by the injured nerve. The symptoms may be accentuated by efferent sympathetic activity involving vasomotor and glandular function. The pain is temporarily arrested by analgesic blocking of the stellate ganglion.

REFERENCES

1. Ochea J.L., Torebjork, H.E.: Pain from skin and muscle. *Pain,* suppl. 1, 1981, p. S87.
2. Bonica J.J.: *The Management of Pain.* Philadelphia, Lea & Febiger, 1953.
3. Wolff H.G., Wolf S.: *Pain,* ed 2. Springfield, Ill., Charles C Thomas, Publisher, 1958.
4. Dalessio D. J.: *Wolff's Headache and Other Head Pain,* ed. 3. New York, Oxford University Press, 1972.
5. Quinn J.H.: Glossodynia. *J.A.D.A.* 70: 1418–1421, 1965.

9

Pains of Dental Origin

THE TEETH OCCUPY A UNIQUE structural and functional position in that they are visceral structures that function as part of the musculoskeletal system. This, perhaps, helps to explain some of the enigmatic behavior of dental pain. Tooth pulps serve as isolated organs, each an individual in its own right. The sensory capabilities of dental pulpal tissue simulate that of other visceral structures; pain of pulpal origin simulates other visceral pains. The connections of the teeth to the bone, however, constitute musculoskeletal structures—fibrous joints constructed in such a manner as to convert masticatory pressure into traction on the alveolar bone. These true joints, termed *gomphosis,* are structurally similar to other fibrous joints in which tractive forces predominate. The mechanoreceptors in periodontal ligaments are similar to those of other fibrous joints, although they differ considerably from the proprioceptors of synovial joint ligaments, tendons, and muscles.[1] Their nerve cell bodies are located in the mesencephalon along with the other masticatory proprioceptors, and serve to inhibit the action of elevator muscles which constitute the driving force of masticatory function.[2-4] The uniqueness of teeth and their alveolar attachment is that visceral structures function as an integral segment of the musculoskeletal system. The sensory behavior, including dental pain, constitutes a mixture of visceral and musculoskeletal characteristics (Fig 9–1).

The unique innervation of teeth is pointed up by a recent observation in two cancer patients who had undergone trigeminal tractotomy along with rhizotomy of the ninth and tenth cranial nerves and of several cervical spinal nerves to control intractable face pain. Both patients displayed analgesia or hypalgesia throughout the cutaneous trigeminal distribution; *yet they continued to maintain normal sensory response to dental stimulation.*[5] It should be noted that, while facial input is represented almost exclusively in the subnucleus cau-

OROFACIAL PAIN SYNDROMES

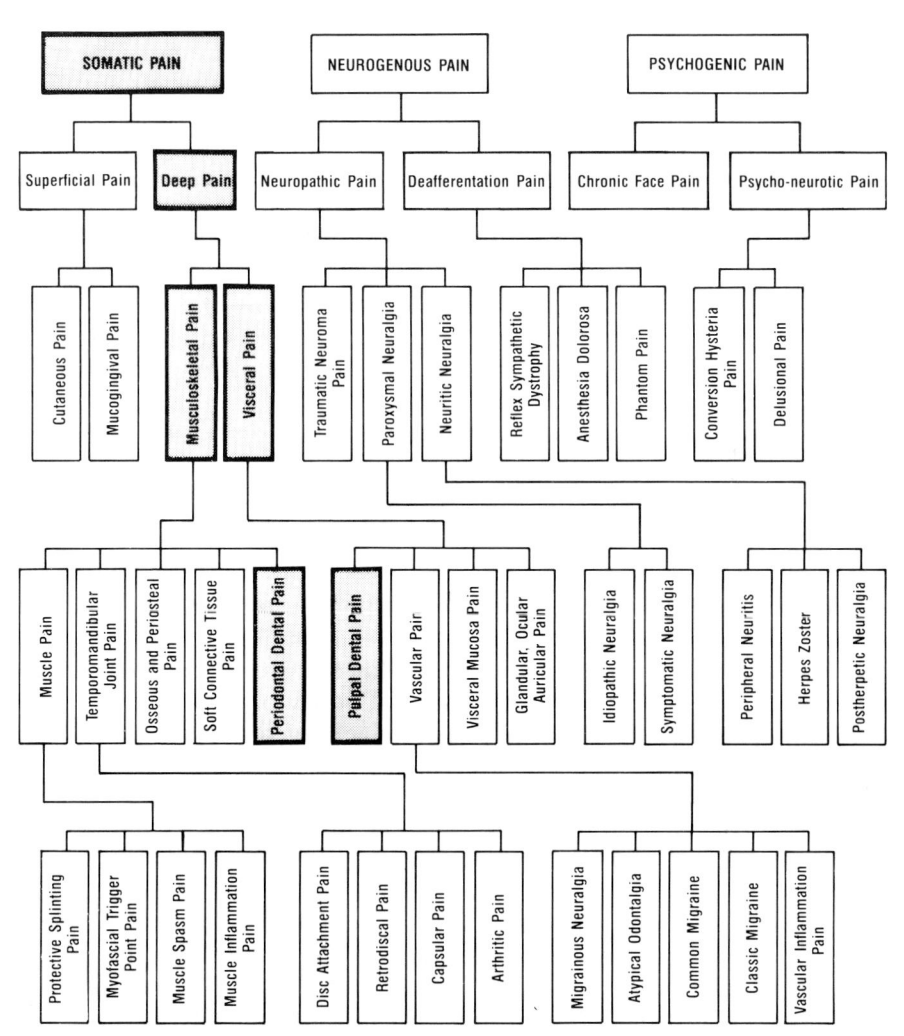

Fig 9-1.—Chart showing classification relationship of dental pains to other orofacial pain syndromes.

dalis, nociceptive input from the oral cavity has a double representation in subnucleus oralis and caudalis.[6] It should be noted that sensory innervation of the teeth is strictly ipsilateral.[7] Except for pain emanating from midface structures, sensory manifestations from the oral cavity are not expressed contralaterally or bilaterally.

degree of masticatory dysfunction as a by-product of the initiating odontogenous pain. Although the masseter is most frequently involved, any muscle innervated by the trigeminal nerve can become spastic in this spreading pain phenomenon. This includes not only the other chief masticatory muscles but also the mylohyoid, anterior digastric, tensor palati, and tensor tympani muscles as well. So a variety of muscle symptoms may occur and persist as a direct result of dental pain.

Occasionally, local autonomic effects may accompany odontogenous pain. Edema of the ipsilateral eyelids, injection of the conjunctiva, lacrimation, and ipsilateral nasal congestion may complicate the symptom picture. These effects are directly dependent on the primary pain source and in due time disappear when the initiating pain is eliminated. Such autonomic symptoms may greatly confuse the clinical problem unless they are recognized and correctly evaluated by the examiner. They may be confused with disease involving the eye, nose, and maxillary sinus.

EFFECT OF TOPICAL ANESTHETIC.—As with all deep pain sources, the effect of applying a topical anesthetic at the site of discomfort is negligible. Analgesic blocking, however, is an effective tool for differentiating primary from secondary pains if they involve different nerve trunks. It is the method of choice for isolating the nerve that mediates the primary odontogenous pain.

Since pulpal pain is of the visceral category, and periodontal pain is musculoskeletal in type, it is necessary to describe them as separate entities even though at a clinical level "tooth pain" may include components of both.

STIMULUS-INDUCED PULPAL PAIN

The sensory capabilities of the dental pulp are predominantly, but not exclusively, nociceptive.[8] The dental pulp also senses thermal stimuli and tingling.[9] It has recently been determined that, under specially controlled circumstances, pulpal receptors may give rise to nonnociceptive impulses that have some sensory function other than the mediation of painful sensation.[10] It is thought that nonpain sensations of the pulp are mediated by a distinct population of afferents that are not nociceptive.[11] The pulp contains both fast and slowly conducting neurons.[12] There is conclusive evidence for the presence of a significant C-fiber population in tooth pulps that can be activated by electrical stimulation.[13] The innervation density of the dental pulp is calculated to be about 15 times that of skin.[14] The mediation of sensory impulses from the dental pulp to the subnucleus caudalis as well as to the more rostrally located subnucleus oralis has been confirmed.[15, 16]

The visceral character of pulpal pain is displayed particularly in its clinical behavior. The pain is of threshold type, as compared with the graduated response exhibited by musculoskeletal pain. No response occurs until threshold level is reached. Pulpal pain responds to noxious stimulation that is unrelated to ordinary masticatory movements. It responds to impact, shock, thermal and chemical irritants, and direct exploration, but not to ordinary masticatory function. The pain is nearly nonlocalizable by the subject.

PAINS OF PULPAL ORIGIN

Pulpal pains may be classified as acute, chronic, recurrent, or mixed with periodontal elements. A basic clinical feature of pulpal pain is that it does not remain the same indefinitely. Generally it resolves, becomes chronic, or proceeds to involve the periodontal structures by direct extension through the apex of the tooth root. Rarely does it remain unchanged for long periods.

ACUTE PULPAL PAIN.—Perhaps the most typical of all visceral pain is acute pulpal pain. It is so completely nonlocalizable by the patient that its source often cannot be determined subjectively. Objective evidence such as deep caries, erosion into the pulp chamber or root canal, fracture or splitting may immediately identify the offending tooth. If such evidence is lacking, and especially if more than a single tooth could be involved (Fig 9–2), clinical identification of the offending tooth may be difficult if not impossible.

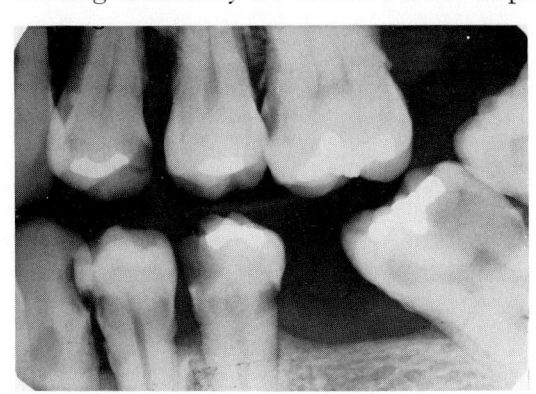

Fig 9–2.—Radiograph showing rampant caries and extensive periodontal disease. Such a situation presents several possible causes of odontogenous pain, pulpal and periodontal.

The cause of acute pulpal pain is noxious stimulation of the pulpal receptors. Normally, tooth structure protects these nerve endings from superficial stimulation so that only extreme surface irritation such as electric stimulation or extremes of thermal change is sensed as pain. If the tooth structure is breached by splitting, a normal pulp may immediately become painful on contact with saliva or air. This occurs especially when masticatory stress tends to "open the split." If the tooth structure is breached by fracture from a dislodged metallic filling, pain results from pressure exerted against the pulp and is increased when additional pressure is brought to bear on the filling by biting against it. Until the pulp becomes inflamed, pain from such cause is intermittent.

The pulp tissue responds to injury whether it be from repeated threshold stimulation of the intact surface, cervical exposure due to gingival recession, repeated irritation of occlusal trauma, breaching of the overlying protective tooth structure due to splitting or fracture, repeated thermal shocks transmitted by metallic fillings, thinning of the overlying tooth structure by erosion or abrasion, traumatic shock, or dental caries. The changes that take place are usually inflammatory. These conditions may be reversible unless congestion occurs, causing pulpal gangrene. Once gangrene occurs, extension to the periodontal tissue through the apical foramen of the root almost invariably takes place. This is especially so if the pulpal inflammation is due to bacterial agents. It should be noted that in multirooted teeth irreversible pulpal changes may occur in one root, with reasonably normal pulp tissue surviving in another. Situations of this type may not occur frequently, but when they do, a confusing symptom picture may result.

The pulpal pains that result from such tissue changes should be understood. As a rule, the pain threshold of all deep receptors and nerve fibers that mediate pain is lowered by inflammation. Thus, the dental pulp that is inflamed is hypersensitive to all stimuli, including electric stimulation, thermal shock, probing, and percussion. Pain may be elicited by application of some or all such stimuli to the tooth. If the tissue change is not too great, application of such stimuli causes pain only for the duration of the noxious stimulation. But if the change is greater, such stimulation may induce toothache. As the inflammatory process progresses, spontaneous toothache may occur with no outside provocation.

Acute pulpal pain may be extremely variable depending on the cause: the type of reaction that occurs in the pulpal tissues; the stimulus applied; the response of the patient; the pain modulation especially imposed by the higher centers as reflected by the mental, emotional, and physical state of the patient at that particular time; and the myriad secondary excitatory effects that take place with pains that are continuous and of sufficient intensity and duration.

Acute pulpal pain may range from occasional hypersensitivity caused by sweets and other minor stimulants to spontaneous violent throbbing toothache of intolerable intensity that cannot be controlled even with narcotic analgesics. It may be induced by many types of irritants or be wholly spontaneous. It may be increased by both heat and cold or increased by heat and relieved by cold. It may be intermittent or continuous. It may be influenced by head or body position. It may relate to the contact of teeth, to the presence or temperature of foods and beverages, or to jaw and head movements. It may be mistaken for sinus headache, sinusitis, earache, neuritis, atypical facial neuralgia, or tic douloureux. It may induce referred pains, areas of secondary hyperalgesia almost anywhere in the face and head, localized autonomic symptoms, and secondary painful muscle spasm in masticatory muscles. It may induce a masticatory pain-dysfunction syndrome or be mistaken for temporomandibular arthritis.

If the pulpal inflammation is great enough to cause severe, continuing toothache, the chance of resolution is extremely low. Under favorable circumstances, resolution does occur. Usually the condition progresses to pulpal gangrene. When this occurs, pain from the pulpal tissues ceases. Such "recovery" from severe toothache should be interpreted as the transition period from pulpal to periodontal involvement. This transition is extremely variable. If the pulpal inflammation is due to infection, the transition is usually rapid, consisting of mixed pulpal and periodontal pains at first and terminating as an acute periodontal abscess (Fig 9–3). If the pulpal inflammation is sterile, all pain may cease and a painless periapical granuloma or radicular cyst may develop (Fig 9–4). All gradations between these extremes may

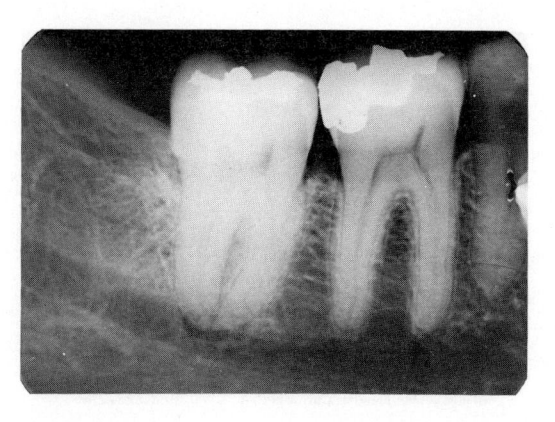

Fig 9–3.—Radiograph showing early periapical radiolucent change (mandibular second molar), indicative of periapical abscess. This tooth was split mesiodistally and had elicited recurrent acute pupal pains on several occasions. As periapical tissues became involved, both pulpal and periodontal pain could be identified. Early in its clinical course, the first molar was suspect, due to the large metallic filling.

Fig 9–4.—Radiograph showing an extensive apical radiolucency involving anterior mandibular teeth. The four incisors were slightly discolored and nonresponsive to thermal and electric stimulation. The condition was painless. History was that of former trauma and acute pulpal pain that soon subsided.

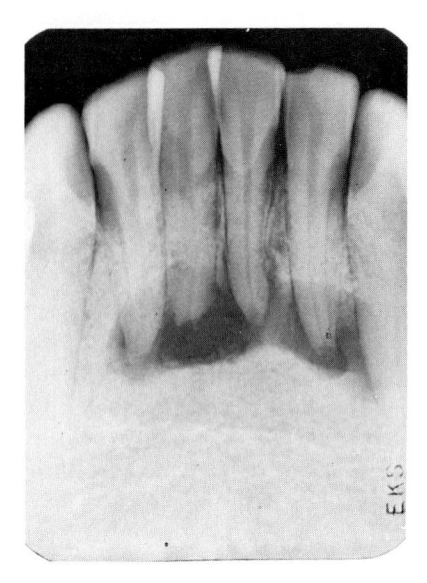

occur. If a multirooted tooth is involved, one root may exhibit symptoms of acute pulpitis, whereas another may show evidence of pulpal gangrene and periapical abscess (Fig 9–5). When this occurs, the symptom picture can become involved indeed.

CHRONIC PULPAL PAIN.—Under certain conditions, injured pulpal tissues may progress from an acute to chronic inflammatory phase, and thus undergo changes that proceed neither to resolution nor to gangrene, but remain indefinitely as what is usually described as chronic pulpitis. The condition that favors this transgression is traumatic injury to a young tooth, especially one with an open expansive root end that is less likely to facilitate congestion and gangrene of the pulp. Such teeth continue to respond to the pulp tester even though considerably

Fig 9–5.—Radiograph showing periapical radiolucent change involving mesial root of mandibular first molar tooth. Clinical symptoms were those of typical pulpal pain and acute periodontal pain occurring simultaneously in the tooth.

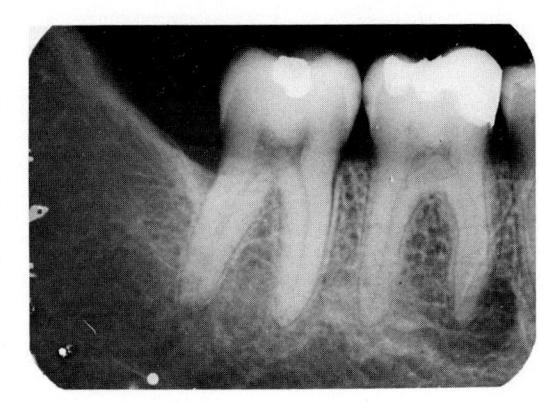

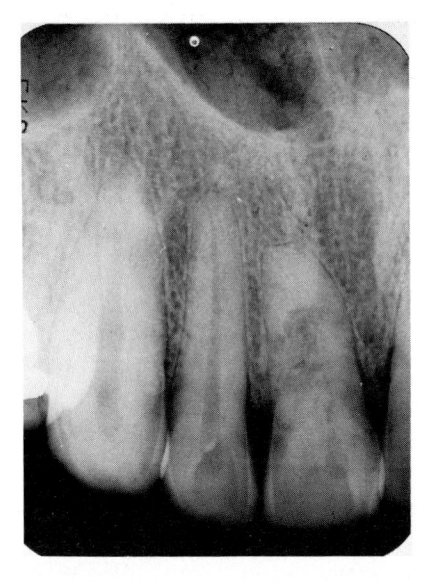

Fig 9-6.—Radiograph showing central radiolucency in maxillary central incisor tooth, indicative of internal resorption. The tooth had normal color and responded positively to electric pulp testing, but considerably less than the adjacent teeth. The patient was 32 years old. There was history of trauma to his tooth 16 years previously, followed by "toothache" which promptly subsided. Presently the tooth is nonsymptomatic.

less responsive than those with normal pulps. Frequently, internal resorption of the tooth occurs (Fig 9-6).

When chronic pulpitis develops, the pain responses change from the extremely variable character of acute pulpal pain to a milder and less variable discomfort that may not be described as pain at all (Fig 9-7). In fact, the tooth may become symptomless unless further injury to it takes place.

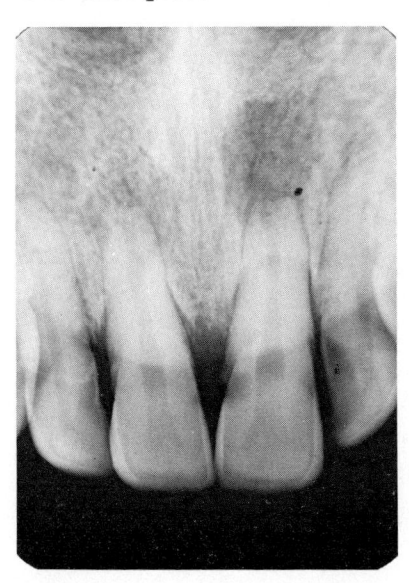

Fig 9-7.—Radiograph showing apical and periapical radiolucency of maxillary central incisors. Both had normal color and responded positively to electric pulp testing, but considerably less so than the adjacent teeth. Both teeth, especially the right incisor, were described as vaguely "uncomfortable," but not "painful."

RECURRENT PULPAL PAIN.—Severe acute pulpal pain is rarely recurrent in the true sense because the inflammation usually goes either to resolution, chronicity, or gangrene. When acute pulpal pain appears to be recurrent, it usually consists of recurring periods of inflammation in a sequential pattern. This may occur when a partially split tooth is opened only by some unusual occlusal stress. Real recurrent pulpal pain ordinarily does not cause toothache but is sensed as recurrent hypersensitivity. Such conditions frequently are associated with changes in vascular pressure or fluid balance. So-called menstrual toothache and high-altitude toothache fall into this category. The offending tooth is usually slightly hyperemic, and the lowered pain threshold becomes symptomatic when the proper environmental conditions prevail. Other instances of recurrent pulpal pain include hypersensitive teeth that are stimulated to the point of pain by such factors as sweets, thermal changes, and occlusal abuse.

MIXED PAIN.—When the transition from pulpal inflammation through gangrene to periapical involvement is rapid, symptoms of both pulpal and periodontal pain may occur. Conversely, when the dental pulp becomes secondarily involved by direct extension from the periodontal structures, mixed symptoms may be evident (Fig 9–8). Also, especially as a result of trauma, both pulpal and periodontal symptoms may occur simultaneously. In all such instances, the cause usually is obvious and the symptoms readily explained.

However, a tooth can present pulpal and periodontal symptoms due to separate and independent causes, and if so, the symptom picture may be confusing. This can occur especially in multirooted teeth. Also, nearby teeth may be simultaneously involved, presenting symptoms that are misleading to examiner and patient alike (Fig 9–9).

Fig 9–8.—Radiograph showing periodontal radiolucency involving the distal root of mandibular second molar tooth. There is extensive interradicular involvement and deep surface resorption into the mesial aspect of the distal root. Clinically, the tooth presented symptoms indicative of a chronic periodontal abscess with more recent symptoms of acute pulpitis. The tooth was responsive to electric pulp testing.

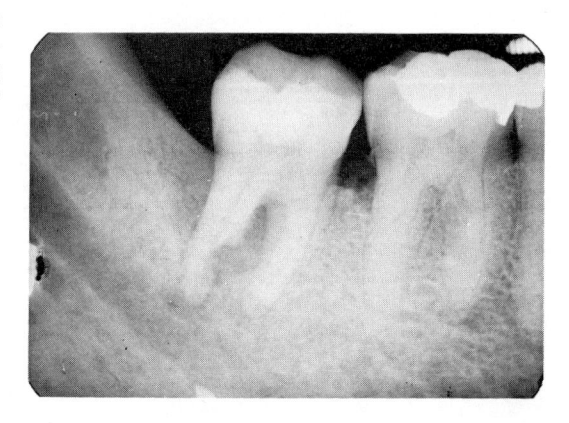

PAINS OF DENTAL ORIGIN 127

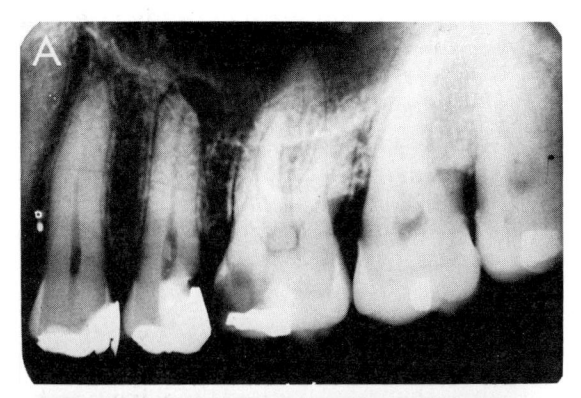

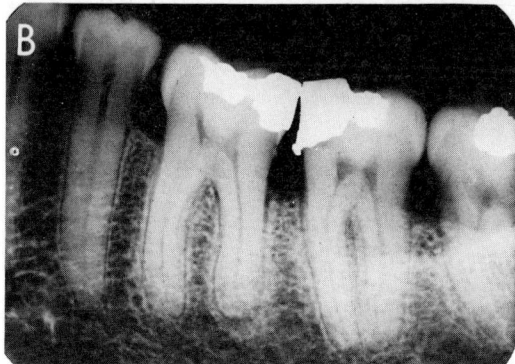

Fig 9-9.—Radiographs showing reasonable cause for pulpal and periodontal pain in adjacent teeth. **A,** maxillary second bicuspid presents periapical radiolucency; first molar has extensive dental caries. **B,** there is evidence of recurrent caries beneath mesial filling in mandibular second molar; distal root of first molar shows slight but definite periapical involvement.

CRITERIA FOR IDENTIFICATION OF PULPAL PAIN.—The examiner should suspect pain as being of pulpal origin when it is difficult for the patient to precisely localize it to a certain tooth. A thorough dental examination becomes mandatory. Obvious possible sources of the pulpal pain should be investigated first. This would include such conditions as primary caries, recurrent caries, defective fillings, cervical exposure, erosion, abrasion, split or fractured teeth, and deep or massive dental restorations, as indicated by clinical and radiographic findings. When a suspicious tooth is located, an attempt to induce or increase the pain by noxious stimulation of that tooth by chemical, thermal, mechanical, or electric irritants should be made. If pain is induced by applying heat to the tooth, cold should be applied to see if the pain is relieved. The examiner should carefully isolate the tooth with celluloid strips when applying thermal or electric irritants to prevent conduction to an adjacent tooth, especially if contacting metallic fillings are present. If the pain can be influenced by local irritation, the tooth should be anesthetized locally to see if anesthesia promptly and completely arrests the pain and prevents stimulation by applied irritants. If such is the case, the offending tooth has been satisfactorily identified.

With no lead as to which tooth is the source of pain—if indeed it is a tooth—the examiner is obliged to be suspicious of every tooth on the side on which there is pain—maxillary and mandibular. Each tooth should be tested by inspection, probing, palpation, percussion, thermal shocking, and electric stimulation to determine if *one tooth* is considerably more responsive than others. Systematic analgesic blocking should be done, first to determine if the pain site is maxillary or mandibular, and then, more accurately, the individual teeth.

Broad conclusions can be drawn as to whether the pain arises from maxillary or mandibular structures. If analgesic blocking fails to arrest the pain promptly and completely for the duration of anesthesia, a conclusion that the pain does not arise from dental structures is justified. If such blocking is accurately effective, the conclusion that the pain is initiated in structures thus anesthetized is usually correct—but it does not necessarily follow that the pain is in fact odontogenous.

If the pain is shown to arise from the dental area but a particular tooth cannot be identified as the offending source, it is wise to wait for pain localization to occur through the process of transition from pulpal to periodontal pain, as previously discussed. Eventually, localized tenderness should identify the proper tooth, probably within a few days or weeks.

Radiographic examination does not identify the source of pulpal pain other than to give clues as to its cause (Fig 9–10). Electric pulp testing has value when done along with other forms of pulpal stimulation but has very limited value by itself. The history, descriptive characteristics, and clinical behavior are extremely important in the diagnosis of pulpal pain. Recognition of secondary excitatory effects is essential, and the importance of an understanding of how such

Fig 9–10.—Radiograph of extensive dental caries involving maxillary second molar distally. The patient presented symptoms of acute pulpal pain without evident clinical cause. Although extensive, the carious lesion was obscured clinically by the third molar.

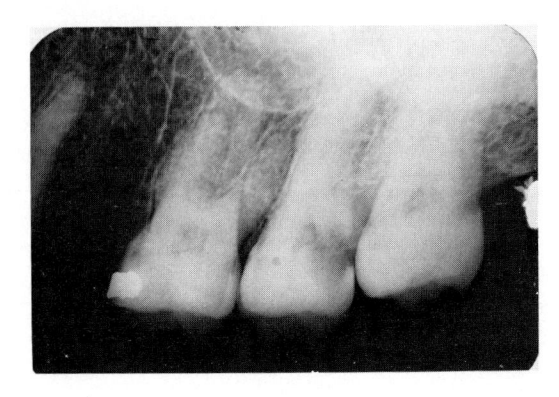

effects relate to the primary pain source cannot be overemphasized. This is especially true regarding secondary painful muscle spasms.

OBSCURE CAUSES OF PULPAL PAIN.—There are several fairly common causes of pulpal pain that are clinically difficult to recognize. Perhaps the most common of these is the mesiodistally split tooth, the margins of which are obscured by adjacent teeth and the presence of which is not radiographically visible. Another common cause is an occlusal filling that is slightly dislodged in a pulpal direction. Recurrent caries obscured both clinically and radiographically by an overlying dental restoration may be the etiologic factor. Still another cause is mechanical abrasion of the root of a tooth due to the presence of an adjacent impacted tooth (Fig 9–11). Abrasions can penetrate the substance of the root until the contents of the root canal are exposed. Another very obscure cause of pulpal involvement is direct extension from a periodontal pocket via an aberrant lateral root canal. Hematogenous infection of the dental pulp has been reported.

All such possibilities should be considered and explored when pain appears to be truly odontogenous but the cause obscure. Occasionally, direct exploration of the tooth is justified if the pain is severe and the patient is unwilling to wait for natural localization. The risk of opening an innocent dental pulp may be justified in order to establish a positive diagnosis. This is better than the more radical approach—that of extracting such a tooth on a presumptive diagnosis. At least, endodontic measures can be used to salvage the tooth if a mistake is made.

STIMULUS-EVOKED PERIODONTAL PAIN

The teeth are united to the alveolar bone by fibrous joints, the periodontal ligaments comprising the flexible, fibrous portions. The

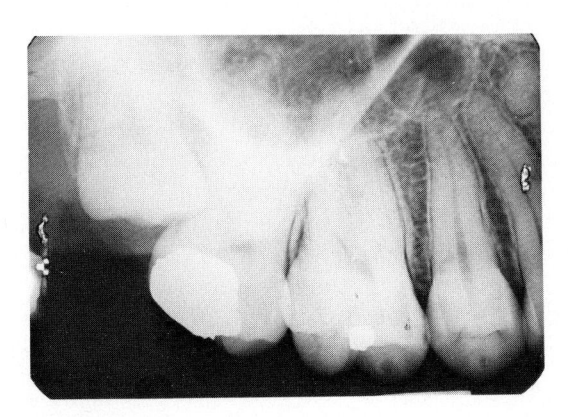

Fig 9–11.—Radiograph of impacted maxillary third molar that had abraded into root of the second molar. The patient presented symptoms of acute pulpal pain emanating from second molar. The tooth was sacrificed. The abraded area involved nerve canal of distobuccal root.

collagenous fibers that connect the cementum to the alveolar cortex are arranged in an oblique fashion so as to convert the pressures entailed in masticatory strokes into traction forces on the bone. The sensory receptors include free nerve endings and mechanoreceptors. When stimulated by pressure on the tooth, the mechanoreceptors exert inhibitory influence on masticatory elevator muscle action. The nonspecialized receptors have good sense of localization so that nociceptive impulses are tooth related. These react to varying degrees of stimulation so that the response to provocation is graduated and localizable. All such sensations are closely related to the requirements of masticatory function. Periodontal pain is deep somatic pain of the musculoskeletal type.

PAINS OF PERIODONTAL ORIGIN

The receptors of the periodontal ligament are capable of rather precise localization of the stimulus. Therefore, periodontal pain of all types presents no real diagnostic problem because the proper offending tooth is readily identified. This is true whether the pain is in the apical area of the periodontal ligament (usually designated as periapical pain) or in the lateral region of the tooth. *This ability of the periodontal receptors to accurately localize the pain source characterizes all periodontal pains and prevents the uncertainty and mystery attendant on acute pulpal pains*, as previously discussed.

Such localization is identified by applying pressure to the tooth laterally or axially. Under the load of occlusal pressure during chewing, the tooth feels sore or elongated. The discomfort may sometimes be felt when the biting pressure is released rather than while it is sustained. Lateral or axial pressure may be applied to the tooth by the examiner as part of his clinical examination.

A dominant feature of periodontal pain is its propensity to induce central excitatory effects similar to those induced by acute pulpal pains, except that here the primary initiating pain is more readily identified both subjectively and objectively. Widely referred pains throughout the jaws and face, secondary hyperalgesias of both deep and superficial type, and painful spasms involving especially the masticatory muscles are expected symptoms when the initiating pain is of sufficient intensity and duration. Some diagnostic confusion may occur when a cycling secondary myospasm perpetuates itself after the initiating cause has ceased by resolution, treatment, or extraction of the offending tooth. Since such spasms almost invariably involve masticatory muscles, chewing pain and muscle shortening may result. When this is the case, careful history-taking may yield the origin of the complaint.

The causes of periodontal pain are many and varied. It may occur as a *primary periodontal inflammatory condition* due to local cause such as trauma, occlusal overstressing (Fig 9–12), contact with an adjacent embedded tooth, or dental treatment. It may occur as a result of dental prophylaxis, endodontic treatment, orthodontic therapy, preparation and manipulation of teeth for restoration, inadequate opposing occlusal contact, occlusal interference, overcontoured or undercontoured proximal contact points, stresses applied to abutment teeth, and surgical interference of all types. It may result from a *spreading inflammatory reaction* incidental to nearby trauma or the healing of surgical wounds. It may occur as an *acute inflammation of a preexistent chronic periodontal lesion* as a result of infection, injury, food impaction, lowered resistance, or dental treatment (Fig 9–13). It may spread from *pulpal inflammation* either directly through the apical root canal, causing a typical periapical abscess (Fig 9–14), or through an aberrant lateral root canal, causing a lateral periodontal abscess. It may occur by *direct extension* from a nearby inflammatory condition involving an adjacent tooth (Fig 9–15), the maxillary antrum or a spreading osseous infection (Fig 9–16).

When the periodontal pain involves several teeth, especially opposing teeth, the matter of *occlusal overstressing* should be considered. This may occur with little or no evidence of gross disease. Overstressing not only from occlusal interference but from clenching and bruxism may occur.

A condition of occlusal overstressing sometimes accompanies certain orthopedic procedures. Called the *pressure pain syndrome*, this

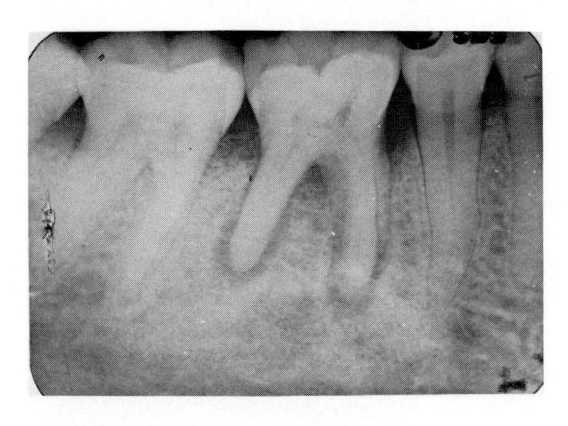

Fig 9–12.—Radiograph of mandibular first molar showing extensive radiolucency around tooth roots. The tooth was in "traumatic" occlusion.

132 OROFACIAL PAINS

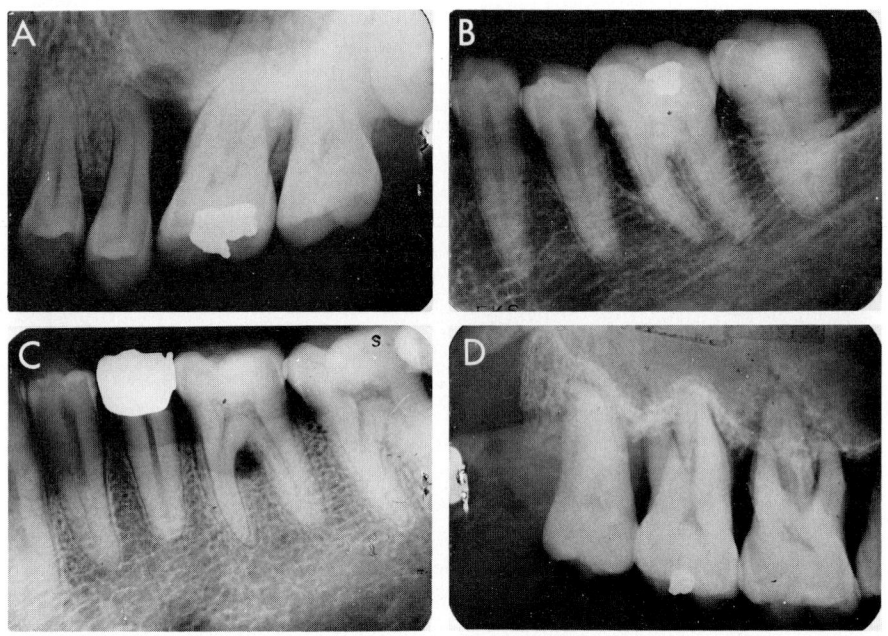

Fig 9–13.—Radiographs showing periodontal lesions of various types: **A,** deep periodontal pocket associated with elongation of maxillary second bicuspid. **B,** buccally located periodontal lesion involving mandibular first molar. **C,** interradicular lesion involving mandibular first molar. **D,** extensive generalized periodontoclasia.

Fig 9–14.—Radiograph showing periapical radiolucency involving maxillary central incisor. This condition followed pulpal inflammation.

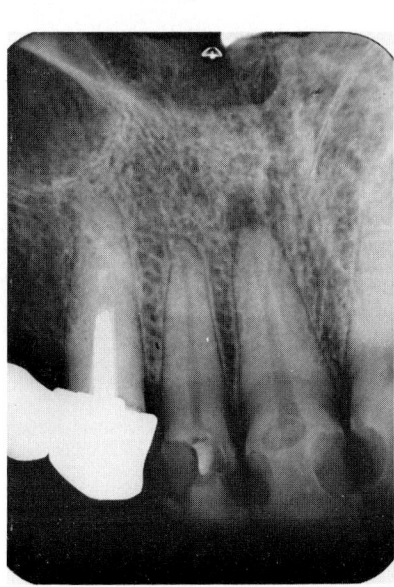

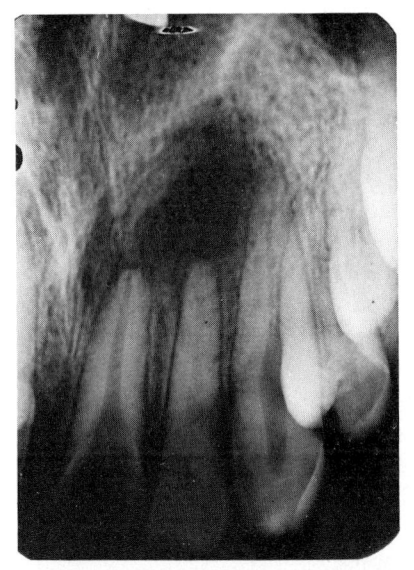

Fig 9–15.—Radiograph of maxillary incisor area showing diffuse radiolucency centered from incisors. Central and lateral incisors had been injured several years before.

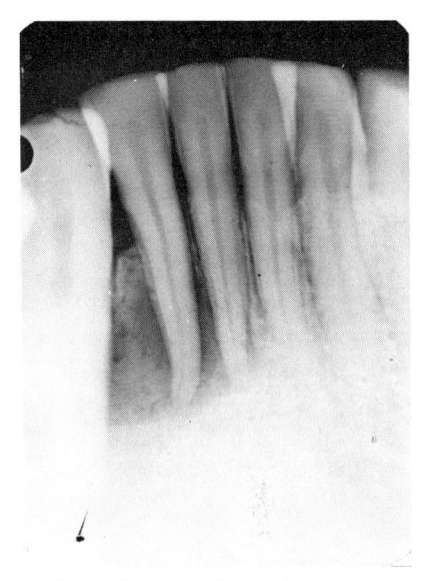

Fig 9–16.—Radiograph of mandibular incisor area showing diffuse radiolucency due to spreading osseous infection.

condition causes pain, and sometimes slight mobility, in the opposing posterior teeth bilaterally.[17] Overstressed teeth may be associated with muscle and temporomandibular joint symptoms and may become part of a general masticatory pain problem. Lack of posterior occlusal support may magnify such symptoms both in the overstressed remaining teeth and in the rest of the masticatory system. Inadequate posterior occlusal support may occur not only from missing teeth, loose posterior teeth, injudicious occlusal grinding, or inadequate replacement, but also from resorption of the supporting ridge beneath a posterior extension saddle of a partial denture. Overstressing of posterior teeth may occur as a result of decreased vertical height of the mandibular ramus due to osseous fracture or degenerative change in the temporomandibular joints.

With multirooted teeth, one root may be periapically or periodontally involved, whereas another can show symptoms of pulpal pain, causing a symptom complex that is confusing indeed. Sometimes the location of the electrode of the pulp tester on the tooth may give some indication of the conditions present.[18] Radiographic evidence may add confirmation.

SECONDARY EFFECTS OF DENTAL PAIN

Being of the deep somatic category, odontogenous pain has the propensity to induce a variety of secondary central excitatory effects. Most acute dental pains have a component of referred pain that is felt in one or more adjacent teeth of the same arch, in teeth of the opposing arch, or in both. Ordinarily, such reference does not cross the midline except when the site of primary pain is located at or close to the midline. Reference to another major division of the trigeminal nerve usually follows a vertical laminated pattern as discussed in chapter 5. Referred dental pain is frequently felt as headache. It may be felt in the orbital and frontal area, in the maxillary sinus region, in the auricular and preauricular parts, or throughout the face. Sometimes, an acute pulpitis will cause pain that radiates throughout the entire face and head with no subjective localization of the primary site at all. The variable, spontaneous, nonlocalizable, and pulsatile qualities of acute pulpal pain together with its secondary effects can simulate almost every known pain syndrome of the face and head.

Secondary hyperalgesia is also a common manifestation of dental pain. It may be expressed superficially as an area of touchy gingiva, skin, or scalp. It may be felt as other tender teeth. Deep secondary hyperalgesia sensed as palpable tenderness may be misdiagnosed as an area of inflammation or myospasm. This is likely to involve the temporal and masseter areas especially.

It is not unusual for dental pain to induce secondary autonomic effects expressed as nasal congestion, lacrimation, and puffy swelling of the eyelids or other areas of loose facial skin. Such symptoms may be misdiagnosed as sinusitis or cellulitis.

Secondary spasm in muscles innervated by the trigeminal nerve may be induced by dental pain. Such involvement of digastric or mylohyoid muscles may cause symptoms in the floor of the mouth and upper cervical region. If the tensor palati muscle is involved, palatal soreness, difficulty with swallowing, and eustachian tube symptoms may occur. If the masticatory muscles are involved, a masticatory pain-dysfunction syndrome may result. It should be noted that if such a secondarily induced muscle condition develops into a cycling myospasm, it becomes wholly independent of initiating cause, and can remain as a separate clinical entity for long periods after the etiologic factor has disappeared.

Perhaps the most confusing complication of dental pain is the induction of myofascial trigger points in muscles innervated by the trigeminal nerve. Such trigger points tend to remain long after the initiating pain has disappeared. As such, they can cause an orofacial complaint for long periods, sometimes in a recurrent, episodial pattern. It should be noted that the zone of reference from such a trigger point frequently is at or near the location of the primary pain that initiated it. Thus, continuing pain at the "toothache site" may be experienced despite adequate dental therapy for the original cause of pain. Clear diagnostic thinking and skillful use of examining techniques may be required to resolve such issues.

TOOTHACHES OF NONDENTAL ORIGIN

Before undertaking any definitive treatment for "toothache," two questions should be answered:
1. Does the pain in fact emanate from a tooth?
2. Is this *the tooth* that is responsible for it?

Toothache, in contrast to *tooth pain,* suggests severity, spontaneity, and nonlocalizability. Odontogenous toothache suggests pulpal rather than periodontal cause. It is essentially a single-tooth condition. Although the site of origin of pulpal pain may be most difficult to locate at first, it usually is only a matter of time (a few days or a few weeks) before it either resolves or progresses via the apical foramen to involve periodontal tissues, thus identifying its location. If prevailing conditions do not permit this passage of time, direct exploration of the suspicious tooth may become a justifiable dental risk.

It is always exasperating to search for the cause of an elusive, obscure dental pain. It is disheartening when such a complaint continues to plague the patient in spite of painstaking efforts to pin it down. It is devastating to institute good definitive therapy, only to have the pain defy and mock you.

The proper defense against mistakes in diagnosis of dental pain comprises knowledge and care: (1) *knowledge* of the mechanisms of pain, the clinical characteristics of various categories of pain, the points of differentiation by which pains are classified and identified, the behavior characteristics of odontogenous pains in particular, and the cardinal warning signs displayed by toothaches of nonodontogenous origin; and (2) *care* that definitive dental treatment is not initiated until all doubt has been resolved.

The general clinical characteristics displayed by toothache of pulpal origin are as follows:
1. The pain has a basic dull, *depressing* quality even though it may escalate as or be punctuated by exacerbations of bright, stimulating pain. The pain may cause some degree of withdrawal,

lassitude, malaise or depression. The pain usually has a pulsatile quality due to the confinement of inflammatory exudate within the rigid walls of dentin.
2. The site of pain (where it is felt) is nonlocalizable subjectively and poorly localizable objectively. It may or may not indicate the true site of origin. The incidence of pain relates more to oral environmental influence than to occlusal function.
3. The pain is spontaneous or provoked, not triggered. Variability is characteristic. It does not relate faithfully to the initiating stimulus in location and intensity, usually being more widespread and of greater intensity than the stimulus. Summation does not occur.
4. Symptoms of central hyperexcitability are commonplace, especially if the pain is continuous. Referred pains, areas of secondary hyperalgesia, autonomic signs, and myospastic activity in otherwise normal structures are expected associated symptoms. Secondary myofascial trigger point pain may persist after the initiating pulpal pain ceases.
5. Dental pulps cause pain individually. Inflammatory pulpal pain follows a time frame sequence (pulpal-to-periodontal) that is characteristic. Adequate local dental cause is identifiable. Analgesic blocking of the individual tooth arrests the primary and associated referred pain.

Toothaches of nondental origin that do not stem from pulpal or periodontal sources occur frequently and must be clearly differentiated from true odontogenous pains. Several orofacial pain syndromes may cause toothache of this type. It is the responsibility of the dental examiner to identify such pains so that proper management can be provided.

TOOTHACHE REFERRED FROM MUSCLES.—Although all deep pains in the head and neck have the propensity to induce secondary referred pain felt as toothache, those of muscle origin are most numerous. The masseter and temporalis muscles are the chief offenders. Myogenous toothache is nonpulsatile and less variable than that of pulpal origin. Being referred, it is not arrested by analgesic blocking of the tooth where the pain is felt. It is arrested only by locating the muscle that constitutes the site of primary pain and by anesthetizing that source of nociceptive input. A good understanding of the muscular genesis of pain and of the overall behavior of musculoskeletal pain syndromes is prerequisite to good management of such toothache complaints (Case No. 9–1).

Oral and Facial Pain
DR. WELDEN E. BELL
8226 DOUGLAS AVENUE
DALLAS, TEXAS

Name: Female age 43

HISTORY

QUALITY	DURATION	LOCALIZATION	AFFECTED BY	LOCAL EFFECTS
(Mild) Severe	Bright (Dull)	(Continuous) Intermittent Recurrent	Localized (Diffuse) Radiating Spreading	Face Movement (Jaw Movement) Tongue Movement Swallowing Head Position	Sensory: Hyp(esthesia Hyper)esthesia Pare(sthesia Dys)esthesia	Special Sense: Visual Au(ditory Olf)actory G(ustatory)
Spontaneous Triggered Induced Paroxysmal (Steady)	— — Pricking Itching Burning (Aching) Pulsating	Momentary Minutes Hours Day long (Protracted)	Body Position Activities Tension Fatigue Secondary Pain	(Time of Day)	Motor: W(eakness) Con(traction) S(pasm)	Autonomic: Ocu(lar Signs) Nasal (Signs) Cuta(neous Signs) Ga(stric Signs)

Location
Inception
Initial pain

Mild to severe variable but protracted continuous steady dull aching pain diffusely located in the left mandibular teeth, jaw, and ear. The pain is usually worse in the early morning and seems to be aggravated by mandibular movement and use.

Duration, clinical course
Therapeutic response
Physical and emotional background
Trauma, infection, etc.
Medications in use

The complaint began about two months ago and has been present ever since. During the two months that preceded this complaint, endodontic treatment was done on the LL4 and a fixed bridge replacing LL5-6 was made. This prosthesis was adjusted occlusally several times and then remade. The new bridge became loose on the LL7 abutment and at that time the present complaint began. It has continued in spite of recementing the bridge, removing the bridge, capping the abutments temporarily, treating the LL7 endodontically, and using antibiotics.
There is no history of prior illness, infection, or trauma. She is medically negative for cause. No medications other than analgesics are presently used.

B/P 118/78   Neurological Survey   Psychological Survey

EXAMINATION

Oral
TM joints
Muscle system
Diagnostic blocks
Diagnostic drugs
Trial therapy

Orally: Clinically and radiographically negative for cause of pain. The LL4 and LL7 capped with aluminum crowns. LL5-6 missing. No hyperalgesia of the teeth or gingiva. All left mandibular and maxillary teeth not endodontically treated respond normally to electric pulp testing.
TM joints: Well within normal limits clinically.
Muscle system: Acute palpable tenderness in the left masseter muscle.
Local anesthetic blocking of the left mandibular nerve failed to stop the pain. Analgesic blocking of the left masseter muscle arrested the dental, mandibular, and auricular pain completely.

Opinion: Deep somatic myofascial pain emanating from the left masseter muscle is being sensed as referred pain in the left mandible and ear. This is interpreted as a central excitatory effect. The initiating cause of the myofascial pain appears to relate to the prior dental experience and likely began as muscle splinting. There is no evidence that the pain arises from dental or oral causes, nor is it an expression of masticatory dysfunction per se.

DIAGNOSIS

Left mandibular "toothache" and jaw pain referred from the masseter muscle.

Case No. 9–1.—Heterotopic pain, felt as toothache, referred from the masseter muscle.

TOOTHACHE OF CARDIAC ORIGIN.—Dentists particularly should be aware of the incidence of jaw and tooth pain that occurs as a secondary manifestation of cardiac pain input.[19] Although other clinical evidence of cardiac distress (such as substernal chest discomfort and left arm and neck pain) is usually present, sometimes the dental symptoms may be the only ones of which the patient complains when he comes to the dentist with what he thinks is a "dental problem." Great care should be exercised in such situations. Lack of adequate dental cause for the pain complaint should always be an alerting sign. Failure of analgesic blocking to arrest the pain promptly and completely is confirming evidence that the primary source of pain is not the tooth. It should be noted that anesthesia is usually quite adequate for dental therapy; therefore, unless the question "Does the tooth still hurt?" is asked, the dentist may not be aware that it did not arrest the toothache. In all cases where pain is an issue and analgesic blocking is used, the patient should be carefully questioned about the effectiveness of the maneuver in arresting the pain (Case No. 9–2).

TOOTHACHE OF VASCULAR ORIGIN.—Classic and common migraine frequently cause pain that is felt as toothache. Usually no management problem arises because such headaches are readily diagnosed, and additional pains about the face and mouth cause little concern on the part of patient or doctor.

Migrainous neuralgia and other migraine variants are a different matter. These syndromes generally are not well understood. Most accompanying toothaches are mistaken for true odontogenous pains and treated as separate entities. Unfortunately, in migrainous neuralgia several characteristics may mislead both patient and doctor:

1. The syndrome is spontaneous, variable, and pulsatile—characteristics that simulate pulpal pain.
2. It may follow illness, sinusitis, dental treatment, surgery, or trauma, appearing to be a complication of a former experience.
3. It very frequently is felt initially in teeth (the maxillary canine and premolar usually) as toothache so convincingly that dental treatment may be undertaken without hesitation even when only minor dental cause can be located.
4. It may undergo remission following dental treatment, although recurrence is characteristic with vascular pains. It may spread to adjacent teeth, opposing teeth, or the entire face.
5. It may induce autonomic effects manifested as nasal congestion, lacrimation, and edema of the eyelids and face, which may be mistaken for sinusitis or dental abscess.

This rather typical behavior of vascular migraine variants should be well understood to prevent unnecessary therapy and the accompanying frustration felt by patient and dentist alike. *To be suspicious of the presence of vascular pain is the key to diagnosis.* Dental treatment, even palliative and quite innocuous, may offer the patient reason to

Oral and Facial Pain
DR. WELDEN E. BELL
8226 DOUGLAS AVENUE
DALLAS, TEXAS

Name	Male age 61		Age	Date		
	QUALITY	DURATION	LOCALIZATION	AFFECTED BY		LOCAL EFFECTS
HISTORY	(Mild)	Bright	Continuous	Localized	Sensory:	Special Sense:
	Severe	(Dull)	Intermittent	(Diffuse)	Hypesthesia	Visual
			Recurrent		Hyperesthesia	Auditory
				Face Movement	Paresthesia	Olfactory
			Radiating	Jaw Movement	Dysesthesia	Gustatory
	Spontaneous		Spreading	Tongue Movement		
	Triggered	Pricking	Momentary	Swallowing		Autonomic:
	Induced	Itching	Minutes	Head Position	Motor:	Ocular Signs
		Burning	Hours	Body Position	Weakness	Nasal Signs
	Paroxysmal	(Aching)	Day long	Activities	Contraction	Cutaneous Signs
	(Steady)	Pulsating	(Protracted)	Tension	Spasm	Gastric Signs
				Fatigue		
			Secondary Pain	Time of Day		

HISTORY

Location — Mild continuous variable protracted steady dull aching pain diffusely
Inception   located in the left mandible as "toothache" and preceded by left shoulder
Initial pain   discomfort being treated as bursitis by his physician.
Duration, clinical course   The complaint in the shoulder began three days ago as a variable vague
               but more or less continuous pain. He went to his physician who diagnosed the
Therapeutic response   complaint as bursitis and initiated some therapy. Two days later, the left
               "toothache" pain began even though patient had been edentulous for about 20
Physical and emotional years. Thinking the mandibular pain stemmed from the dentures, the physician
background   advised a dental examination. His dentist made a dental radiograph of the LL8
Trauma, infection, etc. area and saw part of a deeply impacted LL8 tooth. He, therefore, referred
               him for removal of the tooth on an emergency basis.
Medications in use   No medications are presently being taken except aspirin for pain.

EXAMINATION

B/P 155/85   Neurological Survey   Psychological Survey

Oral — Orally: A normal-appearing edentulous mouth with satisfactory artificial
       dentures is seen. There is no local hyperemia in the denture-bearing areas.
TM joints   There is no palpable discomfort in the LL8 area orally nor in the left sub-
       mandibular triangle. Bilateral oblique radiographs of the mandible revealed
Muscle a deeply impacted LL8 tooth, apparently covered completely with bone, having
system no coronal radiolucency indicative of dental caries, and exhibiting no osseous
       changes around the tooth. Mandibular functioning is clinically normal in all
Diagnostic respects. There is no dental, oral or masticatory cause for the complaint.
blocks TM joints: Clinically normal.
       Muscle system: Clinically negative for cause of pain.
Diagnostic
drugs   Analgesic blocking of the left mandibular nerve did not arrest the pain.

Trial Medical consultation advised. Telephone report that electrocardiogram
therapy indicates cardiac muscle damage. Medical diagnosis of cardiac pain made.

       Opinion: The shoulder pain mistaken for bursitis and the mandibular pain
       mistaken for "toothache" were not associated with appreciable chest discomfort.
       It is presumed, therefore, that the primary cardiac muscle pain was wholly
       inhibited and only the secondary central excitatory effects were felt by
       the patient.

DIAGNOSIS

Cardiac muscle pain referred as mandibular toothache.

Case No. 9–2.—Heterotopic pain, felt as toothache, referred from the cardiac muscle.

blame the dentist for aggravating the problem if not actually initiating it (Case 13–1).

Vascular pain occasionally is manifested with toothache as the only symptom. In recent years this has been described under the name of *atypical odontalgia*.[20-22] Although this new term for well-known *vas-*

cular toothache is unfortunate because it is nondescriptive, it has served to alert the dental profession to this important clinical entity that has been so misdiagnosed and mistreated in the past. The absence of other better-known clinical characteristics of vascular pain has made the diagnosis difficult. The chief indications of this syndrome that mimics real odontogenous toothache are (1) the absence of adequate local dental cause, (2) the tendency for it to be periodic and recurrent, and (3) the patient's ability to precisely locate the painful tooth. Confirming evidence consists of identifying the presence of a vascular pain syndrome by the use of carotid pressure, ergotamine tartrate testing, or trial therapy. Diagnostic analgesic blocking may yield confusing data because sometimes it reduces the pain; sometimes it does nothing; sometimes it increases the pain.

Unfortunately, dental therapy often induces a remission of the pain, thereby deluding the dentist into thinking that the condition is in fact a dental one and that a proper treatment has been applied. With recurrence, additional dental therapy may be performed without realizing that it is futile and may be harmful.

"SINUS HEADACHE" TOOTHACHE.—Pain arising from the nasal mucosa as the result of viral or allergic rhinitis is prone to be expressed as referred pain throughout the maxilla and maxillary teeth in the form of toothache. It may also display autonomic signs that are mistaken for symptoms of maxillary sinusitis. The so-called sinus headache may cause management problems because of the tooth pains.

Diagnostically, analgesic blocking of the tooth proper by infiltration at the apex of the tooth in question does not arrest the toothache if it is referred from the nasal mucosa, whereas topical anesthesia of the nasal mucosa effectively arrests it. Again, *suspicion that the dental pain is referred is the key to diagnosis* (Case No. 14–1).

NEUROGENOUS TOOTHACHE.—*Neuritic pains* arising in the maxillary and mandibular divisions of the trigeminal nerve can cause dental pains along with other neurologic symptoms such as hyperesthesia, hypoesthesia, anesthesia, paresthesia, muscular tics, weakness, and paralysis as well as autonomic and special sense aberrations, depending on the fiber content at the site of neuropathy. Neuritis of the superior dental plexus due to extension from maxillary sinusitis may cause toothache in and around one or more maxillary teeth. Such pain is persistent, nonpulsatile, and burning. If the accompanying maxillary sinusitis is non-symptomatic as to pain—and it may be—diagnosis may not be easy. *The key usually is to recognize accompanying neurologic signs* that involve other teeth or nearby structures served by the same nerve (Case No. 15–7). Similar toothache in the mandibular teeth may occur as an expression of neuritis of the inferior alveolar nerve from direct trauma, dental sepsis, or surgery (Case No. 15–8).

Tic douloureux may be felt in the teeth. Unfortunately, analgesic blocking arrests the paroxysms of pain and may lead to a mistaken diagnosis of odontogenous pain. Also, dental therapy, especially if a local anesthetic block is used, may induce a remission, leading both patient and dentist to assume that the diagnosis is correct and that a proper treatment has been done. When the condition recurs, additional forms of dental therapy may be employed, thus compounding the mistake (Case No. 15–5).

Peripheral deafferentation is another neurogenous condition that may cause tooth pain. It may follow injury due to trauma, tooth-pulp extirpation, tooth extraction, or oral surgery that entails cutting or crushing of afferent neurons. Such pain is usually mistaken for a post-traumatic or postoperative complication. It rather closely simulates neuritic dental pain, from which it should be differentiated. Phantom pains may also be due to deafferentation. The diagnosis is confirmed by analgesic blocking of the stellate ganglion (Case No. 15–12).

PSYCHOGENIC INTENSIFICATION TOOTHACHE.—All conditions that alter the effectiveness of the endogenous antinociceptive system may permit ordinarily nonnociceptive impulses to be transmitted and felt as pain. As a result, teeth may become unduly sensitive or actually painful. They may hurt when touched, moved, pressed, stressed through occlusal use, or subjected to stimulants such as tooth brushing, flossing, thermal changes, or ingestion of sweets. In such situations, many or all of the teeth may become painful. This is usually the warning sign—*pain in many teeth without adequate local dental cause.*

Clinical characteristics cannot be used to determine psychogenesis of pain. Rather, it is the degree to which departure from usual anatomical and physiologic behavior becomes evident that should cause suspicion in such conditions. Inadequacy of local dental cause is the best key. Persistence and chronicity without organic justification and nonphysiologic response to therapeutic efforts constitute confirming evidence.

CARDINAL WARNING SIGNS.—Toothaches of nondental origin require accurate diagnostic identification of the true cause of the patient's pain. The most important step toward proper management is *suspicion that the pain is not of dental origin.* The cardinal warning signs of toothache of nondental origin are as follows:
1. Spontaneous multiple toothaches
2. Inadequate local dental cause for the pain
3. Stimulating, burning, nonpulsatile toothaches

4. Constant, unremitting, nonvariable toothaches
5. Persistant, recurrent toothaches
6. Failure of toothache to respond to reasonable dental therapy[23]

TOOTH PAIN FROM SECONDARY HYPERALGESIA

Stimulation-evoked tooth pain that simulates pain of periodontal origin may occur as the result of deep somatic pain input located elsewhere in the trigeminal area. This manifestation of secondary hyperalgesia is a central excitatory effect. It differs from spontaneous toothache due to referred pain from similar cause in that this tooth pain is provoked by manipulation or functional activities. As such, it is localized and can be confused with true odontogenous pain of periodontal origin, from which it should be differentiated.

Secondary hyperalgesia expressed as "tender teeth" is commonplace. It occurs with pharyngeal and nasal mucosa pains in particular. Similar phenomena, however, occur with other dental pains, especially those of pulpitis.

The differential diagnosis depends chiefly on failure to find adequate local dental cause. Confirmation may be done by analgesic blocking of the site of pain. Primary periodontal pain is arrested while secondary hyperalgesic pain is not.

REFERENCES

1. Willis R.D., DiCosimo C.J.: The absence of proprioceptive nerve endings in the human periodontal ligament: The role of periodontal mechanoreceptors in the reflex control of mastication. *Oral Surg.* 48:108–115, 1979.
2. Hannam A.G.: The response of periodontal mechanoreceptors in the dog to controlled loading of the teeth. *Arch Oral Biol.* 14:781–791, 1969.
3. Anderson D.J., Hannam A.G., Matthews B.: Sensory mechanisms in mammalian teeth and their supporting structures. *Physiol Rev.* 50:171–195, 1970.
4. Cody E.W.J., Lee R.W.H., Taylor A.: A functional analysis of the components of the mesencephalic nucleus of the fifth nerve in the cat. *J. Physiol.* 226:249, 1972.
5. Young R.F.: Effect of trigeminal tractotomy on dental sensations in humans. *J. Neurosurg.* 56:812–818, 1982.
6. Azerad J., Woda A., Albe-Fessard D.: Physiological properties of neurons in different parts of the cat trigeminal sensory complex. *Brain Res.* 246:7, 1982.
7. Wilson S., Fuller P.M., Winfrey J.: Histochemical evidence for strictly ipsilateral innervation of maxillary canine teeth in cats. *Exp. Neurol.* 70:138, 1980.
8. Sessle B.J.: Is the tooth pulp a "pure" source of noxious input? in Bonica J.J., Liebeskind J.C., Albe-Fessard D.G. (eds.): *Advances in Pain Research and Therapy.* New York, Raven Press, 1979, vol. 3, pp. 245–260.

9. Mumford J.M., Bowsher D.: Pain and protopathic sensibility: A review with particular reference to the teeth. *Pain* 2:223–243, 1976.
10. Chatrian G.E., Fernandes de Lima J.M., Lettich E., et al.: Electrical stimulation of tooth pulps in humans: II. Qualities of sensation. *Pain* 14:233–246, 1982.
11. McGrath P.A., Gracely R.H., Dubner R., et al.: Nonpain and nonpain sensations evoked by tooth pulp stimulation. *Pain* 15:377–388, 1983.
12. Narhi M., Jyvasjarvi E., Hirvonen T, et al.: Activities of heat-sensitive nerve fibers in the dental pulp of the cat. *Pain* 14:317–326, 1982.
13. Narhi M., Virtanen A., Huopaniemi T., et al.: Conduction velocities of single pulp nerve fiber units in the cat. *Acta Physiol Scand.* 116:209, 1982.
14. Rozza A.J., Beuerman R.W.: Density and organization of free nerve endings in the corneal epithelium of the rabbit. *Pain* 14:105–120, 1982.
15. Nord S.G.: Responses of neurons in rostral and caudal trigeminal nuclei to tooth pulp stimulation. *Brain Res. Bull.* 1:489, 1976.
16. Vyklicky L., Keller O., Jastreboff P., et al.: Spinal trigeminal tractotomy and nociceptive reactions evoked by tooth pulp stimulation in the cat. *J. Physiol.* (Paris) 73:379–386, 1977.
17. Levenson M.F.: Relieving intraoral pressure generated during orthopedic treatment. *J. Prosthet. Dent.* 49:546–548, 1983.
18. Mumford J.M.: *Toothache and Related Pain.* Edinburgh, Churchill/Livingstone, 1973.
19. Graham L.L., Schinbeckler G.A.: Orofacial pain of cardiac origin. *J.A.D.A.* 104:47–48, 1982.
20. Rees R.T., Harris M.: Atypical odontalgia. *Br. J. Oral Surg.* 16:212–218, 1979.
21. Brooke R.I.: Atypical odontalgia. *J. Oral Surg.* 49:196–199, 1980.
22. Kreisberg M.K.: Atypical odontalgia: Differential diagnosis and treatment. *J.A.D.A.* 104:852–854, 1982.
23. Bell W.E.: Toothaches of nonodontogenic origin. *J. Calif. Dental Assn.*, May 1976, pp. 50–58.

10

Pains of Muscle Origin

MYOGENOUS PAINS THAT EMANATE from the orofacial structures are classified as musculoskeletal pains of the deep somatic category (Fig 10–1). The general features exhibited by muscle pain include those of deep somatic pain, namely, (1) the pain has a dull, depressing quality; (2) subjective localization is variable and somewhat diffuse; (3) the site of pain may or may not identify the correct location of the source of pain; (4) response to provocation at the site of pain is fairly faithful in incidence and intensity, but not in location; and (5) central excitatory effects often accompany the pain. To these features are added characteristics peculiar to musculoskeletal pain, namely, (1) the pain relates reasonably to the demands of function; (2) manual palpation at the site of pain, or functional manipulation, effects a graduated response; and (3) subjective localization varies in accordance with the need for proprioceptive guidance to control and execute useful movements. Myogenous pains are further characterized by more or less labile clinical behavior manifested as suddenness of onset, rapidity of change, recurrence, and variability.

No doubt pain of muscle origin is the most frequent cause of suffering about the neck, head, and face. Since odontogenous pain is the most frequent oral pain, a good rule to follow in diagnosing pains about the face and mouth is initially to assume that the pain is dental until proved otherwise, then muscular until proved otherwise. The possibility of orofacial pain being of muscle origin should be taken into account with every complaint. Even when the primary cause is not muscular, central excitatory effects tend to be expressed in the muscles, making this a frequent complication accompanying other sources of pain.

Muscle pain emanates from the skeletal muscles, tendons, and fascia. It is said to result from stretching, forceful or sustained contraction, ischemia, and hyperemia,[1] as well as from trauma and inflammatory factors. Some muscle pain arises from the blood vessels within the

OROFACIAL PAIN SYNDROMES

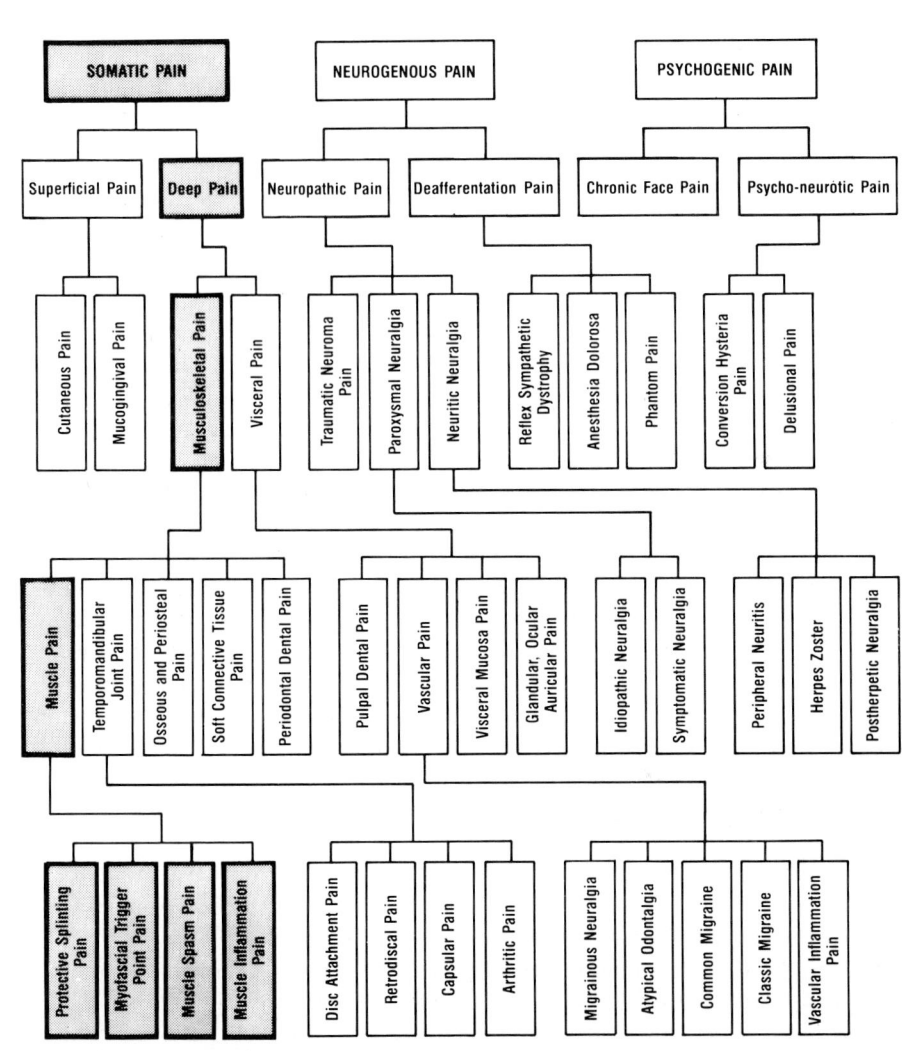

Fig 10–1.—Chart showing classification relationship of muscle pains to other orofacial pain syndromes.

muscles and fascial sheaths.[2] Myofascial genesis of pain accounts for other discomforts of muscle origin.[3]

Muscle pain usually is felt as a nonpulsatile, variable, aching sensation, sometimes having a boring quality. This more constant background discomfort may escalate to or be punctuated by sharper, more severe lancinating pains occurring both spontaneously and in response to stretching, contraction, manipulation, or manual palpation. Sometimes the pain is no more than a feeling of pressure. At other times it may increase to excruciating intensity. It may be transitory or persistent, constant, intermittent, or recurrent. Its behavior is labile—characterized by suddenness of onset and rapidity of change. It follows no time frame unless of inflammatory origin. Accompanying dysfunction may be expressed as tightness and weakness, or it may relate to impairment of muscle function such as stiffness, rigidity, swelling, or shortening. Palpable muscle tenderness, the effect of massage and manipulations on pain intensity, and the fact that movement and functioning modify the pain and stiffness are clinical indications of the presence of muscle pain.[4]

Myogenous pains of different types may involve muscles of the mouth, face, and neck, the symptom-complex depending on the kind, number, and location of muscles involved and the degree to which they are affected. The likelihood of secondary central excitatory effects should be considered. When the primary pain remains relatively silent, the secondary referred pain may constitute most of the complaint. Referred pain from muscles can be the source of considerable diagnostic confusion. For example, more or less silent pain arising in the sternomastoid muscle may be felt in and about the ear as earache or as temporomandibular joint pain. Cardiac muscle pain may be referred to the mandible.

Manual palpation and analgesic blocking techniques offer the best means of identifying and accurately locating the site of origin of muscle pain. Injection of a local anesthetic into inflamed tissues (e.g., myositis) is contraindicated.

According to the symptoms displayed, a muscle pain can usually be classified as one of four clinical types; namely, (1) protective muscle splinting pain, (2) myofascial trigger point pain, (3) muscle spasm pain, and (4) muscle inflammation pain.[5] Since therapy is different for each of these clinical manifestations, accurate differential diagnosis is essential. Transitional phases between these types of pain may be encountered.

GENERAL FEATURES OF MUSCLE PAIN

The stimulation of skeletal muscle tissue induces dull, aching pain felt deeply and diffusely in a broad region of the muscle. It is mediated by group III (A-delta fibers) and group IV (C-fibers) afferent neurons. Sharp pain and itching are not felt. A crescendo of intensity indicates some temporal summation.[6] Regardless of the true source of muscle pain, movements that actively stretch the muscle, or increase its isometric tension, increase the patient's awareness of pain. If *passive* movement is painful, one or more antagonists should be suspected of containing an abnormally tender muscle region.[7]

Significant preauricular pain can be induced by vigorously thrusting the mandible forward for a period of five minutes.[8] In such an experiment, it is important to note that, although referred pain in the preauricular area is felt, palpable tenderness and limitation of jaw function are not produced. Masticatory pain can be induced in the laboratory situation by clenching the teeth for 30 minutes.[9] Recent experiments with such induced pain indicate that pain is not explained on the basis of ischemia alone. Nor is the timing of pain necessarily due to the cumulative effect of EMG activity.[10]

It has long been known that an EMG "silent period" occurs in the masticatory elevator muscles immediately after occlusal contact. That the periodontal mechanoreceptors provide the stimulus that excites reflex inhibitory influence on elevator muscle contraction is shown by the fact that locally anesthetizing the contacting teeth prevents the induction of this silent period.[11] Since the effect of stimulating periodontal mechanoreceptors is inhibitory on elevator muscle action, occlusal relationships offer an unacceptable hypothesis for the initiation of bruxism.[12] Pain has a similar inhibitory effect on elevator muscle action. Threshold stimulation of the dental pulp induces an EMG silent period of 18 to 20 msec duration in the masseter muscle.[13] The masseteric silent period can also be initiated by electrical stimulation of the skin in the region of infraorbital or mental nerves.[14] McGrath et al[15] have concluded, however, that the masseteric inhibitory period cannot be considered a reliable correlate of pain. Although it has been observed that such a silent period is prolonged in patients with symptoms of mandibular pain or dysfunction, which returns to normal with treatment,[16] the individual variation in silent periods makes it impossible to establish criteria for normal or abnormal silent period duration. Although useful in clinical research, at this time silent period determination has no real value in clinical pain diagnosis.[17]

It should be noted that, although painful muscles frequently show excessive EMG activity, the therapeutic reduction of such activity does not in itself lead to a reduction in pain.[18] It is also interesting to note that, although headache is frequently a secondary central excitatory effect of myogenous pain,[19] deep muscle pain can also induce a *deficit* in cutaneous nociception that is not reversed by naloxone and which immediately ceases when analgesic blocking arrests the primary pain input.[20]

PROTECTIVE SPLINTING PAIN

Muscle splinting is a reflex protective mechanism whereby skeletal muscles become hypertonic and painful when contracted. The motivation is to stabilize the threatened part and to protect it from further injury or insult. Pain with contraction and an associated feeling of muscle weakness discourage and minimize functioning of the part. Since the real cause of discomfort and dysfunction may be unknown to the patient, considerable apprehension and alarm may result. The muscular dysfunction consists of (1) tightness of the muscle(s) involved, (2) inhibitory influence of pain when the muscle is contracted, and (3) a feeling of muscle weakness (pseudoparalysis). These symptoms are sufficient to identify accurately the origin of the pain, even though its cause and significance may not be understood.[5]

Ordinarily, since this is a protective mechanism, the splinting disappears promptly when the cause no longer exists. If splinting is protracted, however, the muscle may become spastic. When this occurs, a cycling peripheral myogenous pain source is created and may persist indefinitely as a separate and independent local pain problem.

When masticatory muscles are involved, masticatory pain and dysfunction become evident. This occurs frequently as a result of tension, unusual use, clenching, bruxism, illness, pains in other areas, occlusal interference, changes in the oral or occlusal environment, oral consciousness, interference with normal joint functioning, local anesthesia about the mouth, dental therapy, and dental and oral discomforts of all types.

MYOFASCIAL TRIGGER POINT PAIN

Although the myofascial genesis of pain was introduced into medical literature in 1952 by Travell and Rinzler,[3] the health professions have been slow to grasp the full import of this common cause of human suffering. For reasons that still are not fully understood, certain skeletal muscles develop trigger sites within the muscle, its fascial sheath, or its tendinous attachment. When such sites, known as *myofascial trigger points*, are stimulated either spontaneously or by normal functioning, a variety of symptoms may result ranging from painless restriction of movement to agonizing incapacitating pain.[21] In medical literature, this condition is frequently referred to as *fibrositis*, even though it is neither "fibrous" nor "inflammatory." The term *myofascial* has definite meaning, namely, that trigger point phenomena account for the pain complaint. The term should not be used to designate muscle pain in general, nor should it be used to indicate the presence of muscle spasm activity per se.

A myofascial trigger point is a hyperirritable locus within a taut band of skeletal muscle, located in the muscular tissue or in its associated fascia or tendon. The spot is painful on compression and can evoke characteristic referred pain and autonomic phenomena.[21] An active trigger point causes pain, most of which is heterotopic. This may occur spontaneously or during functional movements. A latent trigger point is nonpainful, but it may cause some restriction of movement and weakness of the affected muscle. As such, they may remain indefinitely. Latent trigger points may be activated by shortening, by chilling while fatigued, and by certain viral illnesses.[21]

Postural and masticatory muscles are the ones most frequently affected. The heterotopic pain usually occurs within the same dermatome, myotome, or sclerotome as the generating trigger point. Trigger points are activated especially by overloading, fatigue, trauma, chilling, visceral disease, arthritis, and emotional distress. Secondary trigger points may develop in synergistic muscles while satellite trigger points may occur within the pain reference zone.[21]

A muscle affected by myofascial trigger points shows no increased EMG activity at rest. Myospasm per se is not a part of myofascial pain. Such a muscle, however, can become spastic, especially if it is painfully stretched. Therefore, muscle spasm may occur as a sequela to preexistent myofascial pain. Minor muscular dysfunction may be displayed. This consists of stiffness and weakness that is noticed especially following periods of inactivity. The resistance to stretch is not due to myospasm; the weakness is not due to a motorneuron deficit. These phenomena are more akin to protective muscle splinting than to CNS-induced tonic contraction or motor paralysis. No muscle atrophy takes place even in chronic myofascial pain conditions. Symptoms will immediately disappear when trigger points are eliminated by proper therapy. Trigger points do not recover spontaneously; they only become latent. Elimination of a trigger point requires active treatment.[21]

When active myofascial trigger points are stimulated, heterotopic pain is generated. This may project to the peripheral distribution of the motor nerve that innervates the muscle. Usually, however, the heterotopic pain is displayed as spontaneous referred pain and/or stimulation-evoked secondary hyperalgesia as typical central excitatory effects. Such pain is felt in a reference zone that is segmentally related to the site of primary pain input—the trigger point. The reference zones for various muscles frequently involved have been charted for many years (Fig 10–2). Since the trigger point primary pain source usually is entirely silent, the patient has no subjective symptoms that help the examiner locate the source of pain. By comparing the heterotopic pain with the known reference zones, one can readily locate the muscle that is responsible for the pain. The charts therefore become essential to diagnosis. The trigger point is then identified by manual palpation. Compression of the trigger site elicits local myalgia. It may or may not accentuate the secondary heterotopic pain. Confirmation of the diagnosis is by therapeutic trial.[21]

There has been considerable speculation concerning a possible relationship between acupoints and myofascial trigger points. Although 71% of acupoints fall within a radius of 3 cm of the more familiar trigger points, there appears to be no relationship between them. Nor are they related to the motor points where nerves enter muscles or to myoneural junctions. Trigger points are more variable in location than these anatomical structures.[21]

Tissue studies of trigger point sites have yielded very little useful information. Mild dystrophic changes similar to those seen with ischemia have been identified. Vigorously active trigger points are more likely to display degenerative muscle effects.[21] Some changes have been identified in long-standing trigger point sites.[22,23] But on the whole, the local tissue changes thus far identified are hardly sufficient to account for trigger point phenomena. It has been conjectured that myofascial pain may result rather from sensitization of trigger point nociceptors by some algogenic substance.[21] It is known that an increased temperature differential exists at such sites, suggestive of increased metabolism, decreased circulation, or both.[21] It is also known that bradykinin is released in muscle tissue during ischemic episodes.[24]

MASSETER MUSCLE.—Trigger points located at sites in the superficial layer of the masseter muscle refer to the posterior mandibular and maxillary teeth, the jaw, and the face (Fig 10–3). Toothache is a common complaint from this source. The deep portion refers to the ear and temporomandibular joint area. Earache and preauricular pain thought to be emanating from the joint are common complaints. Moderate restriction of opening associated with ipsilateral deflection of the midline incisal path may be observed. Tinnitus described as a "low roaring noise" may occur from deep masseter trigger points. The muscle is accessible for manual palpation to identify trigger sites.

TEMPORALIS MUSCLE.—The reference zone of the temporalis muscle includes all the maxillary teeth and upper face (Fig 10–4). Headache and toothache are the common complaints. Restricted opening

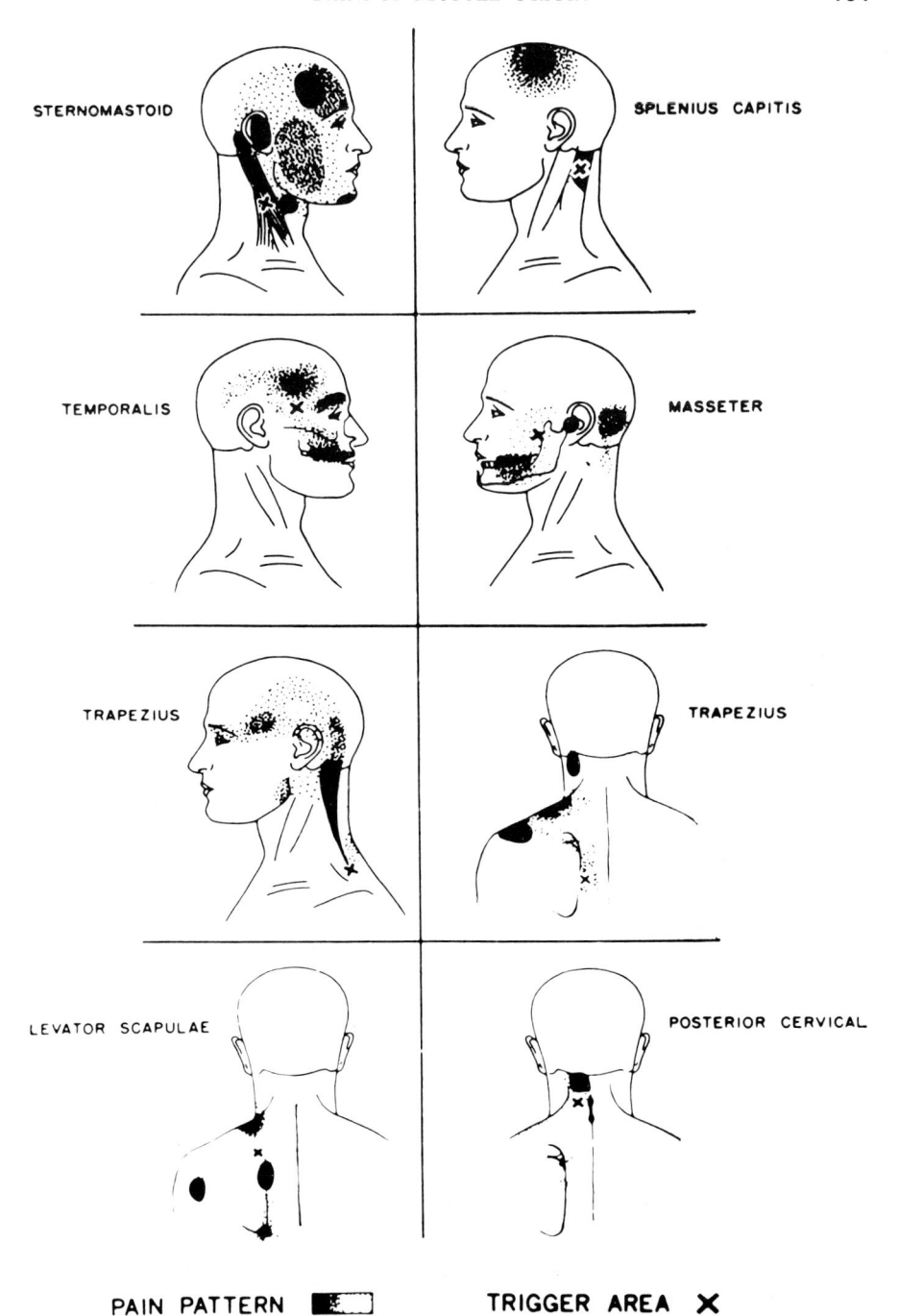

Fig 10–2.—Schematic representation of reference zones of myofascial pains emanating from cervical and facial muscles. (From Travell J., Rinzler S.H.: The myofascial genesis of pain. *Postgrad. Med.* 11:425, 1952. Copyright by McGraw-Hill Book Co. Reproduced with permission.)

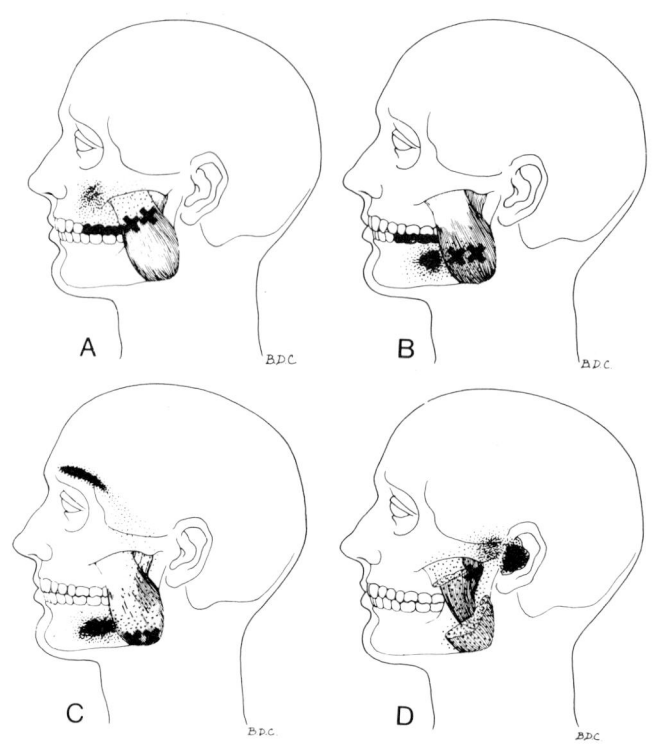

Fig 10–3.—The *X*s locate trigger points in various parts of the masseter muscle. Solid black shows essential reference pain zones; stippled areas are spillover pain zones. **A,** superficial layer, upper portion. **B,** superficial layer, midbelly. **C,** superficial layer, lower portion. **D,** deep layer, upper part. (From Travell J.G., Simons D. G.: *Myofascial Pain and Dysfunction.* Baltimore, Williams & Wilkins Co., 1983. Reproduced with permission.)

is rarely displayed. The muscle is accessible for manual palpation to identify trigger sites.

MEDIAL PTERYGOID MUSCLE.—The reference zone for the medial pterygoid muscle includes the posterior part of the mouth and throat as well as the temporomandibular and infra-auricular areas (Fig 10–5). Throat and postmandibular (infra-auricular) pain is the common complaint. Eustachian tube symptoms may be displayed. Moderate restriction of mouth opening associated with contralateral deflection of the midline incisal path may be observed. The muscle is only partially accessible for intraoral manual palpation to identify trigger sites. Functional manipulation therefore may be needed for this purpose. To stretch the muscle requires an opening effort; to contract the muscle requires biting effort.

PAINS OF MUSCLE ORIGIN 153

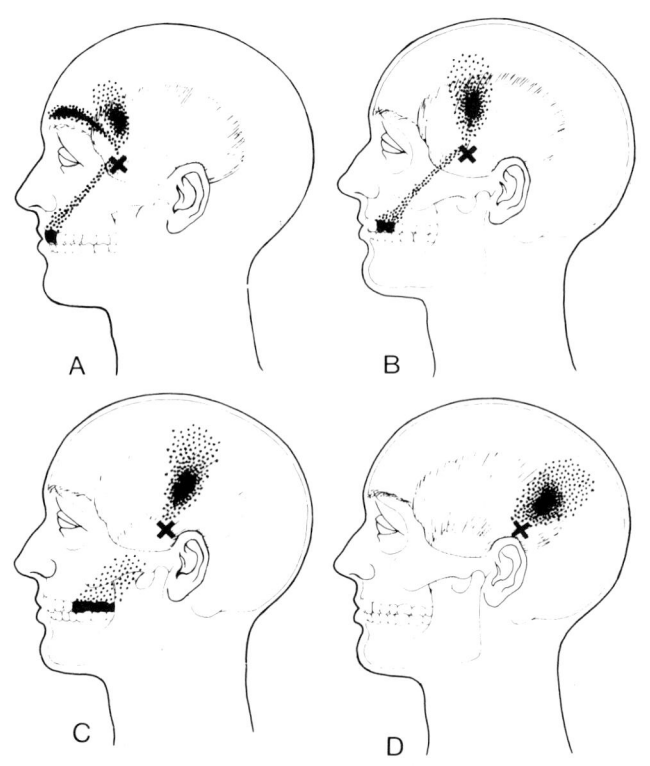

Fig 10-4.—Referred pain patterns from trigger points (*X*s) in the temporalis muscle. **A,** anterior fibers. **B,** and **C,** middle fibers. **D,** posterior fibers. (From Travell J.G., Simons D.G.: *Myofascial Pain and Dysfunction.* Baltimore, Williams & Wilkins Co., 1983. Reproduced with permission.)

INFERIOR LATERAL PTERYGOID MUSCLE.—Trigger points in the inferior lateral pterygoid muscle refer to the temporomandibular joint area (Fig 10-6). The pain complaint from this source is temporomandibular. Slight acute malocclusion may be sensed as disocclusion of the ipsilateral posterior teeth and premature occlusion of the contralateral anterior teeth. Since this muscle is inaccessible for palpation,[25] functional manipulation is required to help identify the presence of myofascial pain. To stretch the muscle requires clenching the teeth firmly in maximum intercuspation; to contract the muscle requires protruding the jaw against resistance.

SUPERIOR LATERAL PTERYGOID MUSCLE.—Trigger points in the superior lateral pterygoid muscle refer to the zygomatic area (Fig 10-6). No dysfunction is observed unless there is extensive degenerative change in the temporomandibular joint sufficient to permit anterior

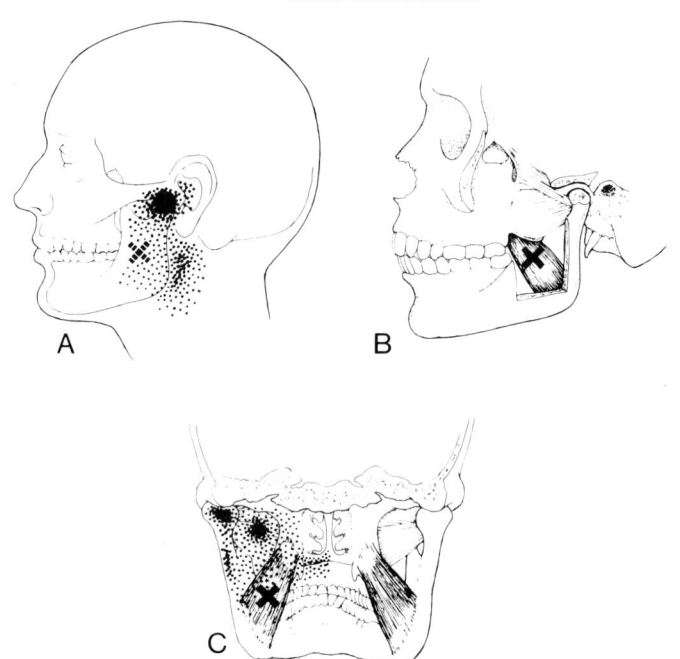

Fig 10-5.—Referred pain pattern and location of responsible trigger point (*X*) in the medial pterygoid muscle. **A,** external areas of pain to which patient can point. **B,** anatomical cutaway to show location of trigger point. **C,** coronal section showing internal areas of pain. (From Travell J.G., Simons D.G.: *Myofascial Pain and Dysfunction.* Baltimore, Williams & Wilkins Co., 1983. Reproduced with permission.)

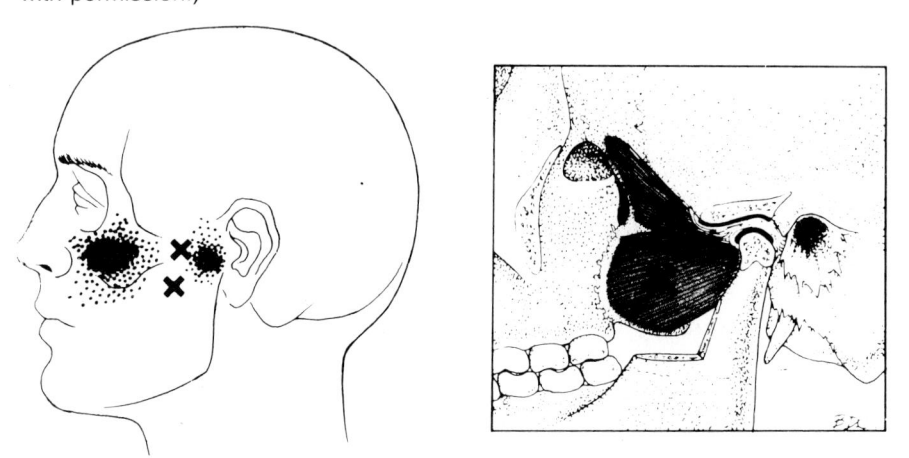

Fig 10-6.—Referred pain patterns of trigger points (*X*s) in the superior and inferior lateral pterygoid muscles. (From Travell J.G., Simons D.G.: *Myofascial Pain and Dysfunction.* Baltimore, Williams & Wilkins Co., 1983. Reproduced with permission.)

displacement of the articular disc. Diffuse pain in the malar area is the usual complaint. Since this muscle is inaccessible for manual palpation,[25] functional manipulation is required to identify the presence of myofascial pain. To stretch the muscle requires clenching the teeth firmly in maximum intercuspation; to contract the muscle requires biting hard against an object between the teeth.

ANTERIOR DIGASTRIC MUSCLE.—Trigger points in the anterior belly of the digastric muscle, which is the trigeminal-innervated part, refer pain to the mandibular incisor area (Fig 10–7). No dysfunction is observed. This muscle is accessible for manual palpation to identify trigger points.

STERNOCLEIDOMASTOID MUSCLE. —The reference zone from the superficial sternal division of the sternocleidomastoid muscle is throughout the entire face and head (Fig 10–8). A great variety of face pain and headache complaints may arise from this source. The deeper clavicular division refers to the ear, postauricular area, and frontal region. Earache, temporomandibular pain, and frontal headache are common complaints. This muscle is a frequent source of so-called tension headache. Postural vertigo may be displayed. The muscle is accessible for manual palpation to identify trigger sites.

TRAPEZIUS MUSCLE.—The reference zone for trigger points in the upper part of the trapezius muscle is along the posterolateral part of

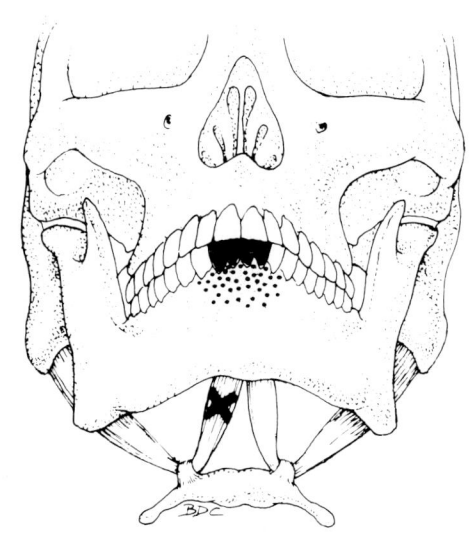

Fig 10–7.—Referred pain pattern of trigger point (X) in anterior belly of digastric muscle. (From Travell J.G., Simons D.G.: *Myofascial Pain and Dysfunction.* Baltimore, Williams & Wilkins Co., 1983. Reproduced with permission.)

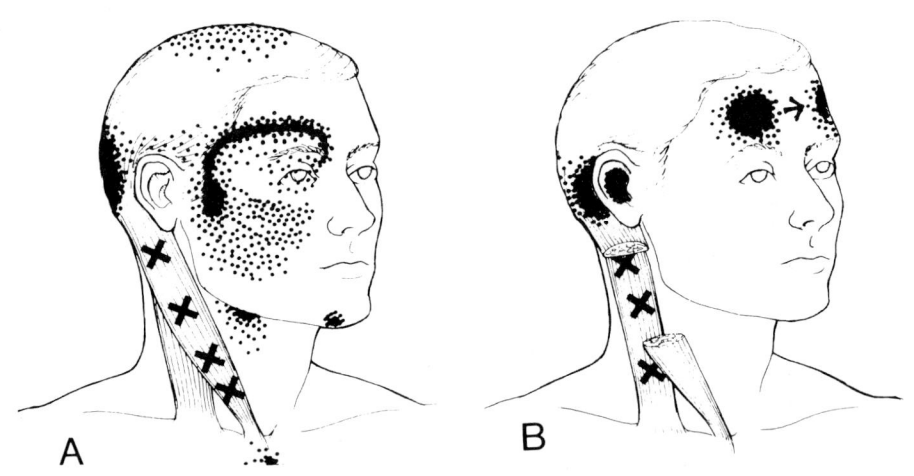

Fig 10–8.—Referred pain patterns with locations of corresponding trigger points (*X*s) in the sternocleidomastoid muscle. **A**, superficial sternal division. **B**, deep clavicular division. (From Travell J.G., Simons D.G.: *Myofascial Pain and Dysfunction*. Baltimore, Williams & Wilkins Co., 1983. Reproduced with permission.)

the neck, the postauricular area, the mandibular angle, and the temple (Fig 10–9). This is a major source of so-called tension headache. It should be noted that tension headache (muscle contraction headache) is due neither to excessive muscular tension nor to muscle contraction because there is no statistically significant difference in the EMG

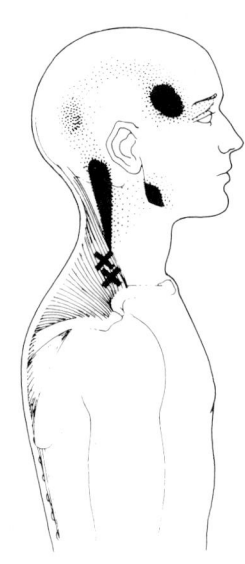

Fig 10–9.—Referred pain patterns and location of trigger points (*X*s) in upper part of the trapezius muscle. (From Travell J.G., Simons D.G.: *Myofascial Pain and Dysfunction*. Baltimore, Williams & Wilkins, Co., 1983. Reproduced with permission.)

activity between such muscles and nonheadache controls.[26, 27] This muscle is accessible for manual palpation to identify trigger sites.

OCCIPITOFRONTALIS MUSCLE.—The frontalis portion refers as frontal headache; the occipital portion refers as lateral cranial and postocular headache (Fig 10–10). This is another major source of tension headache. The muscle is accessible for manual palpation to identify trigger sites. The splenius capitis, splenius cervicis, posterior cervical muscles, and suboccipital muscles are other sources of tension headache.[21]

MUSCLES OF FACIAL EXPRESSION.—Trigger points in the orbicularis oculi muscle refer down through the nose and upper lip; those of the zygomaticus major muscle refer upward along the inner canthus of the eye to the midforehead; those in the platysma muscle refer diffusely in the mandibular region (Fig 10–11). These muscles are all accessible for manual palpation to identify trigger sites.

It should be noted that nonspastic myofascial trigger point pain emanating from muscles innervated by cervical spinal nerves often induce heterotopic pain in the orofacial and head regions. Spontaneous referred pain is usually felt as headache. It is possible, however, that such reference be felt in other structures as earache, toothache, or masticatory pain. Stimulation-evoked secondary hyperalgesia is also a common form of heterotopic pain that occurs secondarily to cervical

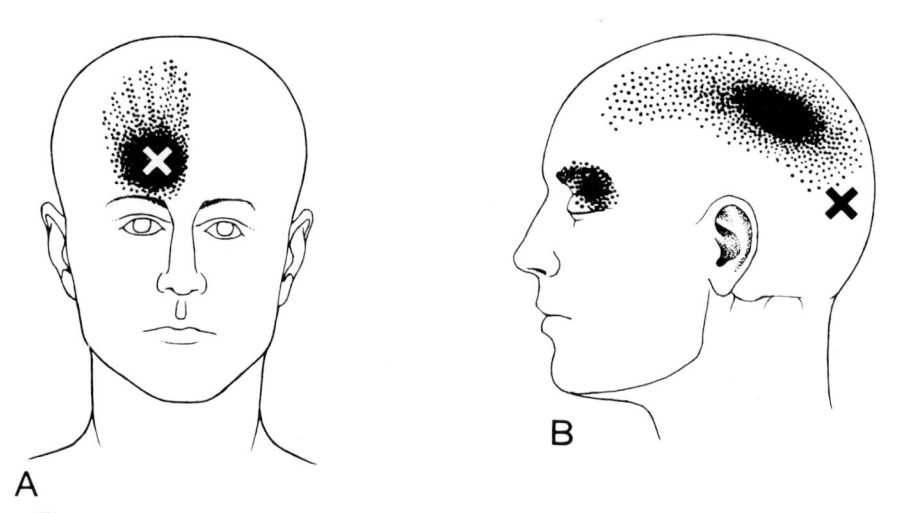

Fig 10–10.—Pain patterns referred from trigger points (*X*s) in the occipitofrontalis muscle. **A,** frontalis belly. **B,** occipitalis belly. (From Travell J.G., Simons D.G.: *Myofascial Pain and Dysfunction.* Baltimore, Williams & Wilkins Co., 1983. Reproduced with permission.)

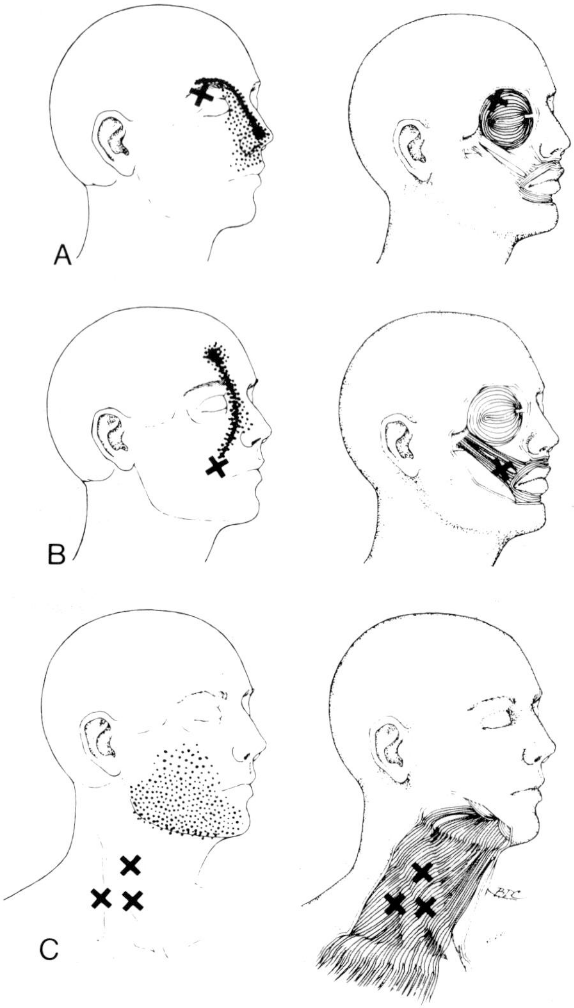

Fig 10–11.—Pain patterns and trigger points (*X*s) from which pain is referred in muscles of facial expression. **A,** orbital portion of orbicularis oculi muscle. **B,** zygomaticus major muscle. **C,** platysma muscle. (From Travell J.G., Simons D.G.: *Myofascial Pain and Dysfunction.* Baltimore, Williams & Wilkins Co., 1983. Reproduced with permission.)

nociceptive input. Thus, areas of touchy skin or scalp may occur. Frequently, however, deeper areas of palpable tenderness that are accentuated by masticatory function may occur. Such heterotopic manifestation of cervical pain may be mistaken for true masticatory pain. Caution therefore should always be exercised when cervical and masticatory pains are felt concurrently. When this occurs, it behooves the dental examiner to be prepared to do at least a cursory clinical examination of the neck.

Such an examination entails observation of the neck contours for deviation or straightening of the neck, rotation or tilting of the head, or elevation of the shoulder. The *mobility* of the neck should be tested both actively and passively for freedom of movement, pain, and crepitation. Tenderness and muscle spasm can be determined by *palpation*. *Sensory evaluation* of neck pain sources as identified by dermatome distribution is important on the basis that cervical nerve pain is felt superficially in the shoulder, outer arm, and hand, whereas thoracic nerve pain is commonly felt in the axillary region and inner arm. *Deep tendon reflexes* and *motor evaluation* of the shoulder and arm should be done, keeping in mind that motor innervation of the deltoid, biceps, triceps, and wrist muscles is from the cervical spinal nerves. Lastly, *radial pulse* changes with postural maneuvers of the arms should be tested.

Such a clinical examination may reveal not only the presence of pain sources in the neck but may help to pinpoint which cervical spinal nerves are involved. It should be noted that upper cervical spinal nerves are more likely sources of pain that refer or spread to the masticatory region than are lower ones. This examination may produce sufficient evidence to warrant an orthopedic consultation.

Among neck conditions that the dentist should be familiar with are the following:

1. Chronic cervical muscle spasm
2. Acute cervical strain
3. Osteoarthritis of the cervical spine and intervertebral disc disease
4. Scalenus anticus syndrome[28]

Secondary effects of muscle pain include not only reference of pain, as previously discussed, but also the development of myospastic activity in other muscles, giving the syndrome a pattern of spreading pain. A nonspastic cervical pain syndrome may by central hyperexcitability secondarily induce spasm of masticatory muscles. This then leads to a typical masticatory pain-dysfunction syndrome, the symptoms of which may become dominant. As such, the very real masticatory dysfunction problem may cause the patient to consider this to be his total complaint when in fact it is no more than a secondary effect of the antecedent neck problem. Masticatory pain-dysfunction syndromes of this type, which represent only a portion of a larger pain syndrome, require astute diagnostic and therapeutic management in order to avoid failure and chronicity.

Nonspastic myofascial pain may take on myospasm activity, changing the whole symptom picture. The usual clinical characteristics of myofascial pain continue, and to this is added sustained contraction of the muscle itself. Local muscle spasm pain and muscular dysfunction become part of the symptom complex. The subject becomes aware of the location of these symptoms even though he may not understand the etiologic factors or significance. When myofascial pain becomes spastic, the term *myofascial pain-dysfunction syndrome* applies.

MUSCLE SPASM PAIN

By definition,[29] muscle spasm is a sudden, involuntary contraction of a muscle or group of muscles, attended by pain and interference with function, producing involuntary movement and distortion. A criterion of spasticity is increased EMG activity in the muscle at rest. Although the initial contraction may be painless, in due time pain usually develops, and with it a cycling mechanism that tends to perpetuate the condition indefinitely after the initiating cause has ceased. It seems evident that the factors of duration and constancy are important in initiating the cycling mechanism that characterizes painful muscle spasm. Once the spasm becomes well established, it is likely to continue. Once it becomes painful, it is likely to intensify and spread. Pain results from both contracting and stretching the spastic muscle (Fig 10–12).

The incidence of muscle spasm relates to local causes such as minor strain, abuse, and fatigue, as well as to less obvious causes such as muscle splinting, preexistent nonspastic myofascial pain syndromes, and central excitatory effects secondary to deep pain input elsewhere. Owing to the local muscle pain and muscular dysfunction, the site of origin of spasm pain is fairly well known. There may still be additional referred pain whose site of origin is unknown to the patient. He may not understand the cause or significance of the pain and dysfunction, however. Dysfunction consists of rigidity if contraction is isometric and shortening if it is isotonic. The total symptom picture includes local pains, muscular dysfunction, and a variety of secondary central excitatory effects.

As previously mentioned, the incidence of muscle spasm seems to follow one of three preexistent conditions, namely, (1) muscle splinting activity, (2) continuing input of deep somatic pain, or (3) preexistent myofascial trigger point activity. Most local conditions, such as strain and abusive use, that terminate in myospasm go though a protective muscle splinting phase. The generation of muscle spasm as a central excitatory effect of deep somatic pain is well established and documented.[4] The transition of myofascial trigger point pain into myospasm occurs most frequently by painfully stretching the affected muscle.[21]

Pain-Dysfunction Syndrome

Initially introduced into the literature by Schwartz[30] in 1956 under the name *temporomandibular joint pain-dysfunction syndrome*, the condition was described as *painful spasm* of the masticatory muscles

PAINS OF MUSCLE ORIGIN   161

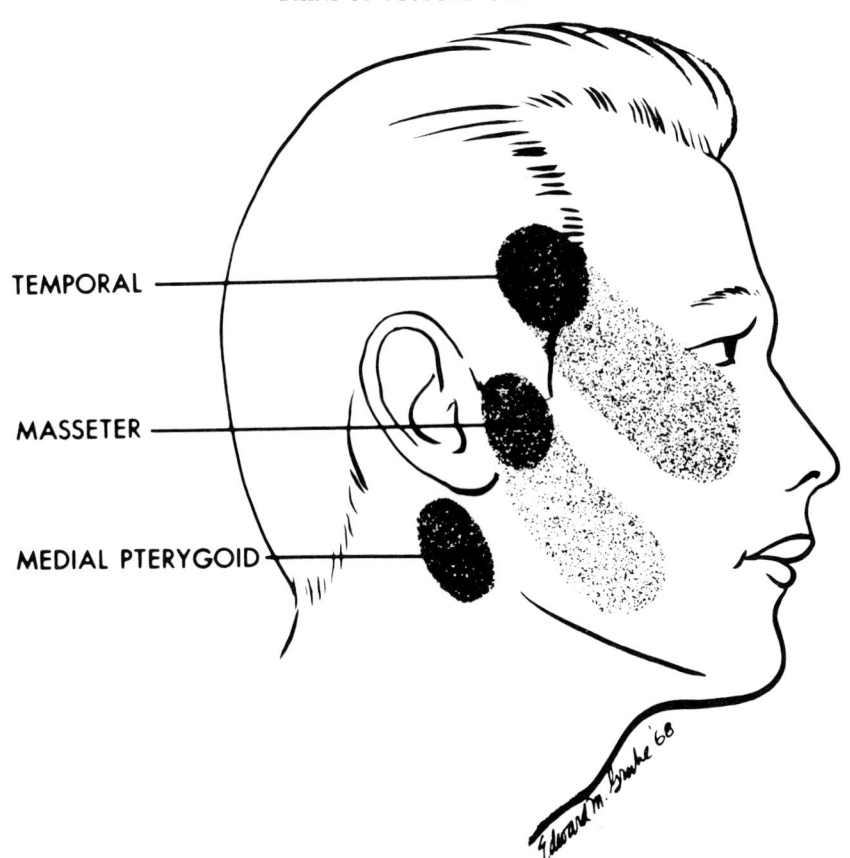

TEMPORAL

MASSETER

MEDIAL PTERYGOID

Fig 10–12.—Schematic drawing showing areas of distribution of masticatory muscle pain. Darker shading represents areas where pain is more frequently felt; lighter shading indicates possible areas of diffusion and spreading. (From Bell W.E.: Clinical diagnosis of the pain-dysfunction syndrome. *J.A.D.A.* 79:154–160, 1969. Copyright by the American Dental Association. Reproduced by permission.)

accompanied by dysfunction of the muscle(s) involved. Schwartz considered that limitation and incoordination of mandibular movements were the chief criteria of dysfunction, and he specifically differentiated this clinical entity from organic disturbances of the joints, which present similar signs and symptoms. This important new concept of temporomandibular joint disease fundamentally altered the clinical management of many masticatory pain problems.

Since the introduction of this syndrome, much investigation has taken place, and many authors have discussed the subject. Experimental evidence through EMG studies has helped confirm early clinical impressions. The importance of emotional tension has been substantiated by several well-controlled studies.[31-36]

The term *myofascial pain-dysfunction (MPD) syndrome* was introduced by Laskin[35] in 1969. This term was used on the premise that the condition constituted a myofascial trigger point mechanism—which no doubt many times it does. The masticatory myospasm disorder that this term is used to designate frequently does not stem from a preexistent trigger point mechanism, but occurs from other antecedent causes. Local conditions such as muscle fatigue and proprioceptively induced muscle splinting that terminate as myospasm are known causes of this muscle disorder. It also frequently results from deep somatic pain input such as otitis media, or from vascular pain syndromes and cervical pain sources of many types. In the dental literature, the term has largely lost its meaning when we see it frequently used to designate all types of temporomandibular disorders, even structural joint disease.

It is of real clinical importance that the dental examiner be able to recognize the pain-dysfunction syndrome and *clearly differentiate it from structural joint disease.*[37, 38] The therapist should be extremely cautious in the application of irreversible alteration of the occlusion until such a differential diagnosis has been made. Too frequently, permanent alteration of occlusal surfaces of the teeth by selective grinding or occlusal reconstruction is undertaken to relieve a complaint of painful malocclusion with little or no attempt to determine if the source of pain is arthralgic or myalgic. Too much cannot be said against hasty definitive therapy for all masticatory pain problems. Adequate differential diagnosis as an essential prerequisite to treatment should form the foundation for the management of all orofacial pain complaints.

The masticatory pain-dysfunction syndrome is initiated as a spasm of one or more masticatory muscles. If the spasm persists, it becomes painful—hence the origin of masticatory pain. If the spasm persists, the shortened muscle(s) alters mandibular movements—hence the origin of the masticatory dysfunction. The location, severity, and duration of pain depend on which muscles are painfully contracted and to what degree. The total suffering relates to how the condition is reacted to by the individual. Much of the clinical behavior of the pain depends on reference and spreading. Thus, *clinical evaluation of the pain requires thorough understanding of the mechanisms of pain and the special peculiarities of deep somatic pain behavior.* The masticatory dysfunction likewise depends upon which muscles are shortened and to what degree. Thus, *clinical evaluation of the dysfunction requires thorough understanding of oral and masticatory physiology.*

The masticatory pain-dysfunction syndrome may result from local strain and abuse as well as from tension, clenching, and bruxism. It may develop from protracted splinting or from preexistent nonspastic myofascial involvement of the muscle. It may be a manifestation of central hyperexcitability from deep pain input elsewhere in the head and neck region. It may relate to occlusal disharmony or interference with joint function. It may occur secondarily as a central excitatory effect from true arthralgia.

Spasm of Elevator Muscles

Spasm of an elevator muscle restricts opening movement to the extent of the shortened muscle, but does not appreciably restrict protrusive or contralateral excursion except that due to the inhibitory effect of pain. The mandibular incisal path is deflected to the *affected side* when the masseter or temporal is shortened unilaterally. It is deflected to the *opposite side* when the medial pterygoid is shortened unilaterally. *Deflection does not occur when both masseter and medial pterygoid are shortened unilaterally or with any combination of bilateral muscle shortening.* Deflection of protrusive excursion does not occur except that due to pain inhibition.

Interference during mandibular movement occurs when the spasm increases the passive interarticular pressure sufficiently to alter the normal functioning of the articular disc. This may be identified as noise, sensations of functional interference, deviations of the incisal path, and altered movements.

Some ill-defined acute malocclusion may occur, more readily sensed subjectively by the patient than witnessed objectively by the examiner.

The pain of elevator muscle spasm occurs when the patient attempts to open the mouth, chew food, or clench the teeth. The clenching pain is not decreased by biting on a tongue blade placed between the teeth on the painful side and usually is increased by biting on a tongue blade placed on the opposite side. Pain with opening is due to stretching the spastic muscle. Pain with chewing food and clenching the teeth is due to contracting the spastic muscle. Pain with ipsilateral excursion is usually temporal in origin. If discal interference becomes traumatic, some arthralgic pain may result.

All the pain experienced by the patient is extra-articular except when secondary discal interference induces arthralgia. The location of the discomfort felt by the patient may be wholly inaccurate as a means of identifying its source. The overriding painful sensation is usually described as having a dull, aching quality. Spontaneous lancinating pains may occur—shooting to the ear, temple, or face. Such pains may also relate to chewing and opening. Palpable tenderness over the joint is frequently masseteric in origin. Infra-auricular, post-mandibular, and pharyngeal discomfort is usually medial pterygoid in origin. Temple discomfort is usually temporal in origin. Earache is usually masseteric in origin. Although secondary referred pains may be felt widely over the auricular, preauricular, infra-auricular, temporal, and facial areas, such pain is rarely described as located in the postauricular, occipital, or cervical areas unless cervical muscles are simultaneously involved. Headache may occur.

The intensity of elevator muscle spasm pain relates to stretching or contracting the spastic muscle(s). It is characterized by an intimate and accurate relationship to masticatory function. Pain in the individual muscles can be identified by skillful manual palpation, and the source accurately confirmed by analgesic blocking.

Radiographic evidence of elevator muscle spasm is extremely reliable. Although the joints present a normal appearance structurally, the condylar movement in open position is considerably restricted compared with that of contralateral position, which is usually normal unless inhibited by pain or restricted by disc jamming. This radiographic evidence is seen unilaterally *when the mandibular incisal path deflects to the affected side* (Fig 10–13). It is seen bilaterally *when such deflection does not occur* (Fig 10–14). As a general rule, little or no evidence of occlusal disharmony is radiographically identifiable.

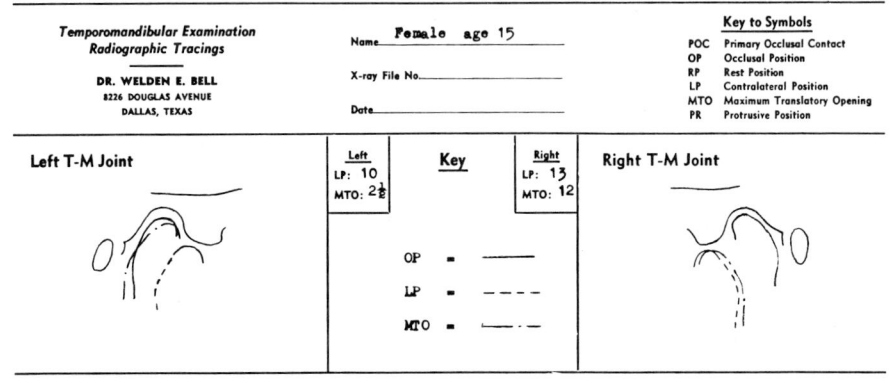

Fig 10–13.—Radiographic tracings illustrating a masticatory pain-dysfunction syndrome expressed as unilateral spasm of left masseter muscle only. Note that all findings are essentially normal except the restricted movement of left condyle in MTO compared with LP. Clinically deflection of the incisal path to the affected side is seen.

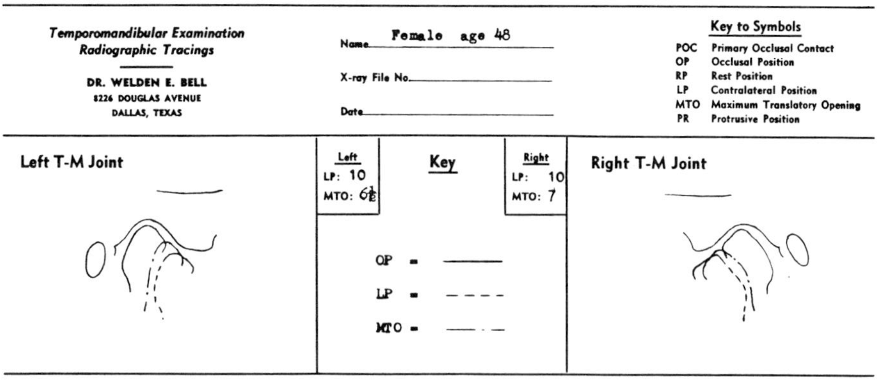

Fig 10–14.—Radiographic tracings illustrating masticatory pain-dysfunction syndrome expressed as multiple involvement of elevator masticatory muscles. Note that all findings are essentially normal except for restricted condylar movement in MTO bilaterally. Clinically, no deflection of the incisal path is seen.

To summarize, the pain of elevator muscle spasm may be felt in and about the ear, temple, and face. Pain increases with opening, chewing food, and clenching the teeth, the latter pain not being reduced by biting on a tongue blade ipsilaterally and usually being increased by biting on a tongue blade placed on the opposite side. The masticatory pain is accompanied by restriction of opening. Deflection of the incisal path depends on the muscles involved. There is minimal restriction of lateral and protrusive movements except when caused by the inhibitory influence of pain or secondary disc jamming. Interference with mandibular movements occurs when the spasm appreciably increases the passive interarticular pressure, causing disc noise, sensations of interference, deviations of the incisal path, and altered movements. Acute malocclusion may be sensed subjectively but is difficult to observe objectively. The pain sources are identified by manual palpation and arrested by analgesic blocking of the muscles in painful spasm. Radiographically, condyle movement with opening is restricted, whereas that of contralateral excursion is normal except as inhibited by pain or disc jamming (Fig 10–15). Unilateral restriction is accompanied by incisal path deflection. It is to be noted that the radiographic interarticular space does not decrease in width under biting stress (Case No. 10–1).

Spasm of Inferior Lateral Pterygoid Muscle

The lateral pterygoid muscle has been mercilessly incriminated as the cause of numerous temporomandibular complaints. This probably

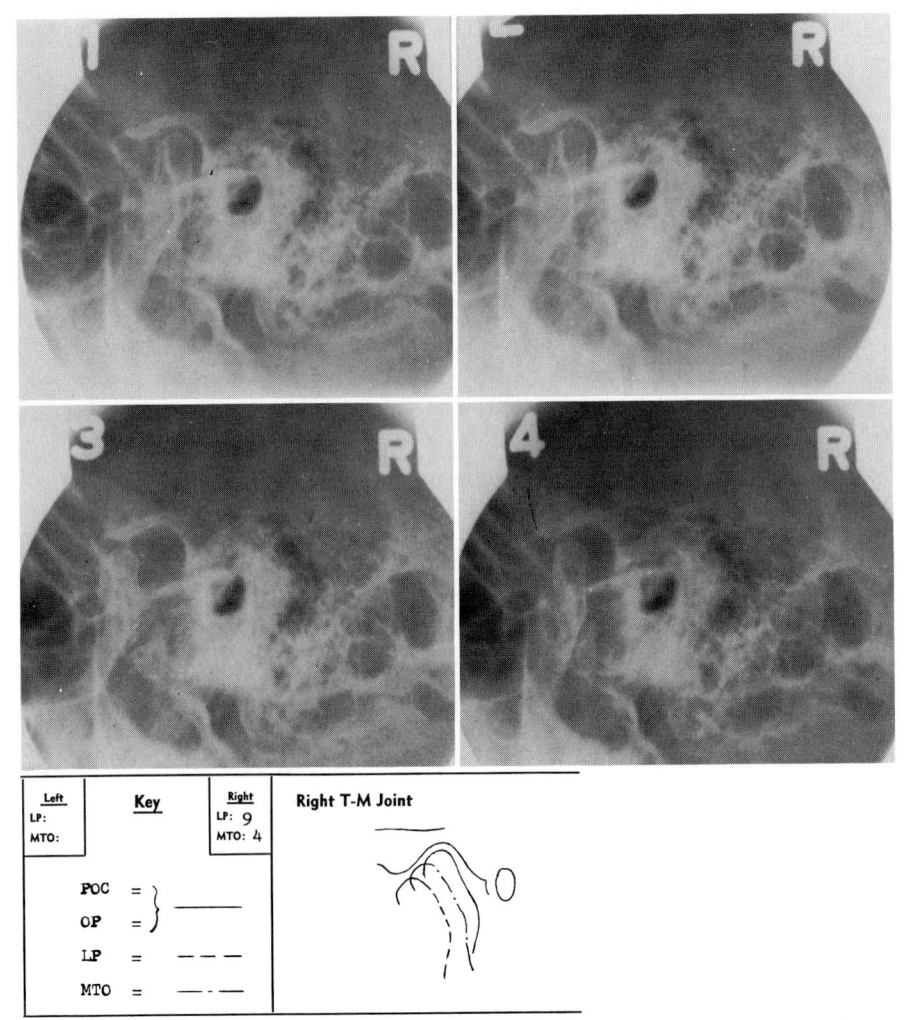

Fig 10–15.—Illustration of radiographic evidence of extracapsular restriction of mouth opening. Note that condyle moves reasonably well in LP but is definitely restricted in MTO. *Top,* radiographs of right temporomandibular joint in POC (**1**), OP (**2**), LP (**3**) and MTO (**4**). *Bottom,* radiographic tracings show that movement of condyle in MTO is considerably less than in LP. (From Bell W.E.: Management of temporomandibular joint problems, in Goldman H.M., Gilmore H.W., Royer R.Q, et al. (eds.): *Current Therapy in Dentistry.* St. Louis, C.V. Mosby Co., 1970, Vol. 4. Reproduced with permission.)

Oral and Facial Pain

DR. WELDEN E. BELL
8226 DOUGLAS AVENUE
DALLAS, TEXAS

Name: Female age 52

	QUALITY	DURATION	LOCALIZATION	AFFECTED BY	LOCAL EFFECTS
HISTORY	(Mild) Severe — Spontaneous Triggered Induced Paroxysmal (Steady)	Bright (Dull) — — Pricking Itching Burning (Aching) Pulsating	(Continuous) Intermittent (Recurrent) — — Momentary Minutes Hours Day long (Protracted)	Localized (Diffuse) — Radiating (Spreading) — Enlarging Migrating — Secondary Pain	Face Movement Jaw Movement Tongue Movement Swallowing (Head Position) Body Position Activities (Tension) (Fatigue) Time of Day	Sensory: Hyperesthesia Hypoesthesia Paresthesia Dysesthesia — Motor: Weakness Contraction (Spasm)	Special Sense: Visual Auditory Olfactory Gustatory — Autonomic: Ocular Signs Nasal Signs Cutaneous Signs Gastric Signs

Location
Inception
Initial pain
Duration, clinical course
Therapeutic response
Physical and emotional background
Trauma, infection, etc.
Medications in use

Mild continuous protracted steady dull aching pain diffusely located in the temporal, preauricular, and occipital areas bilaterally, aggravated by head movements, tension, fatigue, and jaw use.

During the past 6-7 years, patient has had recurring episodes of bilateral occipital and temporal headaches lasting up to 2-3 months and occurring at irregular intervals. They were aggravated by head movements, tension, and fatigue and have been treated as tension headaches by her osteopathic physician. About 8-9 months ago, the present episode began, first intermittently, then becoming constant. During recent months, the pains have been aggravated by chewing and opening widely and she has noticed moderate restriction of opening. Her physician, therefore, has advised a dental examination. She has concomitant neck, finger, arm, and leg complaints but she has been cleared medically and neurologically for cause except minor osteoarthritis of the cervical vertebrae. No medications or therapy presently in use.

B/P 145/85 Neurological Survey   Psychological Survey

EXAMINATION

Oral

TM joints

Muscle system

Diagnostic blocks

Diagnostic drugs

Trial therapy

Orally: No dental or oral cause for the pain is evident clinically or radiographically. The teeth respond normally to electric testing. She has bilateral preauricular pain with opening, sustained clenching, and hard biting eccentrically. Her maximum opening is about 34mm with no deflection. Lateral and protrusive movements are normal. She has moderate diskal noise with extended or strained movements only. There is no discernible occlusal disharmony.

TM joints: Clinically and radiographically normal except for moderate restriction of condylar movement bilaterally with opening. (See tracings.)

Muscle system: Palpable tenderness in the masseter, temporal, medial pterygoid, sternomastoid, occipital, and trapezius muscles bilaterally.

Opinion: The masticatory pain and dysfunction appear to be wholly from muscular causes and intimately related to preexistent muscle pain emanating from the cervical musculature bilaterally. By history, the cervical component antedates the more recent masticatory complaint and the entire symptom complex is highly suggestive of a cervical myofascial pain syndrome that has spread to involve the masticatory muscles. It is presumed that cervical arthritis is a likely predisposing cause and this possibility deserves serious investigation on a medical level. There is no identifiable dental, oral, or masticatory cause for the patient's complaint.

DIAGNOSIS

Masticatory pain-dysfunction syndrome expressed as cycling spasm of the elevator muscles bilaterally, representing secondary spreading from a preexistent cervical myofascial pain syndrome of undetermined origin.

Case No. 10–1, A.—Case chart. Masticatory myalgia, expressed as spasm of elevator muscles (pain-dysfunction syndrome).

stems from lack of understanding of how the muscle is constructed and what its normal functions are. No doubt, the difficulty of adequately examining the muscle clinically has provided good cover for these incriminations. Several hard facts need to be considered in evaluating the effects of this muscle on masticatory symptoms. It should

168   OROFACIAL PAINS

Temporomandibular Examination
Radiographic Tracings

DR. WELDEN E. BELL
8226 DOUGLAS AVENUE
DALLAS, TEXAS

Name: Female age 52

X-ray File No.

Date

Key to Symbols
POC   Primary Occlusal Contact
OP   Occlusal Position
RP   Rest Position
LP   Contralateral Position
MTO   Maximum Translatory Opening
PR   Protrusive Position

Left T-M Joint   Left LP: 12 MTO: 9   **Key**   Right LP: 12 MTO: 8½   Right T-M Joint

POC =
OP =
LP =
MTO =

INTERPRETATION

Both joints were viewed in five positions, four transparietal, one transfacial:
1. Position of primary occlusal contact (POC).
2. Fully occluded position (OP).
3. Contralateral excursion (LP).
4. Maximum opening - 34mm (MTO).
5. Transfacial in protrusive position.

Both joints present well defined smoothly contoured articular surfaces with interarticular spaces of adequate width which do not decrease in width under biting stress. There is no evidence of degenerative joint disease or other structural abnormality.

There is excellent superimposition of POC and OP in both joints indicative of no occlusal disharmony gross enough to cause radiographically visible displacement of either condyle when the teeth are firmly occluded.

Translatory movement in LP is normal and symmetrical in both joints. In MTO, however, there is restricted condylar movement in both joints, indicative of extracapsular restraint, which with the clinical symptoms is interpreted as the effect of shortening of elevator muscles bilaterally.

Case No. 10–1, B.—Radiographic tracings of temporomandibular joints.

be understood first that the upper and lower heads comprise two different muscles.[39] Only the inferior lateral pterygoid muscle protracts the mandible and therefore can act to create acute occlusal disharmony when it is shortened. The superior muscle remains inactive at all times except during power strokes in conjunction with elevator muscle action. Even when shortened, the superior lateral pterygoid muscle cannot disrupt joint functioning in the absence of structural joint disease.

The dearth of muscle spindles reduces the chance of reflex contraction when this muscle is stretched. Then too, the muscle is composed of slow-contracting fibers that resist fatigue and seldom undergo spastic activity. The prime reason that diagnosis of this muscle is so difficult is because it is inaccessible for manual palpation.[25] Despite voluminous testimony to the contrary, the possibility of diagnostically accurate manual or instrument palpation of the muscle is remote.

When the inferior lateral pterygoid muscle shortens due to myospastic activity, acute malocclusion results. This is recognized as disocclusion of the ipsilateral posterior teeth and premature occlusion of the contralateral anterior teeth. The presence of pain sites within the muscle is identified by functional manipulation which consists of stretching and contracting the muscle. To stretch the inferior lateral pterygoid muscle requires clenching the teeth firmly in maximum intercuspation. To contract the muscle requires protruding the jaw against resistance. The pain induced by stretching the muscle is reduced by biting against a tongue blade separator, which prevents intercuspation of the teeth. Unless acute malocclusion can be identified and pain be induced by functional manipulation, a diagnosis of spasm of this muscle is invalid.

When the muscle becomes spastic, little or no discomfort results if jaw movements are moderate and relaxed and if maximum intercuspation is avoided. Extended and forceful opening, protrusion, and contralateral excursion, however, require contraction of the muscle, and pain should be elicited. Extended ipsilateral excursion in some individuals causes stretching of this muscle and therefore may elicit pain. There should be no limitation of any of these movements except as inhibited by pain.

Chewing food requires holding action on the part of the lateral pterygoid muscle and elicits pain proportionate to the resistance of the bolus of food and the vigor of chewing movements. This pain increases as the teeth reach a fully occluded relationship.

Local analgesic blocking of the lateral pterygoid muscle promptly arrests all pain emanating from this source and offers the best clinical means of accurately locating the source of pain.

Radiographically, the primary occlusal contact position of the condyle is slightly anterior to the fully occluded position. This confirms the occlusal disharmony clinically evident and, unless subsequently proved otherwise, should help classify it as acute malocclusion. All other radiographic evidence should fall well within normal limits except for the effect of pain inhibition on translatory movements.

Bilateral spasm of lateral pterygoid muscles causes clinical findings that are essentially the same except bilaterally situated. The acute malocclusion is described as anterior premature contact or overstressing accompanied by bilateral disocclusion posteriorly. Bilateral local analgesic blocking promptly arrests the pain emanating from these muscles. Radiographically, the acute malocclusion may be identified bilaterally, all other radiographic evidence falling well within normal limits except for the effect of pain inhibition. (Unilateral spasm of a lateral pterygoid muscle may give similar radiographic evidence due to sympathetic positioning of the nonsymptomatic condyle.)

To summarize, the pain of lateral pterygoid muscle spasm is usually felt in the joint proper, but this may vary. *It is most severe when the teeth are fully occluded. This is reduced by insertion of a tongue blade between the molar teeth to prevent intercuspation.* Chewing foods is somewhat painful; discomfort is slight with relaxed translatory movement except when extended to maximum range. When so extended, pain may be sensed with all movements. The *masticatory pain is accompanied by acute malocclusion*, but there is no other evidence of masticatory dysfunction except that induced by the inhibitory effect of pain. The *pain is promptly arrested by analgesic blocking of the offending muscle*. Radiographically, the occlusal disharmony is identified if of sufficient magnitude. The joints are otherwise normal radiographically (Case No. 10–2).

Spasm of Elevators and Lateral Pterygoid

Spasm of elevator and inferior lateral pterygoid muscles may occur simultaneously. The symptom complex may become involved, as the characteristics of the two types of conditions blend into a single complaint. The dysfunction is characterized by definite *acute malocclusion*, described as anterocontralateral premature contact if the condition is unilateral and as anterior premature contact in bilateral conditions. This is accompanied by disocclusion of the posterior teeth. The dysfunction is also expressed as *restriction of opening*. The inhibitory effect of pain may add some restriction of protrusive and lateral excursions. When the spasm appreciably increases passive interarticular pressure, normal disc functioning may be interfered with, causing noise, sensations of functional interference, deviations of the incisal path, and disc jamming. Thus all clinical types of masticatory dysfunction symptoms may be observed as part of a complex pain-dysfunction syndrome.

The pain characteristically occurs with opening, chewing food, extended excursions, and clenching the teeth. Insertion of a tongue blade may alter, but usually does not arrest, the pain induced by firmly occluding the teeth. Contralateral placement of the tongue blade usually increases the pain of biting. Relaxed protrusive and lateral movements may not elicit much pain, but forced and extended movements usually increase pain. Pain may be felt in the joint, ear, infra-auricular region, pharyngeal area, and temple and throughout the face. When intracapsular interference is sufficient to induce intrinsic trauma, arthralgic pain may be added to the symptom picture.

Initially, all pain is extra-articular unless early discal interference occurs. The elevator muscle pain is identified by manual palpation.

PAINS OF MUSCLE ORIGIN

Oral and Facial Pain
DR. WELDEN E. BELL
8226 DOUGLAS AVENUE
DALLAS, TEXAS

Name: Female age 20

	QUALITY	DURATION	LOCALIZATION	AFFECTED BY		LOCAL EFFECTS	
	(Mild)	Bright	Continuous	Localized		Sensory:	Special Sense:
	Severe	(Dull)	(Intermittent)	(Diffuse)	Face Movement	Hypesthesia	Visual
			(Recurrent)		Jaw Movement	Hyperesthesia	Auditory
				Radiating	Tongue Movement	Paresthesia	Olfactory
				Spreading	Swallowing	Dysesthesia	Gustatory
	Spontaneous				Head Position		
	Triggered	Pricking	Momentary		Body Position		Autonomic:
	(Induced)	Itching	(Minutes)	Enlarging	Activities	Motor:	Ocular Signs
		Burning	Hours	Migrating	Tension	Weakness	Nasal Signs
	Paroxysmal	(Aching)	Day long		Fatigue	Contraction	Cutaneous Signs
	(Steady)	Pulsating	Protracted	Secondary Pain	Time of Day	(Spasm)	Gastric Signs

HISTORY

Location
Inception
Initial pain
Duration, clinical course
Therapeutic response
Physical and emotional background
Trauma, infection, etc.
Medications in use

Mild variable steady dull aching pain diffusely located in the right ear and preauricular area. It is induced by clenching the teeth, chewing, and other jaw use, and lasts variable periods of time. The pains are intermittent. It is noted that discomfort relates especially to gum-chewing, hard biting, and forceful jaw movements. She complains also of malocclusion of the teeth described as premature contact of the left anterior teeth with disocclusion of the posteriors. When she brings the teeth into full occlusion, she feels the acute pain -- so she avoids it.
The complaint began about two years ago in sudden recurring episodes lasting usually only a few days and then disappearing for variable periods of time. The complaint seemed to be worse especially in the early mornings. The present episode began about six months ago and has remained much the same ever since.

EXAMINATION

B/P   Neurological Survey   Psychological Survey

Oral
TM joints
Muscle system
Diagnostic blocks
Diagnostic drugs
Trial therapy

Orally: The teeth are clinically and radiographically negative for cause of pain individually. Disharmony in the occlusion is evident subjectively. She feels premature touching of the left anterior teeth while the posteriors do not feel to be in firm contact. When she brings all the teeth into firm occlusion, she experiences pain in the right TM area. This can be prevented by biting on a tongue blade to preclude full intercuspation of the teeth. She thinks her occlusion was normal six months ago and relates the malocclusion to her pain complaint.
TM joints: Clinical functioning of the joints is well within normal limits except for the sensation of malocclusion and the right-side pain when she occludes the teeth or moves the jaw forcefully. She opens 45 mm with no deviation or deflection of the incisal path. Protrusive and lateral excursions are adequate and symmetrical. Radiographically, both joints appear to be within normal limits structurally. There is radiographically visible displacement of the right condyle as the teeth are fully occluded from the position of primary occlusal contact (see tracings).
Muscle system: There is no palpable tenderness. The discomfort appears to be wholly subjective. Analgesic blocking of the right lateral pterygoid muscle immediately arrests the pain complaint.
Opinion: The pain is myalgic and arises wholly from the right lateral pterygoid muscle. The malocclusion is acute and relates to muscle spasm.

DIAGNOSIS

Masticatory pain-dysfunction syndrome expressed as cycling myospasm of the right lateral pterygoid muscle. The etiology is presumed to relate to clenching, tension, fatigue, etc.

Case No. 10–2, A.—Case chart. Masticatory myalgia, expressed as spasm of the lateral pterygoid muscle (pain-dysfunction syndrome).

Analgesic blocking may be required to confirm the various sources of pain.

Radiographically, the joints appear normal structurally. The occlusal disharmony induced by lateral pterygoid muscle spasm is identified by anterior displacement of the condyle in primary occlusal contact

Temporomandibular Examination Radiographic Tracings	Name Female age 20	Key to Symbols
DR. WELDEN E. BELL 8226 DOUGLAS AVENUE DALLAS, TEXAS	X-ray File No. Date	POC Primary Occlusal Contact OP Occlusal Position RP Rest Position LP Contralateral Position MTO Maximum Translatory Opening PR Protrusive Position

Left T-M Joint	Left LP: 13 MTO: 18	Key	Right LP: 13 MTO: 19	Right T-M Joint
		POC = ─────── OP = ·········· LP = ─ ─ ─ ─ MTO = ─ · ─ ·		

INTERPRETATION

Both joints were viewed in five positions, four transparietal, one transfacial:
1. Position of primary occlusal contact (POC).
2. Fully occluded position (OP).
3. Contralateral excursion (LP).
4. Maximum opening - 45mm (MTO).
5. Transfacial in protrusive position.

Both joints present well defined, smoothly contoured articular surfaces with interarticular spaces of adequate width which do not decrease in width under biting stress. There is no evidence of degenerative joint disease or other structural abnormality.

There is lack of superimposition of POC and OP in the right joint, there being radiographically visible displacement of the right condyle in a posterior direction when the teeth are firmly occluded. Based on the clinical evidence, it is interpreted that the POC position represents anterior displacement of the condyle due to contraction of the right lateral pterygoid muscle while the occluded position (OP) represents the effect of maximum intercuspation of the teeth.

Translatory movement in LP and MTO in both joints is well within normal limits.

Case No. 10–2, B.—Radiographic tracings of temporomandibular joints.

position compared with the fully occluded position. Translatory movement in open position is restricted compared with that of contralateral position. Lateral excursions are usually normal unless inhibited by pain or arrested by disc jamming (Case No. 10–3).

MUSCLE INFLAMMATION PAIN

Local muscle soreness is the familiar, ordinary variety of muscle pain. Its incidence relates to a local cause that is known to the subject. It therefore usually has no aura of mystery and creates little apprehension. It stems from such factors as unaccustomed use, abusive use, strain, external trauma, and infection. The site of origin of the pain is accurately identifiable by the patient. It is accompanied by dysfunction such as stiffness and swelling.

Any muscle about the mouth and face can become sore. *When masticatory muscles are involved, masticatory pain and masticatory dys-*

PAINS OF MUSCLE ORIGIN

Oral and Facial Pain
DR. WELDEN E. BELL
8226 DOUGLAS AVENUE
DALLAS, TEXAS

Name: Female age 47

QUALITY	DURATION	LOCALIZATION	AFFECTED BY	LOCAL EFFECTS
(Mild) Severe	Bright (Dull)	(Continuous) Intermittent Recurrent	Localized (Diffuse)	Face Movement (Jaw Movement) Tongue Movement Swallowing Head Position Body Position Activities Tension Fatigue Time of Day	Sensory: Hypesthesia Hyperesthesia Paresthesia Dysesthesia Motor: Weakness Contraction (Spasm)	Special Sense: Visual Auditory Olfactory Gustatory Autonomic: Ocular Signs Nasal Signs Cutaneous Signs Gastric Signs
Spontaneous Triggered Induced Paroxysmal (Steady)	Pricking Itching Burning (Aching) Pulsating	Momentary Minutes Hours Day long (Protracted)	Radiating Spreading Enlarging Migrating Secondary Pain		

HISTORY

Location / Inception / Initial pain: Mild continuous protracted variable steady dull aching pain diffusely located in the right ear, preauricular area, face, and temple, aggravated by opening widely, chewing food, and clenching the teeth, and accompanied by acute malocclusion and restricted opening.

Duration, clinical course / Therapeutic response / Physical and emotional background / Trauma, infection, etc. / Medications in use: The patient has had recurring episodes of earache associated with acute upper respiratory infections for several years. About three weeks ago, she had such an episode with continuous severe earache on the right side. After about seven days, she noticed her "bite" was off, she couldn't open normally, and she had pain with opening, chewing, and occluding the teeth. This has become progressively worse even though antibiotic therapy by her ENT physician is said to have cleared the ear completely. He advised examination by her dentist who recognized the trismus and occlusal disharmony but declined to adjust the occlusion pending further investigation of the temporomandibular joints. She has no other physical complaint and takes no medications.

EXAMINATION

B/P 130/80   Neurological Survey   Psychological Survey

Oral / TM joints / Muscle system / Diagnostic blocks / Diagnostic drugs / Trial therapy:

Orally: The teeth clinically and radiographically are normal. She describes premature contact of the left anterior teeth and disocclusion of the posteriors unless she uses effort. When she fully occludes the teeth, there is acute pain in the right TM area. This is decreased by biting on a tongue-blade. Pain also occurs with eccentric biting, forceful lateral and protrusive movements, and opening beyond 20mm. Opening is restricted to 31mm with deflection to the right after 23mm.

TM joints: Both joints are normal structurally and the left joint normal functionally. The right condyle appears to be protruded in primary occlusal contact position and fails to move properly with opening efforts. (See tracings)

Muscle system: There is palpable tenderness in the right masseter and temporal muscles.

Analgesic blocking of the right lateral pterygoid muscle arrested pain induced by fully occluding the teeth and making forceful excursions. Similar blocking of the right masseter and temporal muscles arrested all other pain.

Opinion: The masticatory pain is muscular and stems from the right lateral pterygoid, masseter, and temporal muscles only. The malocclusion is acute and symptomatic of spasm of the right lateral pterygoid muscle. The trismus is due to spasm of the right masseter and temporal muscles. The myospasms occurred as central excitatory effects induced by primary otalgia. Cycling has occurred.

DIAGNOSIS

Masticatory pain-dysfunction syndrome expressed as cycling myospasm of the right lateral pterygoid, masseter, and temporal muscles, secondary to otalgia.

Case No. 10–3, A.—Case chart. Masticatory myalgia, expressed as spasm of elevator and lateral pterygoid muscles (pain-dysfunction syndrome).

function become evident. Sore masticatory muscles may develop as a result of unaccustomed use or minor strain. Examples of this include the following:
1. Unusual yawning, yelling, biting, chewing
2. Strained sleeping position

Temporomandibular Examination	Name	Female age 47		**Key to Symbols**
Radiographic Tracings			POC	Primary Occlusal Contact
			OP	Occlusal Position
DR. WELDEN E. BELL	X-ray File No.		RP	Rest Position
8226 DOUGLAS AVENUE			LP	Contralateral Position
DALLAS, TEXAS	Date		MTO	Maximum Translatory Opening
			PR	Protrusive Position

| Left T-M Joint | Left
LP: 12
MTO: 15 | **Key**

POC = ————
OP = - - - - - -
LP = — — —
MTO = —·—·— | Right
LP: 12
MTO: 8 | Right T-M Joint |

INTERPRETATION

Both joints were viewed in four positions:
1. Position of primary occlusal contact (POC).
2. Fully occluded position (OP).
3. Contralateral excursion (LP).
4. Maximum opening - 31 mm (MTO).

Both joints present well defined smoothly contoured articular surfaces separated by interarticular spaces of adequate width which do not decrease in width under biting stress. There is no radiographic evidence of degenerative joint disease. Both joints appear to be normal structurally.

There is excellent superimposition of POC and OP in the left joint, indicative of no identifiable occlusal disharmony. Translatory movement of the left condyle in LP and MTO is normal.

In the right joint, there is lack of superimposition of POC and OP indicative of gross displacement of the right condyle when the teeth are occluded. The condylar displacement is in a posterior direction. With clinical symptoms of muscle spasm of the right lateral pterygoid, it is presumed that the displaced condylar position is in primary occlusal contact position and the condylar position when the teeth are fully occluded is the correct one. This would be indicative of anterior displacement of the right condyle due to muscle spasm and the occlusal disharmony seen radiographically should be classified as acute and symptomatic.

Translatory movement of the right condyle in contralateral excursion is normal and symmetrical with the left joint, indicative of freedom of movement within the capsule. With opening, however, the condylar movement is restricted, due to extracapsular causes, which with clinical symptoms presented is presumed to be spasm of right-side elevator muscles. Since there is no similar restraint of condylar movement in the left joint, it is concluded that no shortening of the right medial pterygoid muscle has occurred.

Case No. 10–3, B.—Radiographic tracings of temporomandibular joints.

3. Activities involving minor blows, sports, playing a musical instrument, holding objects in the mouth or between the teeth
4. Spontaneous dislocation or near-dislocation
5. Periods of sustained emotional tension
6. Bruxism
7. Muscular contractions associated with intermittent pains (e.g., tic douloureux)
8. Excessive or prolonged opening for dental treatment
9. Use of a local anesthetic, especially mandibular anesthesia

10. Intubation for general anesthesia
11. Minor strains of all types

Myositis of masticatory muscles may result from very minor strains and changes in the environmental situation such as inadvertently increasing the vertical dimension beyond rest position.

Perhaps the most common condition that elicits pain and altered masticatory function from extracapsular causes other than the pain-dysfunction syndrome is myositis of masticatory muscles. Inflammation of an elevator muscle causes local inflammatory pain, swelling, and restriction of mandibular movement. *The familiar trismus associated with dental sepsis, injury, surgery, or needle abscess typifies this condition.* Painful restriction of opening and mandibular immobilization are characteristic. Swelling is usually present. Clinical symptoms of localized infection such as regional lymphadenitis, elevation of body temperature, and malaise may become evident if sepsis is the initiating cause. Muscles most frequently involved are the medial pterygoid and the masseter. Sepsis spreading into the infratemporal fossa may involve the temporal muscle. Pain is increased with movements of the muscle, especially stretching to open the mouth. Low-grade infection and chronic inflammatory conditions may cause prolonged mandibular dysfunction with minimal pain.

Masticatory myositis may occur as a result of trauma. External blows and violence of different types, as well as needle trauma from mandibular local anesthetic injections, may initiate muscle inflammation. Muscular strain from forceful reduction of spontaneous dislocation constitutes another cause. *Sometimes myospasm terminates as myositis* (Case No. 10–4).

Myositis usually can be distinguished from myospasm by the presence of localized inflammation and swelling. The resulting masticatory dysfunction is due to immobilization of the muscle from inflammatory exudate rather than from tonic contraction. Some dysfunction relates to the inhibitory influence of the pain. Diagnostic analgesic blocking is not only unnecessary but contraindicated owing to the inflammatory process. Radiographic examination should reveal normal joints in all respects except for the clinically obvious restriction of mandibular movement. Interference with mandibular movements and acute malocclusion are usually minimal. It should be noted that myositis may terminate as muscular contracture (Case No. 10–5).

Other inflammatory myogenous pains are fasciitis, tendinitis, and bursitis. Fasciitis is an inflammatory condition of the muscle sheath that occurs in conjunction with, and is diagnostically inseparable from, inflammation of the body of the muscle. Although myofascial pain is not inflammatory, it may be designated *myofasciitis* for administrative

Oral and Facial Pain
DR. WELDEN E. BELL
8226 DOUGLAS AVENUE
DALLAS, TEXAS

Name: Male age 67

HISTORY

QUALITY	DURATION	LOCALIZATION	AFFECTED BY	LOCAL EFFECTS
(Mild) / Severe	Bright / (Dull)	(Continuous) / Intermittent / Recurrent	Localized / (Diffuse)	Face Movement / (Jaw Movement) / Tongue Movement / Swallowing / Head Position / Body Position / Activities / Tension / Fatigue / Time of Day	Sensory: Hypesthesia, Hypoesthesia, Paresthesia, Dysesthesia / Motor: Weakness, Contraction, Spasm	Special Sense: Visual, Auditory, Olfactory, Gustatory / Autonomic: Ocular Signs, Nasal Signs, Cutaneous Signs, Gastric Signs
Spontaneous / Triggered / Induced / Paroxysmal / (Steady)	Pricking / Itching / Burning / (Aching) / Pulsating	Momentary / Minutes / Hours / Day long / (Protracted)	Radiating / Spreading / Enlarging / Migrating / Secondary Pain		

Location / Inception / Initial pain: Mild continuous protracted steady dull aching pain diffusely located in the left face, temple, and jaw, accompanied by marked trismus, and aggravated by attempting to open the mouth for chewing.

Duration, clinical course / Therapeutic response / Physical and emotional background / Trauma, infection, etc. / Medications in use: The complaint occurred as a postoperative complication following the removal of the LL8 tooth about 30 days ago. Prior to extraction, there was moderate soreness in the LL8 area but no acute pain or trismus. The removal of the tooth was described as a difficult and painful experience. Swelling and pain in the LL8 region followed the surgery and after about 3-4 days trismus occurred restricting mouth opening to about 10mm or less. Generalized pain, localized swelling, and inability to open the mouth have persisted. No therapy other than the application of heat and suggestions to encourage jaw use has been prescribed.

Presently, no medications are in use.

EXAMINATION

B/P 155/85 Neurological Survey Psychological Survey

Oral / TM joints / Muscle system / Diagnostic blocks / Diagnostic drugs / Trial therapy:

Orally: The remaining teeth cannot be adequately examined clinically. Radiographically, a lateral oblique film of the mandible shows no osseous change and the LL8 alveolus appears normal. There is localized swelling and tenderness in the LL8 area intraorally, moderate tenderness in the left submandibular triangle, and slight swelling and tenderness above the left zygomatic arch. Opening is restricted to about 8mm with little or no deflection and accompanied by pain in the left temporal and postmandibular areas. Lateral and protrusive movements are moderately restricted and painful.

TM joints: Both joints appear normal structurally. The restricted condylar movement is interpreted as representing the effect of myositis of the left temporal and medial pterygoid muscles. (See tracings.)

Muscle system: Palpable tenderness in the left temporal muscle area. The left medial pterygoid muscle is not accessible for palpation. The left masseter muscle appears to be clinically normal.

Opinion: The history, clinical course, and present clinical and radiographic symptom complex indicate that inflammation in the left pterygomandibular space followed the surgical removal of the LL8 tooth. As this progressed superiorly, the left infratemporal space also became involved, hence the swelling above the left zygomatic arch. Some inflammation still persists as evidenced by intraoral and suprazygomatic symptoms. The left medial pterygoid and temporal muscles appear to be inflamed also.

DIAGNOSIS

Trismus due to myositis of the left temporal and medial pterygoid muscles.

Case No. 10-4, A.—Case chart. Masticatory myalgia, expressed as inflammation of elevator muscles (masticatory myositis).

or insurance purposes.[21] Tendinitis is an inflammatory condition of a tendon or tendon-muscle attachment. Abusive use and trauma are the most frequent causes. Bursae are sac-like antifriction structures that facilitate muscle movements especially when bidirectional. A bursa is found at the hamular process of the sphenoid bone to facilitate tensor

PAINS OF MUSCLE ORIGIN 177

Temporomandibular Examination
Radiographic Tracings

DR. WELDEN E. BELL
8226 DOUGLAS AVENUE
DALLAS, TEXAS

Name __Male age 67__

X-ray File No. _____

Date _____

Key to Symbols
POC Primary Occlusal Contact
OP   Occlusal Position
RP   Rest Position
LP   Contralateral Position
MTO Maximum Translatory Opening
PR   Protrusive Position

Left T-M Joint

Left	Key	Right
LP: 8		LP: 10
MTO: 2		MTO: 3

POC = ⎫
OP = ⎬ ————
LP = --- ---
MTO = — - —

Right T-M Joint

INTERPRETATION

Each joint was viewed in four transparietal positions:
1. Position of primary occlusal contact (POC).
2. Fully occluded position (OP).
3. Contralateral excursion (LP).
4. Maximum opening - 8mm (MTO).

Both joints present well defined smoothly contoured articular surfaces with interarticular spaces that do not decrease in width under biting stress. There is no radiographic evidence of degenerative joint disease or other structural abnormality.

There is satisfactory superimposition of POC and OP in both joints, indicative of no occlusal disharmony gross enough to cause radiographically visible displacement of either condyle when the teeth are firmly occluded.

Translatory movement in LP appears to be slightly restricted as judged by the location of the crest of the articular eminence. This restriction appears to be more in the left joint than in the right.

Translatory movement in MTO is severely restricted in both joints, being slightly more restricted in the left than the right.

With the history, clinical course, and current clinical findings, this restriction of condylar movement is interpreted as being induced by inflamed left temporal and medial pterygoid muscles. No doubt some of the restriction represents the effect of pain inhibition.

Case No. 10–4, B.—Radiographic tracings of temporomandibular joints.

palati muscle action. One lies beneath the tongue. Several facilitate muscle action involving the hyoid bone. Bursitis is an inflammatory condition of a bursa and usually results from trauma.

MASTICATORY PAINS OF MUSCLE ORIGIN

Temporomandibular disorders frequently display the symptom of pain—masticatory pain. Arthralgic masticatory pain emanates from temporomandibular joints; myalgic masticatory pain emanates from muscles of mastication. Myogenous masticatory pains may be representative of the various types of muscle pain. Since the treatment for the different types of muscle pain is not the same, accurate differential

Oral and Facial Pain
DR. WELDEN E. BELL
8226 DOUGLAS AVENUE
DALLAS, TEXAS

Name: Female age 42

HISTORY

QUALITY	DURATION	LOCALIZATION	AFFECTED BY	LOCAL EFFECTS
(Mild) Severe	Bright (Dull)	(Continuous) (Diffuse) Localized	Face Movement Jaw Movement	Sensory: Hypesthesia Hyperesthesia Paresthesia Dysesthesia	Special Sense: Visual Auditory Olfactory Gustatory
Spontaneous Triggered (Induced) Paroxysmal (Steady)	Intermittent Recurrent Pricking Itching Burning Aching Pulsating	Radiating Spreading Momentary Minutes Hours Day long (Protracted)	Tongue Movement Swallowing Head Position Body Position Activities Tension Fatigue Time of Day		Enlarging Migrating Secondary Pain	Motor: Weakness Contraction Spasm	Autonomic: Ocular Signs Nasal Signs Cutaneous Signs Gastric Signs

Location
Inception
Initial pain
Duration, clinical course
Therapeutic response
Physical and emotional background
Trauma, infection, etc.
Medications in use

Recurrent episodes of mild continuous protracted steady dull aching pain diffusely located in the right auricular and preauricular area, induced by attempts to open the mouth beyond 22 mm, and preceded by progressive restriction of opening during painless as well as painful periods.

The complaint began about ten years ago as recurrent episodes of right "earache" lasting a few days and disappearing. She has been aware of some progressive restriction of opening she thinks was initiated by a painful experience of right joint dislocation about 25 years ago. Prior to that, she had "loose noisy joints". About two years ago, her ENT physician found the ears to be normal and suggested it was a right joint condition. Her physician has since treated her for arthritis periodically without significant change in the complaint. Recently, she had an episode of earache following minor dental treatment, so her dentist referred her for a TM joint examination. Presently, she takes no medications.

EXAMINATION

B/P 120/80   Neurological Survey   Psychological Survey

Oral
TM joints
Muscle system
Diagnostic blocks
Diagnostic drugs
Trial therapy

Orally: She presents no dental or oral cause for the pain. There is minor palpable tenderness of the right masseter muscle and increasing discomfort as she tries to open beyond 22mm. There is no pain with other movements. Her opening is restricted to 22mm with deflection to the right. Protrusive and lateral movements are within normal limits.

TM joints: Both joints appear to be structurally normal. There is restriction of right condylar movement with maximum opening, interpreted as indicative of contracture of the right masseter muscle. (See tracings.)

Muscle system: Moderate tenderness and shortening of the right masseter muscle.

Opinion: Recurrent mild myositis due to injudicious stretching of preexistent myofibrotic contracture of the right masseter muscle presumed to be related etiologically to an experience of painful dislocation of the right temporomandibular joint some 25 years ago. The contracture appears to be progressive.

DIAGNOSIS

Painful extraarticular adhesions that restrict mouth opening. (Muscle contracture involving the right masseter muscle.)

Case No. 10–5, A.—Case chart. Masticatory myalgia, expressed as inflammation of elevator muscles (inflamed myofibrotic contracture).

diagnosis is essential to effective therapy. The clinical differentiation of these types is as follows:

1. Protective splinting pain

Local muscle pain induced by actively contracting the muscle, usually accompanied by a feeling of weakness. Dysfunction con-

Temporomandibular Examination Radiographic Tracings DR. WELDEN E. BELL 8226 DOUGLAS AVENUE DALLAS, TEXAS	Name Female age 42 X-ray File No. Date	Key to Symbols POC Primary Occlusal Contact OP Occlusal Position RP Rest Position LP Contralateral Position MTO Maximum Translatory Opening PR Protrusive Position
Left T-M Joint	**Left** **Key** **Right** LP: 13 LP: 11 MTO: 17 MTO: 6 POC = OP = LP = - - - MTO = -·-·-	**Right T-M Joint**

INTERPRETATION

Both joints were viewed in four positions:
1. Primary occlusal contact (POC).
2. Fully occluded position (OP).
3. Contralateral excursion (LP).
4. Maximum opening -- 22mm (MTO).

Both joints present well defined smoothly contoured articular surfaces with interarticular spaces of adequate width which do not decrease in width under biting stress. There is no radiographic evidence of any degenerative joint disease or other structural abnormality.

There is excellent superimposition of POC and OP in both joints, indicative of no occlusal disharmony gross enough to cause radiographically visible displacement of either condyle when the teeth are fully occluded.

Translatory movement in the left joint is entirely normal. In the right joint, movement in LP is normal indicative of no capsular or intracapsular restriction of condyle movement. In MTO there is definite restriction of movement that is extraarticular in location. This is interpreted to represent shortening of an elevator muscle that is laterally situated in relationship to the right condyle -- namely, the masseter. By history, clinical course, and description of the present complaint, it is believed that these findings relate to preexistent myofibrotic contracture of the right masseter muscle presumed to be reactive to an experience of painful dislocation of the right joint some 25 years ago. The recurrent episodes of right auricular and preauricular pain appear to be due to mild myositis of this muscle induced by injudicious attempts to stretch it in order to open the mouth beyond 22mm interincisal distance.

Case No. 10-5, B.—Radiographic tracings of temporomandibular joints.

sists of the inhibitory influence of painful use and the sensation of weakness.

2. **Myofascial trigger point pain**
   Heterotopic pain felt elsewhere, expressed as referred pain or secondary hyperalgesia. Dysfunction consists of stiffness and weakness especially after periods of inactivity.
3. **Muscle spasm pain (pain-dysfunction syndrome)**
   Local muscle pain induced by contracting or stretching the muscle. May be accompanied by heterotopic pains. No pain is felt with passive movements. Dysfunction due to shortened or rigid muscle.

11

Temporomandibular Joint Pains

PAINS THAT EMANATE from the structures of the temporomandibular joint are of the deep somatic category. As such, they display the clinical characteristics of deep somatic pain. Additionally, they are of the musculoskeletal type and therefore display the features that identify such pains, namely (1) there is a strong relationship to the demands of function; (2) the pain is accentuated in a graduated manner by manual palpation or functional manipulation at the site of pain; and (3) subjective localization of the pain varies in accordance with the need for proprioceptive guidance to control and execute useful movements (Fig 11–1).

Arthralgic pain can arise only from pain-sensitive structures of the joint and its ligaments. Normally, the pressure-bearing articular surfaces as well as the articular disc are noninnervated and therefore are incapable of initiating sensory response of any kind, including nociception. Proprioceptive input needed for functional guidance does not come from the articular surfaces, but from proprioceptors located in the ligaments and muscles. Arthralgic pain that emanates from a nonarthritic temporomandibular joint must arise from structures that are innervated, namely, (1) the collateral discal ligaments that attach the articular disc to the medial and lateral poles of the mandibular condyle (Fig 11–2); (2) the retrodiscal tissue that lies between the disc and the posterior wall of the capsule (Fig 11–3); and (3) the joint capsule itself, which includes the strong temporomandibular (lateral) ligament that reinforces the lateral wall (Fig 11–4).[1] Therefore, depending on the structure from which the pain emanates, nonarthritic temporomandibular arthralgia may be identified as (1) disc-attachment pain, (2) retrodiscal pain, or (3) capsular pain—or some combination of the three. Arthritis comprises a fourth source of arthralgia which may be identified as arthritic pain.

It should be noted that most arthralgia is related to functional abuse and trauma which may be accompanied by inflammation. Thus, ar-

OROFACIAL PAIN SYNDROMES

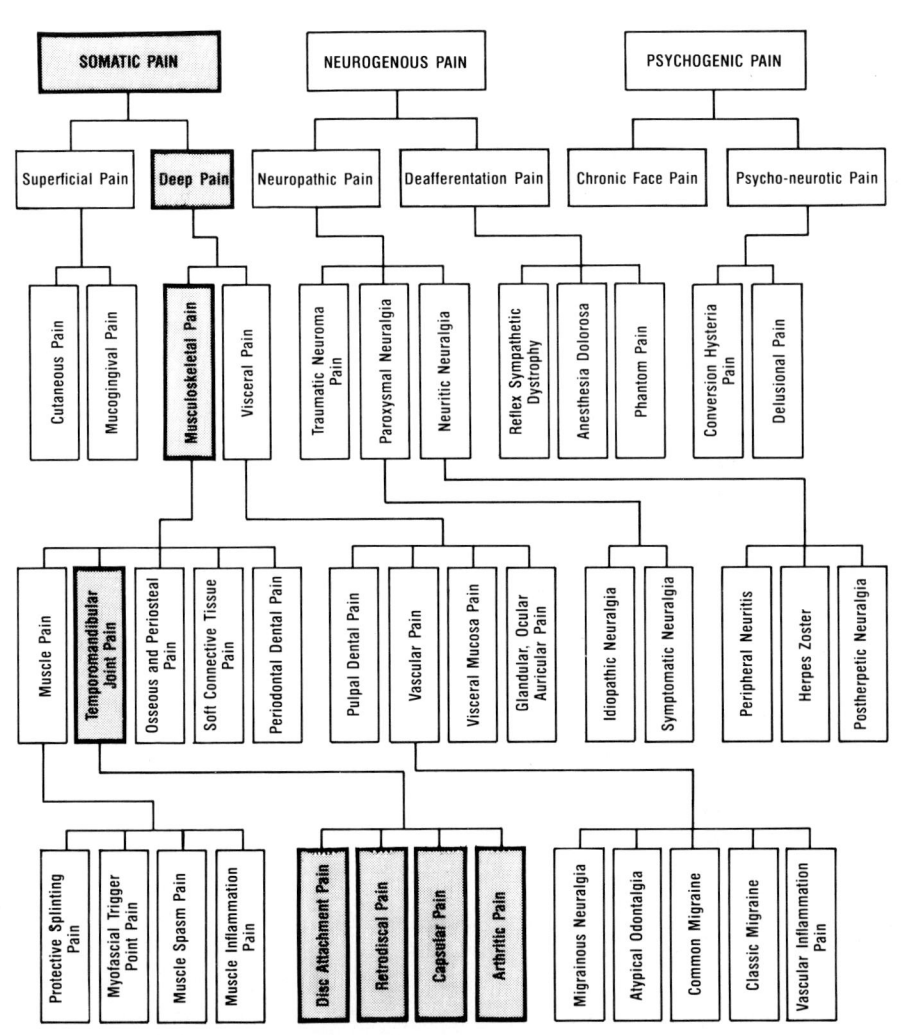

Fig 11–1.—Chart showing classification relationship of temporomandibular joint pains to other orofacial pain syndromes.

thralgia frequently displays clinical characteristics of inflammatory pain which are influenced by the location, degree, and phase of inflammation present. Such pains exhibit features that depend on local provocation and functional manipulation as well as on the extent and confinement of inflammatory exudate. As long as joint pain occurs

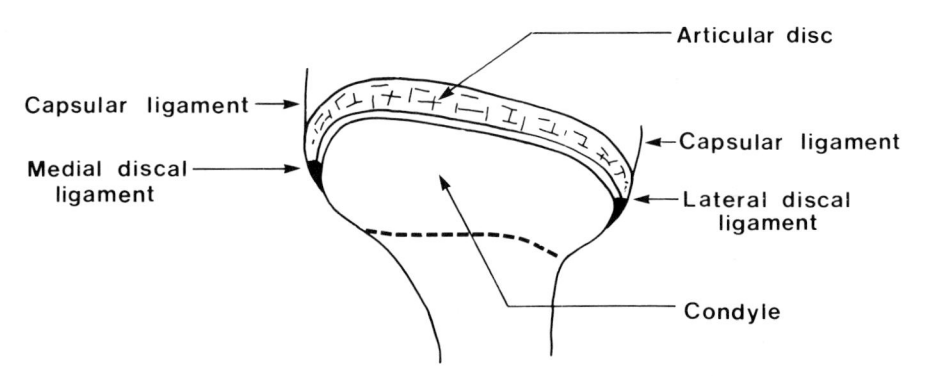

Fig 11–2.—Schematic representation of discal ligaments that attach articular disc to medial and lateral poles of mandibular condyle.

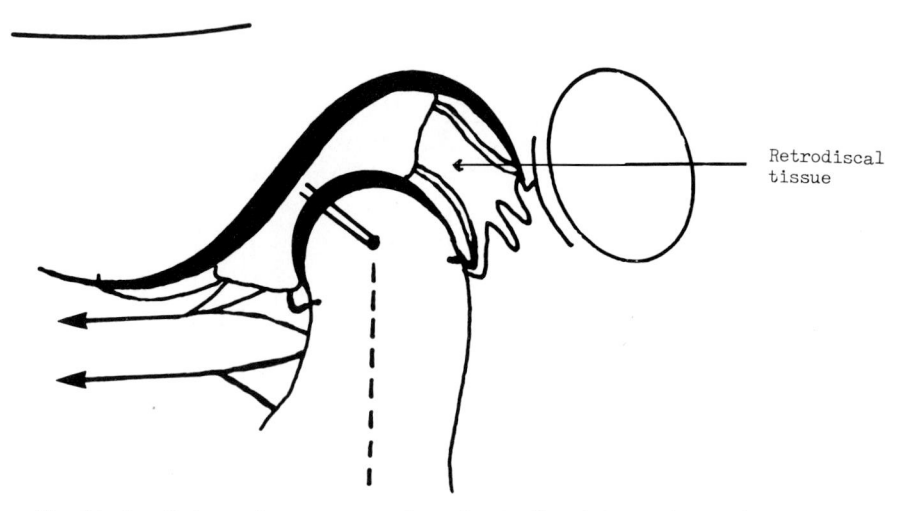

Fig 11–3.—Schematic representation of retrodiscal tissue located posterior to articular disc in the temporomandibular joint.

intermittently, it remains diffusely localized to the joint region and does not initiate secondary central excitatory effects. If arthralgia becomes continuous, however, a variety of secondary effects may become evident such as referred pains, headaches, secondary hyperalgesias expressed as areas of deep palpable tenderness, and spastic activity in the musculature.

The ligamentous structures of the joint (disc-condyle attachments, joint capsule, and temporomandibular ligament) are innervated for proprioceptive function. They therefore are particularly responsive to such biomechanical factors as pressure, traction, stress, strain, torque, and movement. If such mechanical influence becomes noxious, pain results.[2] It should be noted that both proprioceptive and nociceptive responses are dependent upon the presence of *normal* neural structures.[3] As ligamentous deterioration takes place, proprioceptive response, as well as pain, diminishes. It is a paradox that decreasing pain emanating from such structures may be indicative of a worsening condition of the ligaments from which it arises. It is important that this be kept in mind when evaluating the seriousness of joint pains. It should also be noted that proprioceptive responses are answered by skeletal muscle activity. Muscle splinting is a normal protective reaction of muscles in response to altered proprioceptive input. Therefore, muscle pain of the protective splinting type may accompany noxious biomechanical forces that affect the joint. Again, such response depends on *normal* innervation of the ligamentous structures of the joint. Acute muscle effects are indicative of normally functioning proprioceptors and therefore identify a lesser degree of deterioration in the ligaments. As deterioration takes place due to continued functional abuse and trauma, such muscle effects are less likely to occur.

It should be recognized that masticatory pain emanates from masticatory muscles, from pain-sensitive structures of the temporomandibular joints, or from both. Effective therapy depends on accurate identification of pain source. It is therefore of considerable importance that, not only should myalgia be distinguished from arthralgia, but, the type of myalgia or arthralgia be correctly identified. (For diagnostic criteria by which different kinds of muscle pain can be recognized,

Fig 11–4.—Schematic representation of outer oblique and inner horizontal portions of temporomandibular (lateral) ligament that reinforces the joint capsule laterally.

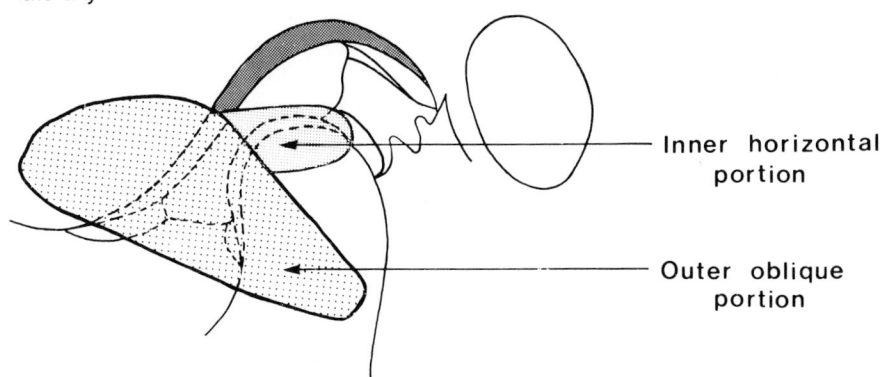

refer to chapter 10.) Arthralgia emanating from the temporomandibular joints may be classified as follows:
1. Disc attachment pain
2. Retrodiscal pain
3. Capsular pain
4. Arthritic pain

DISC ATTACHMENT PAIN

Normally, movements between condyle, articular disc, and eminence-fossa during mastication and speech are smooth, relatively silent, and painless. Strained or overextended excursions may cause interference. Hypermobile joints are noisy when opened too widely but less so when moved protrusively. The normal joint does not elicit pain unless interference is such that the ligamentous attachments that hold the disc to the lateral poles of the condyle are strained. When this occurs, pain is felt each time interference causes stress on these ligaments. As long as pain is intermittent, secondary effects of central hyperexcitability do not occur. When inflammation is sufficient to cause continuous pain, spreading to involve the capsule soon follows, and central excitatory effects may become evident.

The condyle-disc complex is a movable hinge joint. The complex proper is composed of compatible surfaces shaped to move in one plane only and restricted to hinge movement by the discal ligaments, which cause the disc to follow the condyle wherever it goes. This hinge movement is facilitated by the reciprocal action of the elastic superior retrodiscal lamina opposing the forward pull of the superior lateral pterygoid muscle. Any violation of simple hinge movement between disc and condyle may be damaging.

The condyle-disc complex operates against the eminence-fossa as a freely movable joint. Its movements are restricted only in the outer ranges. All movements therefore are permissible between disc and eminence.

The condyle, disc and eminence remain in sharp contact at all times by muscle tonus plus functional contraction. Displacement of the articulating parts constitutes dislocation.

Subluxation (partial dislocation) is displacement of the articular disc without loss of surface contact between the condyle, disc, and eminence and therefore without collapse of the articular disc space. Luxation (complete dislocation), in contrast, is displacement of the articular disc with loss of surface contact between the condyle, disc, and eminence with resulting collapse of the articular disc space. Apparent separations of the articulating parts as evidenced by radiographic widening of the articular disc space may occur during certain phases of joint action. Although seen as increased width of the interarticular space, sharp contact is maintained as a thicker portion of disc rotates into the "space." This intricate and essential disc action should be understood and appreciated, for it is the key to otherwise inexplicable functional problems of the temporomandibular joint.[4]

Normally the thinnest portion of the disc is centered on the condyle when the interarticular space is minimal, as during maximum intercuspation (so-called centric occlusion). Biting against a bolus of food depresses the condyle, widening the space. When this occurs, the disc is rotated anteriorly by the superior lateral pterygoid muscle, which contracts in conjunction with elevator muscle action. Thus, the thicker posterior part of the disc firmly fills the articular disc space, and adequate stability of the joint is maintained. Then, as the teeth bite through the bolus and the space narrows accordingly, the disc automatically rotates posteriorly, bringing the thinner portion of disc back into position. It becomes fully centered when maximum intercuspation is accomplished. As resting position is assumed, the space increases, with compensating rotation of the disc anteriorly as the result of muscle tonus in the resting superior lateral pterygoid muscle. This permits synovial fluid to bathe the surfaces from which it was expelled by pressure during the biting effort.

Subtle but essential disc rotatory movement is constantly going on. This is in addition to that necessary for keeping the upper surface of the disc in proper contact with the eminence during translatory movement as well as for gross separation of the jaws for opening. *The more steeply inclined the articular eminence, the greater the disc movement required for condylar translation.*

Sensations of interference and abnormal disc sounds relate chiefly to movement of roughened or irregular articular surfaces. Such roughening may result from malformation, trauma, abusive use, or degeneration. Disc interference pain relates chiefly to strain and inflammation of the discal ligaments, which resist abusive movements that tend to displace the disc from the condyle.

Damaged articular surfaces cause interference that tends to displace the disc. The sensations and noises thus generated depend on the location of the damage, the type and degree of surface change, the interarticular pressure present at the time, the velocity of movement, and the inclination of the articular eminence. Pain depends chiefly on the extent of displacement and on the condition of the neural structures that innervate the discal ligaments.

If interference is met during normal translatory movement of the condyle, it may be expressed as varying degrees of sensation, noise, and pain during opening-closing or excursive efforts. If the interference is great enough, jaw movement may be arrested. If compensatory jaw movements are developed to avoid such interference, deviations of the incisal path may be observed. As mentioned above, when the teeth are forced against a firm bolus of food, the effects differ from those of similar unobstructed movements. Interference therefore may be expressed differently.

As the teeth are occluded, translatory movement should cease as primary occlusal contact (so-called centric position) is reached. Any further movement would occur under increasing interarticular pressure, expelling the synovial fluid and permitting frictional attrition of the moving parts. Occlusal disharmony that induces movement in any direction after occlusion of the teeth is potentially damaging to the joint. Pain is felt with maximum intercuspation if disc displacement is great enough. Noise and sensations of interference may not occur until occlusal pressure is released. *Insidious damage to the articular surface may occur.*

Normally after maximum intercuspation, the occlusal pressure is released, allowing the interarticular space to widen. As the disc rotates to compensate for this increase, synovial fluid floods the moving parts and the joint is lubricated. If damaged or roughened, the disc may stick as a result of intercuspation, and the essential disc movement and synovial fluid action cannot take place—or do so too slowly to be efficient. The next translatory movement then begins with the disc dry and stuck. Rotation of the condyle is not resisted and therefore the teeth can be separated to some degree without any problem. But as condylar translation occurs, the discal ligaments tug the disc free. Noise and pain may thus be produced. This condition may be mistaken for *interference* during translatory movement, and the two must be differentiated since treatment is not the same.

As the result of occlusal disharmony or trauma, discal ligaments may deteriorate, and the articular disc may suffer damage. Such change may permit sliding movement between disc and condyle and therefore may predispose to displacement of the disc during normal functional movements. Deterioration in the disc posteriorly predisposes to anterior displacement; deterioration in the disc anteriorly predisposes to posterior displacement. As long as such functional displacement constitutes only subluxation (partial dislocation without collapse of the articular disc space), jamming of the disc may take place with symptoms of interference, noise, pain, locking, or a combination. The timing of such symptoms relative to mouth opening depends on the extent of damage in the joint. Early opening symptoms are indicative of less damage, and discrete symptoms, pain, and muscle splinting may be displayed. Later opening symptoms are usually indicative of more extensive damage, but with it, less discrete symptoms, less discomfort, and fewer muscle effects. If disc jamming is sufficient to arrest jaw movement during the opening effort, so-called closed-lock may be exhibited. If the jamming occurs during the closing effort, so-called open-lock may be evident.

If functional displacement is sufficient to permit luxation (loss of contact of the parts with collapse of the articular disc space), jamming of the disc cannot occur, and discrete symptoms therefore are not displayed. Instead, the symptoms are those of irregular movement and more or less continuous, mild, grating noise, as well as retrodiscitis and a sensation of overstressed ipsilateral posterior teeth when clenched in maximum intercuspation. If the dislocated disc blocks forward movement of the condyle, reduction is impossible, and the dislocation will remain protracted. Posterior dislocations, however, are automatically reduced by the next closing movement of the jaw.[1]

It should be noted that symptoms of disc jamming due to functional displacement occur in response to forces applied to the disc during translatory movements. These forces are (1) anterior traction exerted by the superior lateral pterygoid muscle, and (2) posterior traction exerted by the superior retrodiscal lamina. An understanding of the action of these forces during translatory movements of the condyle is essential to the identification and management of disc interference disorders of the temporomandibular joint.[1]

Pain emanating from the ligamentous attachments of the articular disc to the mandibular condyle is caused by noxious stimulation of those structures. This may be due to external violence. It may result from intrinsic stress and tension on the attachments as they attempt to prevent dislodgment or displacement of the disc from the condyle when discal obstruction takes palce. The term *discitis* is used to describe this condition. It does not imply that the entire disc is inflamed—only the discal attachments, which are innervated and vascularized. The disc proper has no vessels to sustain an inflammatory reaction and no nerve fibers to relay sensation. If pain emanates from the articular disc it must come from the discal attachments. External violence may cause detachment of one or both attachments, thus interfering with normal disc functioning. Intrinsic injury may result from abusive chewing habits, especially if there is already some degenertive change in the disc proper.

Discitis may result from functional obstruction of the disc during translatory movements. Impingement tends to dislocate it from the condyle, causing strain and injury to the attachments. When acute and painful, discitis may spread to involve the capsule also, giving symptoms of capsulitis as well. When less acute, pain occurs only when actual obstruction takes place. This may happen with extended movements, during the course of ordinary translatory movements or as the teeth are firmly occluded. When discal pain occurs in occlusal position as a result of occlusal disharmony, it is appreciably decreased by biting on a tongue blade, which prevents intercuspation (Case No. 11–1).

Radiographically, evidence is available to demonstrate the effect of arrested condylar movement (Figs 11–5 and 11–6). If gross degenerative change has taken place in the articular disc, the radiographic articular disc space may be seen to decrease in width under biting stress (Fig 11–7). If occlusal disharmony is sufficiently gross and occurs in the sagittal plane, it may be visualized radiographically if a precise technique is used (Figs 11–8 and 11–9). Overriding fragments of a fractured articular disc may show a widened articular disc space, while collapse of the disc space may show near contact of the condyle and articular eminence. Tomographic projection is needed to accurately confirm judgments relative to the articular disc space.

The clinical symptoms by which disc attachment pain can be recognized are as follows:
1. The pain occurs intermittently in conjunction with clinically evident disc interference of some type.
2. Pain that occurs in conjunction with occlusal disharmony when the teeth are clenched in maximum intercuspation is reduced by biting against a separator that prevents intercuspation of the teeth.
3. Pain that occurs in conjunction with condylar translatory movements relates specifically to one of the following etiologic groups of disc-interference disorders[1]:
    (a) Excessive passive interarticular pressure.
    (b) Structural incompatibility between the sliding parts.
    (c) Impaired disc-condyle complex function.
4. Protective muscle splinting may be displayed.
5. Dysfunction in the form of interference during mandibular movements is characteristic. If such interference is sufficient to arrest condylar movement, dysfunction in the form of restricted mandibular movement is displayed.
6. Ordinarily, central excitatory effects are not seen. (If the discal ligaments become inflamed, the clinical characteristics of cap-

Temporomandibular Joint Pains

Oral and Facial Pain
DR. WELDEN E. BELL
8226 DOUGLAS AVENUE
DALLAS, TEXAS

Name: Female age 45

HISTORY

QUALITY	DURATION	LOCALIZATION	AFFECTED BY	LOCAL EFFECTS
Mild ✓	Bright	Continuous	Localized		Sensory:	Special Sense:
Severe ✓	*Dull* ✓	*Intermittent* ✓	*Diffuse* ✓	Face Movement	Hypesthesia ✓	Visual ✓
		Recurrent		*Jaw Movement* ✓	Hyperesthesia	Auditory
			Radiating	Tongue Movement	Paresthesia ✓	Olfactory ✓
Spontaneous			Spreading	Swallowing	Dysesthesia ✓	Gustatory
Triggered	Pricking	Momentary		Head Position		
Induced ✓	Itching	*Minutes* ✓	Enlarging	Body Position	Motor:	Autonomic:
	Burning	Hours ✓	Migrating	Activities	Weakness ✓	Ocular Signs
Paroxysmal	*Aching* ✓	Day long		Tension	Contraction ✓	Nasal Signs
Steady ✓	Pulsating	Protracted	Secondary Pain	Fatigue	Spasm ✓	Cutaneous Signs
				Time of Day		Gastric Signs

Location
Inception
Initial pain
Duration, clinical course
Therapeutic response
Physical and emotional background
Trauma, infection, etc.
Medications in use

Mild to severe intermittent steady dull aching pain diffusely located in the right preauricular area, induced by clenching the teeth, and lasting from a few minutes to an hour or longer. The pain is accompanied by sensations of interference and disc noise especially associated with occluding the teeth firmly.
The complaint began about six months ago. On day while chewing, she bit down firmly and sensed a locking of the right joint. As she opened, it popped very loudly and she felt severe sharp pain in the TM area. The noise and pain have occurred with firmly occluding the teeth ever since. Prior to this, she had noisy TM joints with chewing for several years. She remembers no pain or sensations of functional interference, however. She presently has no complaint of restriction of mandibular movements or any recent alteration in her "bite".
She is taking no medications of any kind.

EXAMINATION

B/P 135/80 **Neurological Survey**   **Psychological Survey**

Oral
TM joints
Muscle system
Diagnostic blocks
Diagnostic drugs
Trial therapy

Orally: She is dentally and orally negative for cause of pain except clinical evidence of occlusal disharmony indicated by sensing premature contact of the right bicuspid teeth, a feeling of increased pressure on those teeth in the fully occluded position, and some movement from primary contact to the full occlusal position. She feels right preauricular pain when she clenches the teeth and this is accompanied by a "binding sensation". As she releases the teeth, moderate right disc noise is heard. All this is readily prevented by biting on a tongue blade. Otherwise, masticatory functioning is clinically normal.
TM joints: Both joints present evidence of degenerative change in the articular discs. There is evidence of occlusal disharmony that is interpreted as chronic and likely etiologic. (See tracings.)
Muscle system: No palpable tenderness in the masticatory muscles. All functioning appears to be well within normal limits.

Opinion: The patient appears to have had some minor occlusal disharmony for several years of which she was entirely unaware. Very likely as a result of this, degenerative change has occurred in both articular discs, indicated by "noisy joints" with chewing. A few months ago, she accidentally impinged the right disc with sufficient force to injure its attachments to the condyle, thus causing the symptoms of acute discitis.

DIAGNOSIS

Acute discitis of the right TM joint, due to intrinsic injury.

Case No. 11–1,A.—Case chart. Temporomandibular arthralgia, expressed as disc attachment pain, due to acute discitis.

192   OROFACIAL PAINS

Temporomandibular Examination
Radiographic Tracings

DR. WELDEN E. BELL
8226 DOUGLAS AVENUE
DALLAS, TEXAS

Name __Female age 45__

X-ray File No._____

Date_____

Key to Symbols
POC   Primary Occlusal Contact
OP   Occlusal Position
RP   Rest Position
LP   Contralateral Position
MTO   Maximum Translatory Opening
PR   Protrusive Position

Left T-M Joint

Left	**Key**	Right
LP: 11		LP: 11
MTO: 15		MTO: 14

POC = ─────
OP = ·········
LP = ─ ─ ─ ─
MTO = ─ · ─ ·

Right T-M Joint

INTERPRETATION

Both joints were viewed in five positions, four transparietal, one transfacial:
1. Primary occlusal contact (POC).
2. Fully occluded position (OP).
3. Contralateral excursion (LP).
4. Maximum opening -- 42mm (MTO).
5. Transfacial in protrusive position.

Both joints present well defined smoothly contoured articular surfaces. The interarticular spaces are of minimal width and both decrease in width under biting stress, indicative of degenerative change in the articular discs. This appears to be greater in the right than the left.

There is lack of superimposition of POC and OP in both joints, there being a radiographically visible displacement of both condyles anteriorly when the teeth are firmly occluded. The displacement appears greater in the right than in the left. This is evidence of occlusal disharmony and since it appears to be wholly unconscious it is interpreted as chronic and perhaps etiologic.

Translatory movement in LP and MTO is entirely normal in both joints.

Case No. 11–1,B.—Radiographic tracings of temporomandibular joints.

Temporomandibular Examination
Radiographic Tracings

DR. WELDEN E. BELL
8226 DOUGLAS AVENUE
DALLAS, TEXAS

Name __Female age 52__

X-ray File No._____

Date_____

Key to Symbols
POC   Primary Occlusal Contact
OP   Occlusal Position
RP   Rest Position
LP   Contralateral Position
MTO   Maximum Translatory Opening
PR   Protrusive Position

Left T-M Joint

Left	**Key**	Right
LP: 10		LP: 10
MTO: 16		MTO: 14

OP = ─────
LP = ─ ─ ─ ─
MTO = ─ · ─ ·

Right T-M Joint

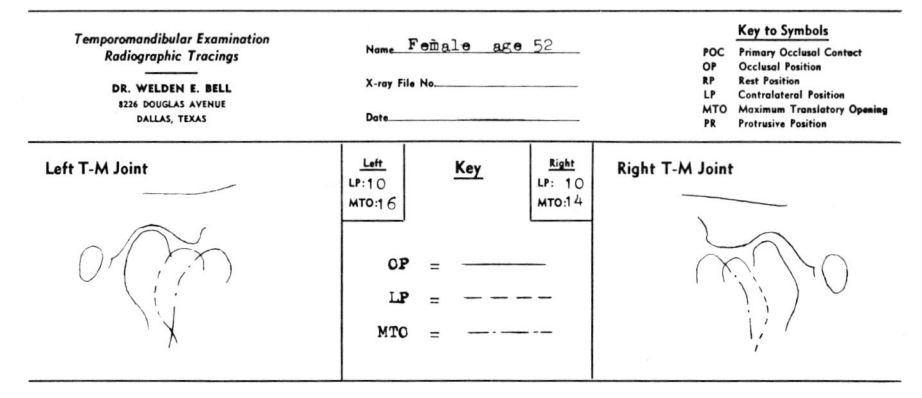

Fig 11–5.—Tracings from temporomandibular radiographs in occlusal position (OP), contralateral excursion (LP), and open position (MTO) to illustrate normal translatory movement of condyles. Note that in LP, the movement is adequate (10 mm or more) and bilaterally symmetric. In MTO it exceeds that of LP and is bilaterally symmetric.

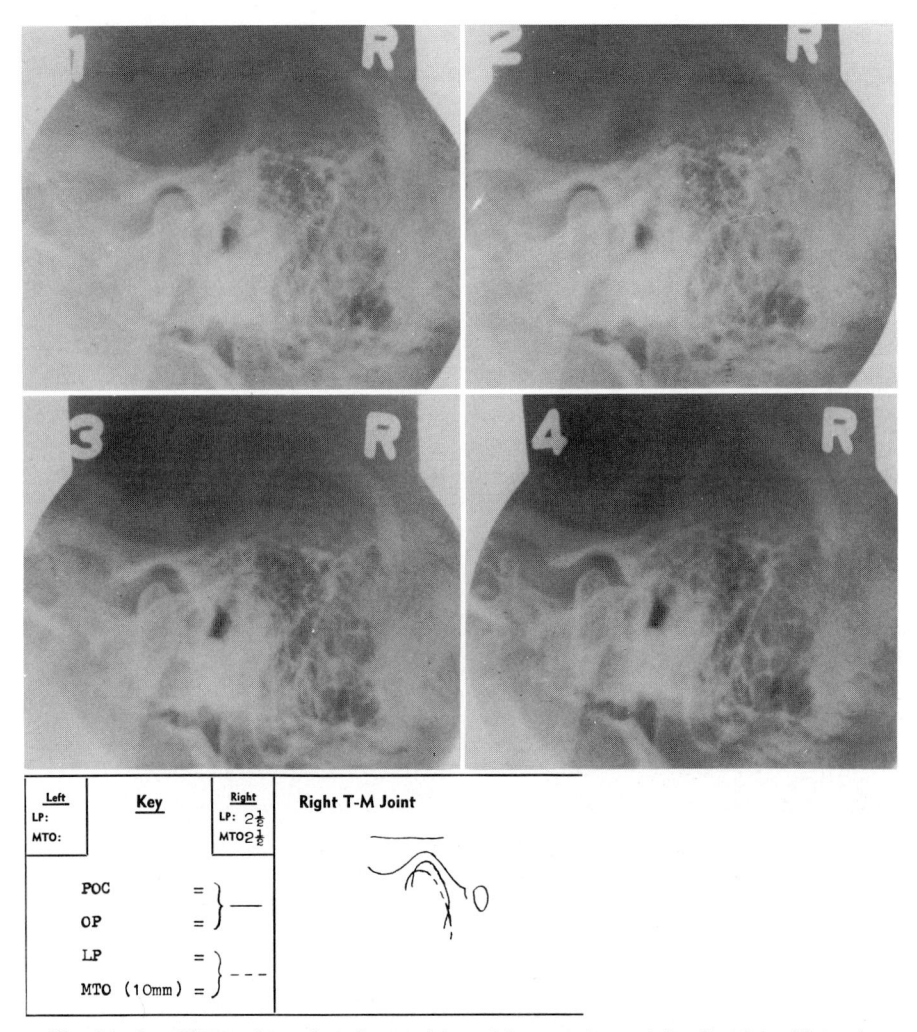

Fig 11-6.—Illustration of radiographic evidence of condylar fixation. Note that condyle fails to move appreciably in either LP or MTO but remains close to OP. *Top,* radiographs of right temporomandibular joint in POC (**1**), OP (**2**), LP (**3**), and MTO (**4**). *Bottom,* radiographic tracings show severe restraint of condylar movement in both LP and MTO.

194 OROFACIAL PAINS

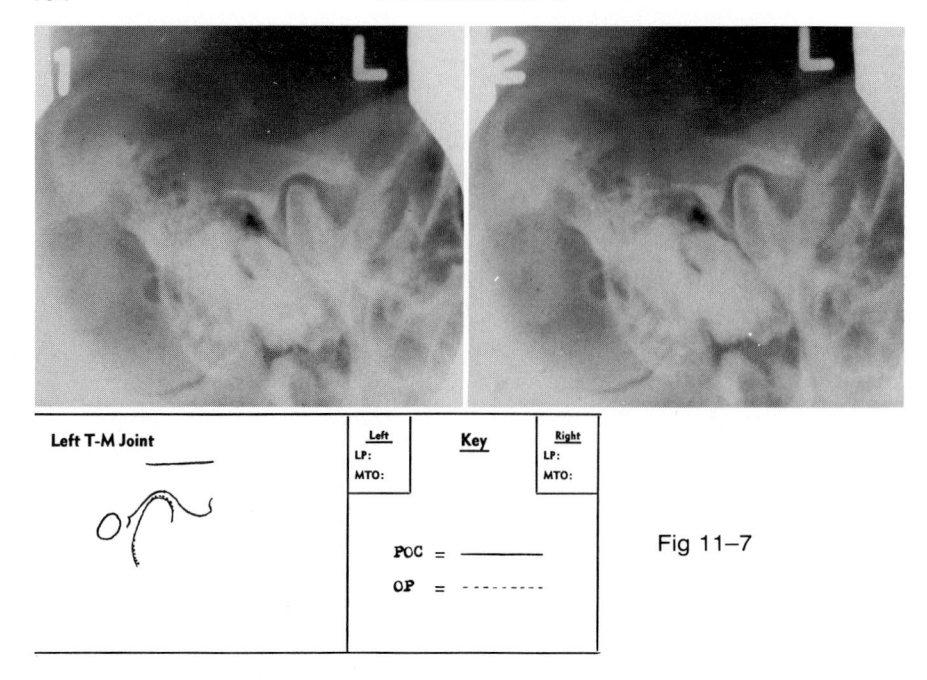

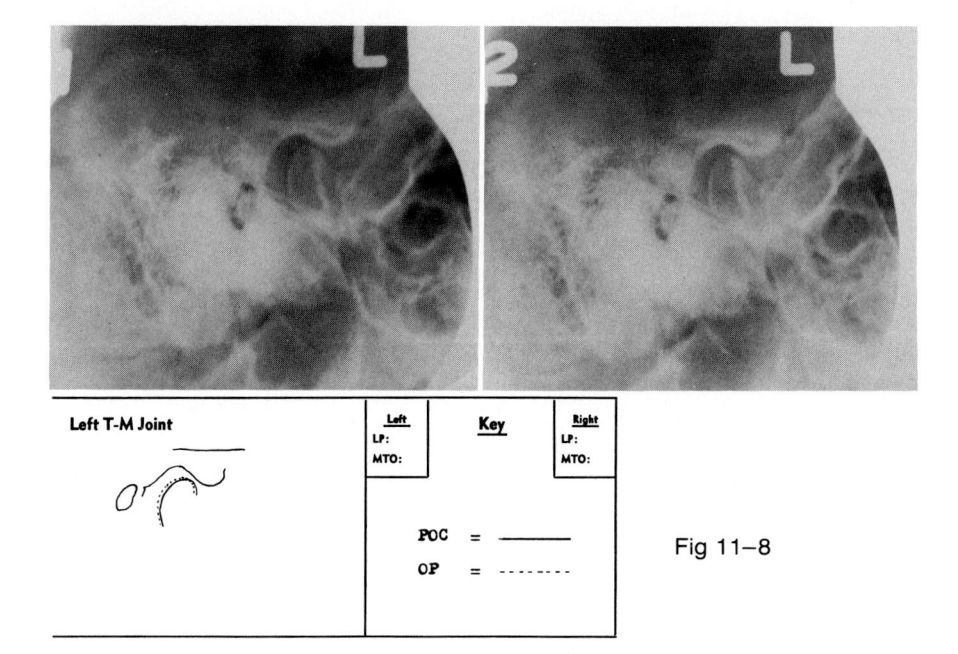

Fig 11–7

Left T-M Joint

Key
Left LP: MTO:
Right LP: MTO:

POC = ———
OP = - - - - - -

Fig 11–8

Left T-M Joint

Key
Left LP: MTO:
Right LP: MTO:

POC = ———
OP = - - - - - -

TEMPOROMANDIBULAR JOINT PAINS 195

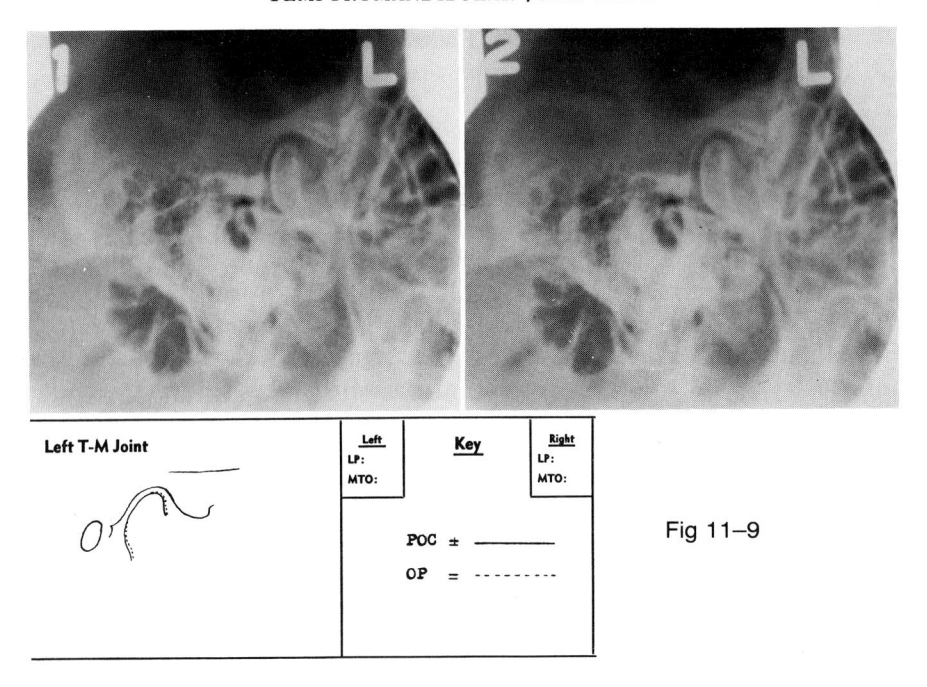

Fig 11-9

Fig 11-7.—Illustration of radiographic evidence of degenerative change in the articular disk. Note decrease in width of interarticular space under biting stress (OP) compared with that of primary occlusal contact (POC). *Top*, radiographs of left temporomandibular joint in POC (**1**) and OP (**2**). *Bottom*, radiographic tracings show change in interarticular space width.

Fig 11-8.—Illustration of radiographic evidence of condylar displacement that could represent either acute (symptomatic) or chronic (etiologic) occlusal disharmony. Note that condylar position when teeth are fully occluded (OP) is posterior to that of primary occlusal contact (POC). In acute disharmony, the POC position is displaced. In chronic disharmony, the OP is displaced. *Top*, radiographics of left temporomandibular joint in POC (**1**) and OP (**2**). *Bottom*, radiographic tracings show condylar displacement.

Fig 11-9.—Illustration of radiographic evidence of occlusal disharmony sufficient to grossly displace condyle anteriorly when teeth are firmly occluded. Note that condyle position in fully occluded position (OP) is anterior to that of primary occlusal contact (POC). *Top*, radiographs of left temporomandibular joint in POC (**1**) and OP (**2**). *Bottom*, radiographic tracings show condylar displacement in fully occluded position.

OROFACIAL PAINS

Oral and Facial Pain
DR. WELDEN E. BELL
8226 DOUGLAS AVENUE
DALLAS, TEXAS

Name Female age 46

HISTORY

QUALITY	DURATION	LOCALIZATION	AFFECTED BY	LOCAL EFFECTS
(Mild) Severe	Bright (Dull)	Continuous (Intermittent) Recurrent	(Localized) (Diffuse)	Face Movement (Jaw Movement) Tongue Movement Swallowing Head Position Body Position Activities Tension Fatigue Time of Day	Sensory: Hypesthesia Hyperesthesia Paresthesia Dysesthesia Motor: (Weakness) Contraction Spasm	Special Sense: Visual Auditory Olfactory Gustatory Autonomic: Ocular Signs Nasal Signs Cutaneous Signs Gastric Signs
Spontaneous Triggered (Induced) Paroxysmal (Steady)	Pricking Itching Burning (Aching) Pulsating	Momentary Minutes Hours Day long Protracted	Radiating Spreading Enlarging Migrating Secondary Pain		

Location. Mild intermittent steady dull aching pain diffusely located in the left preauricular area induced by clenching the teeth and accompanied by acute

Inception
Initial pain malocclusion described as premature contact of the right anterior teeth with disocclusion of the posteriors unless forced into full occlusion.

Duration, clinical course The complaint began a week ago following an automobile accident in which she sustained a heavy blow to the right chin. Radiographs failed to identify a

Therapeutic response mandibular fracture. Being suspicious of an unidentified fracture because of the malocclusion, the oral surgeon placed arch bars and intermaxillary elastics

Physical and emotional background to bring the teeth into normal occlusion. In doing so, however, pain increased until it became intolerable, so he removed the intermaxillary elastics and

Trauma, infection, etc. referred the patient for a TM joint examination.

Medications in use No medications are presently in use.

EXAMINATION

B/P 130/80 **Neurological Survey** **Psychological Survey**

Oral
TM joints
Muscle system
Diagnostic blocks
Diagnostic drugs
Trial therapy

Orally: There is no dental or oral cause for the complaint other than the obvious malocclusion. Deep tenderness in the left joint is sensed with heavy manual palpation and this increases considerably with forced occlusion of the teeth. There is slight discomfort with maximum opening and extended lateral and protrusive movements and the patient senses a feeling of muscular weakness with these movements as well as with attempting to fully occlude the teeth. The occlusal position pain is prevented by biting on a tongue blade to keep the teeth separated. There is no discomfort with eccentric biting or with manually straining the mandible as long as the teeth are slightly separated.

TM joints: Both joints appear to be normal structurally. The left condyle is displaced anteriorly in primary occlusal contact position, interpreted as due to inflammatory swelling of the left retrodiskal pad (retrodiskitis). (See tracings.)

Muscle system: There is no palpable discomfort in any masticatory muscle and no muscular dysfunction of any kind.

Analgesic blocking of the left lateral pterygoid muscle did not arrest the occlusal position pain, confirming that it is not of muscle origin.

Opinion: It is presumed that the blow on the chin forced the left condyle posteriorly and traumatized the retrodiskal pad. The resulting inflammatory swelling displaces the condyle forward and pain results when forced occlusion causes the condyle to press against the inflamed pad.

DIAGNOSIS

Acute retrodiskitis of the left TM joint, traumatic.

Case No. 11-2,A.—Case chart. Temporomandibular arthralgia, expressed as retrodiscal pain, due to trauma.

as further degeneration of the tissue takes place. Retrodiscitis is sometimes improperly referred to as a "posterior capsulitis."

It should be noted that since the retrodiscal tissue is not responsive proprioceptively, protective muscle splinting effects do not occur. Also, the pain is frequently intermittent and therefore does not induce sec-

Temporomandibular Examination Radiographic Tracings	Name Female age 46	Key to Symbols
DR. WELDEN E. BELL	X-ray File No.	POC Primary Occlusal Contact
8226 DOUGLAS AVENUE		OP Occlusal Position
DALLAS, TEXAS	Date	RP Rest Position
		LP Contralateral Position
		MTO Maximum Translatory Opening
		PR Protrusive Position

Left T-M Joint	Left LP: 12 MTO: 17	Key	Right LP: 14 MTO: 18	Right T-M Joint
		POC = ————		
		OP = - - - - -		
		LP = — — —		
		MTO = — · —		

INTERPRETATION

Both joints were viewed in five positions, four transparietal, one transfacial:
1. Primary occlusal contact (POC).
2. Fully occluded position (OP).
3. Contralateral excursion (LP).
4. Maximum opening — 45mm (MTO).
5. Transfacial in protrusive position.

Both joints present well defined smoothly contoured articular surfaces with interarticular spaces of adequate width which do not decrease in width under biting stress. There is no radiographic evidence of any degenerative joint disease or traumatic effect to the osseous structure. The left mandibular ramus and condyle appear to be normal in all respects.

There is excellent superimposition of POC and OP in the right joint. In the left, there is lack of such superimposition indicative of occlusal disharmony of gross proportions. Considering the history, clinical course, and present behavior of the complaint, this disharmony is interpreted as acute in type and represents anterior displacement of the condyle in primary occlusal contact position rather than a displaced attitude of the condyle in the fully occluded position. In the absence of evidence that the displacement is due either to osseous fracture or contraction of the left lateral pterygoid muscle, it is concluded that the condylar displacement is due to inflammatory swelling of the retrodiscal pad or so-called "retrodiscitis".

Translatory movement in LP and MTO is normal in both joints.

Case No. 11–2,B.—Radiographic tracings of temporomandibular joints.

ondary central excitatory effects. Acute retrodiscitis from trauma, however, may induce referred pain and secondary myospastic activity in the masticatory muscles.

The clinical symptoms by which retrodiscal pain can be recognized are as follows:
1. The pain is accentuated by clenching the teeth in maximum intercuspation.
2. Such pain is decreased by biting against a separator that prevents intercuspation of the teeth.
3. The pain is accentuated by forced ipsilateral excursive movement of the mandible.
4. Pain is not induced by resisted protrusion of the mandible.

5. Dysfunction is displayed as acute malocclusion in the resting occluded position. This consists of disocclusion of the ipsilateral posterior teeth with premature occlusion of the contralateral anterior teeth, or disocclusion of the ipsilateral posterior teeth with premature occlusion of the contralateral posterior teeth, or both.
6. Secondary central excitatory effects may be displayed.

CAPSULAR PAIN

Capsular pain results from inflammation of the synovial and fibrous capsules, synovitis and capsulitis. To distinguish between the two is difficult if not impossible clinically. Pain occurs when the inflamed capsule is stretched by translatory movement of the condyle. It is accentuated therefore by protrusion, contralateral excursion, and opening widely. There is palpable tenderness directly over the condyle and sometimes fluctuant swelling as well. Although acute capsulitis may cause restriction in the outer ranges of condylar movement due to swelling, most masticatory dysfunction results only from the inhibitory influence of pain.

Synovitis causes (1) swelling due to effusion within the joint cavity, (2) discomfort with joint movements, and (3) alteration of the synovial fluid. The increased intracapsular fluid may induce a measure of acute malocclusion. In more chronic form, gelation of the synovial fluid may alter joint movements and cause some stiffness, especially after periods of inactivity. This may be accompanied by peculiar joint sounds. Such symptoms usually decrease as normal activity is resumed. Synovitis may result from localized trauma, abusive use, toxemias, specific infection, or as an allergic response. It frequently occurs as a manifestation of arthritis.

Capsulitis may result from acute trauma or from intrinsic strains that injure the capsular ligament (Case No. 11–3). A common cause has to do with inflammatory conditions of the discal ligaments and the temporomandibular ligament as the result of occlusal disharmony that tends to displace the articular disc from the condyle. Bruxism combined with such occlusal disharmony is an important activating factor. Capsulitis may result from habits that entail excessive mandibular movements and from abusive joint hypermobility.

Inflammatory conditions of the capsule may cause varying degrees of capsular fibrosis which may restrict the outer ranges of condylar movement. This condition can be visualized radiographically (Fig 11–10). Ordinarily, capsular fibrosis is entirely painless. If forced by ex-

Oral and Facial Pain

DR. WELDEN E. BELL
8226 DOUGLAS AVENUE
DALLAS, TEXAS

Name Female age 20		Age	Date	
QUALITY	DURATION	LOCALIZATION	AFFECTED BY	LOCAL EFFECTS
(Mild) Severe	Bright **(Dull)**	**(Continuous)** Intermittent Recurrent	Localized **(Diffuse)**	Face Movement Jaw Movement Tongue Movement Swallowing Head Position Body Position Activities Tension Fatigue Time of Day	Sensory: Hypesthesia Hyperesthesia Paresthesia Dysesthesia	Special Sense: Visual Auditory Olfactory Gustatory
Spontaneous Triggered Induced Paroxysmal **(Steady)**	Pricking Itching Burning **(Aching)** Pulsating	Momentary Minutes Hours Day long **(Protracted)**	Radiating Spreading Enlarging Migrating Secondary Pain		Motor: **(Weakness)** Contraction Spasm	Autonomic: Ocular Signs Nasal Signs Cutaneous Signs Gastric Signs

HISTORY

Location
Inception
Initial pain
Duration, clinical course
Therapeutic response
Physical and emotional background
Trauma, infection, etc.
Medications in use

Mild continuous protracted steady dull aching pain diffusely located in the left preauricular area described as deep tenderness to pressure over the left condyle that increases considerably with opening beyond 30mm as well as with extended protrusive and contralateral excursions. There is no complaint of restricted mandibular movements, interference with movements, or acute malocclusion.
    The complaint began about three weeks ago following a volley-ball accident in which she received a sharp blow on the left mandible. She thinks her mouth was partly open at the time. The blow was painful and after 24 hours the left TM joint became acutely sore and slightly swollen. All jaw use was painful and difficult for several days. Then it subsided to about as presently described. When the complaint persisted, she consulted her dentist who promptly referred her for a TM joint examination.
    No medications are presently being taken.

B/P 120/80   Neurological Survey   Psychological Survey

EXAMINATION

Oral

TM joints

Muscle system

Diagnostic blocks

Diagnostic drugs

Trial therapy

Orally: There is no dental or oral cause for the pain nor any evidence of injury to the dentition. She has deep tenderness to pressure over the left condyle. The discomfort increases with all condyle movements that tend to stretch the capsule. She has a feeling of muscular weakness with these movements and they may be slightly inhibited by pain but there is no identifiable occlusal disharmony or masticatory dysfunction of any kind.
    TM joints: Both joints are radiographically normal structurally and functionally except for slight decrease in amplitude of translatory movement in the left joint, interpreted as the effect of pain inhibition. (See tracings.)
    Muscle system: There is no palpable tenderness in any masticatory muscle and no muscular dysfunction.
    Analgesic blocking of the left lateral pterygoid muscle did not arrest the pain, confirming that the discomfort was not muscular.
    Opinion: By history, clinical course, and the present behavioral characteristics of the complaint, it is presumed that the left capsular ligament was traumatized by the blow causing acute immobilizing capsulitis which has now subsided to a subacute nonimmobilizing stage.

DIAGNOSIS

Subacute capsulitis of the left TM joint, traumatic.

Case No. 11–3,A.—Case chart. Temporomandibular arthralgia, expressed as capsular pain, due to trauma.

cessive condylar movement, however, acute capsulitis may result (Case No. 11–4).

Since capsular pain is more or less continuous, some secondary central excitatory effects may be induced. This may be manifested as

Temporomandibular Examination Radiographic Tracings DR. WELDEN E. BELL 8226 DOUGLAS AVENUE DALLAS, TEXAS	Name _Female age 20_ X-ray File No. Date	Key to Symbols POC Primary Occlusal Contact OP Occlusal Position RP Rest Position LP Contralateral Position MTO Maximum Translatory Opening PR Protrusive Position

Left T-M Joint	Left LP: 11 MTO: 13	Key	Right LP: 13 MTO:15	Right T-M Joint

POC = ⎫
OP = ⎭ _____
LP =   - - - -
MTO =   — - —

INTERPRETATION

Both joints were viewed in five positions, four transparietal, one transfacial:
1. Position of primary occlusal contact (POC).
2. Fully occluded position (OP).
3. Contralateral excursion (LP).
4. Maximum opening — 45mm (MTO).
5. Transfacial in protrusive position.

Both joints present well defined smoothly contoured articular surfaces with interarticular spaces of adequate width which do not decrease in width under biting stress. There is no radiographic evidence of any degenerative joint disease or other osseous abnormality or traumatic effect.

There is excellent superimposition of POC and OP in both joints, indicative of no occlusal disharmony gross enough to cause radiographically identifiable displacement of either condyle when the teeth are firmly occluded.

Translatory movements are well within normal limits in both joints in LP and MTO. It appears that such movements in the left joint are slightly less than in the right, interpreted as the influence of pain inhibition.

Case No. 11–3,B.—Radiographic tracings of temporomandibular joints.

referred pain including headache, areas of heterotopic deep palpable tenderness, and secondary myospastic activity in masticatory muscles.

The clinical symptoms by which capsular pain can be recognized are as follows:
1. Palpable tenderness directly over the condyle.
2. Sometimes palpable fluctuant swelling over the joint proper.
3. The pain is accentuated by translatory movements that stretch the capsule.
4. There is no increase in pain by clenching the teeth, nor is there any alteration in pain by biting against a separator.
5. Dysfunction occurs in the form of restricted mandibular movement, especially in extended ranges. Most restriction is due to the inhibitory influence of pain. Joint stiffness and strange joint sounds may occur during the first few movements following pe-

Temporomandibular Joint Pains 203

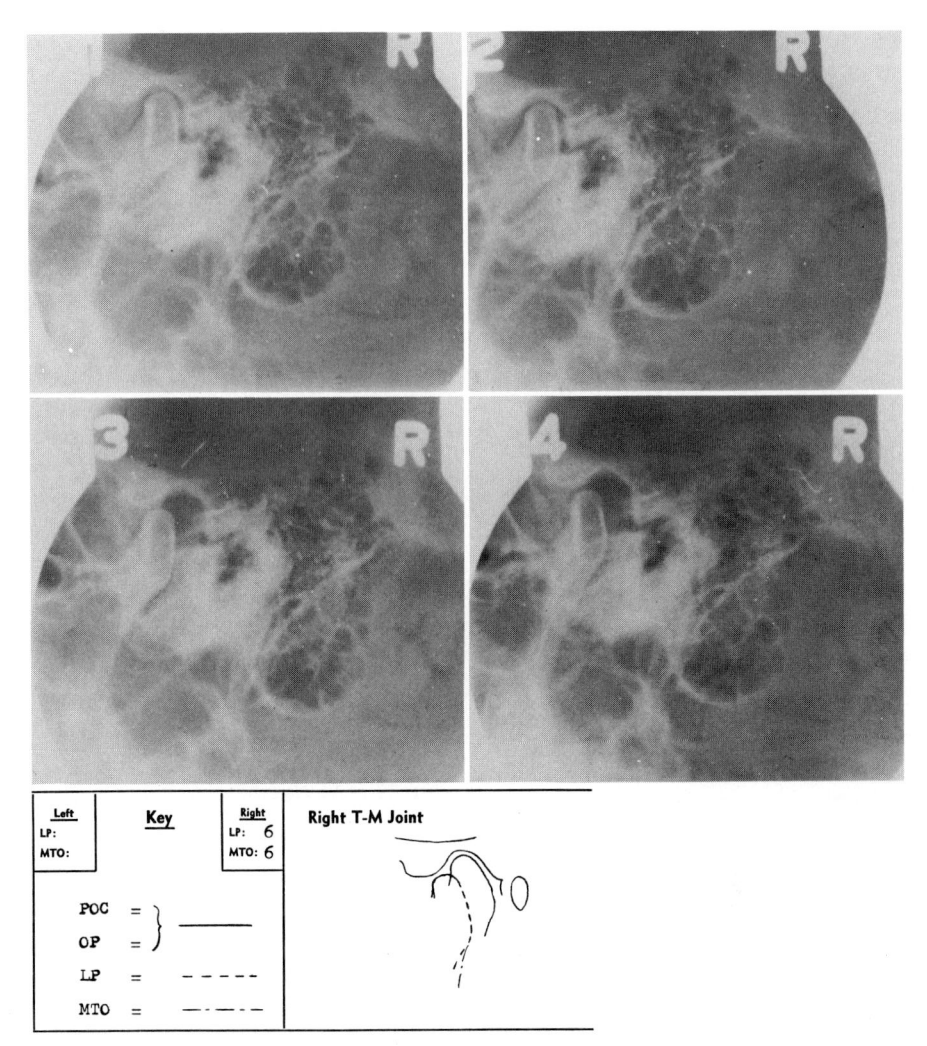

Fig 11–10.—Illustration of radiographic evidence of capsular restraint on condylar movement. Note that condyle moves along upper articular surface to a point definitely short of crest of articular eminence and that this point of restraint is the same in both LP and MTO. *Top*, radiographs of right temporomandibular joint in POC (**1**), OP (**2**), LP (**3**), and MTO (**4**). *Bottom*, radiographic tracings show restriction of condylar movement in both LP and MTO short of articular eminence. (From Bell W.E.: Management of temporomandibular joint problems, in Goldman H.M., Gilmore H.W., Royer R.Q., et al. (eds.): *Current Therapy in Dentistry.* St. Louis, C.V. Mosby Co., 1970, Vol. 4. Reproduced with permission.)

Name	Female age 46			Age	Date	Oral and Facial Pain DR. WELDEN E. BELL 8226 DOUGLAS AVENUE DALLAS, TEXAS
	QUALITY		DURATION	LOCALIZATION	AFFECTED BY	LOCAL EFFECTS

HISTORY

QUALITY		DURATION	LOCALIZATION	AFFECTED BY	LOCAL EFFECTS	
(Mild)	Bright	(Continuous)	Localized	Face Movement	Sensory:	Special Sense:
Severe ✓	(Dull)	Intermittent	(Diffuse)	(Jaw Movement)	Hypesthesia	Visual
		(Recurrent)		Tongue Movement	Hyperesthesia	Auditory
			Radiating	Swallowing	Paresthesia	Olfactory
Spontaneous			Spreading	Head Position	Dysesthesia	Gustatory
Triggered	Pricking	Momentary		Body Position		Autonomic:
(Induced)	Itching	Minutes	Enlarging	Activities	Motor:	Ocular Signs
	Burning	Hours	Migrating	Tension	Weakness	Nasal Signs
Paroxysmal	(Aching)	Day long		Fatigue	Contraction	Cutaneous Signs
(Steady)	Pulsating	(Protracted)	Secondary Pain	Time of Day	Spasm	Gastric Signs

Location
Inception
Initial pain
Duration, clinical course
Therapeutic response
Physical and emotional background
Trauma, infection, etc.
Medications in use

Mild to severe recurring episodes of continuous protracted steady dull aching pain diffusely located in the left preauricular area, induced by forceful or prolonged opening of the mouth, and aggravated by jaw use.
The complaint appears to relate to moderate restriction of opening (about 32mm interincisal distance) which dates from a childhood injury. The present pain complaint began about six months ago following extensive dental treatment that required extended and prolonged opening of the mouth. This was immediately followed by soreness in the left joint area and acute pain with opening fully. The discomfort has been recurrently present ever since, each episode depending on the amount and type of force used to open the mouth beyond her "normal". Her physician has treated her with systemic as well as local injection of corticosteroid medications with only transitory benefit. He then advised "correction of her bite" by her dentist. Finding no occlusal disharmony, he referred her for a temporomandibular joint examination.

B/P 125/80   Neurological Survey   Psychological Survey

EXAMINATION

Oral
TM joints
Muscle system
Diagnostic blocks
Diagnostic drugs
Trial therapy

Orally: Three first molar teeth are missing and the spaces moderately closed leaving considerable mutilation of the dentition, but there is no occlusal disharmony clinically or radiographically identified. She feels sharp pain in the left TM area with opening beyond 28mm and dull tenderness with protrusive and contralateral movements. Opening is restricted to 32mm with slight deflection to the left. Protrusive and contralateral movements appear to be adequate.
TM joints: Both joints appear to be normal structurally and the right joint functionally. There is restriction of left condylar movement that is interpreted as capsular, presumed to be due to preexistent capsular fibrosis or contracture, probably of traumatic origin. (See tracings.)
Muscle system: Essentially negative for cause of pain.

Opinion: Capsular fibrosis has no doubt restricted left condylar movements for many years. When strained by excessive and prolonged opening incidental to required dental treatment, the capsule became inflamed and episodes of capsulitis have continued ever since.

DIAGNOSIS

Painful adhesions that restrict condyle movements. (Capsular fibrosis)

Case No. 11–4,A.—Case chart. Temporomandibular arthralgia, expressed as capsular pain, due to inflamed capsular fibrosis.

riods of inactivity. Acute malocclusion may occur as the result of increased intracapsular fluid.
6. Secondary central excitatory effects may be displayed.

Temporomandibular Examination Radiographic Tracings DR. WELDEN E. BELL 8226 DOUGLAS AVENUE DALLAS, TEXAS	Name Female age 46 X-ray File No. Date	Key to Symbols POC Primary Occlusal Contact OP Occlusal Position RP Rest Position LP Contralateral Position MTO Maximum Translatory Opening PR Protrusive Position

Left T-M Joint	Left LP: 8 MTO: 8	Key	Right LP: 11 MTO: 15	Right T-M Joint

POC = ⎫
OP = ⎬ ─────
LP =   - - -
MTO =   — · —

INTERPRETATION

Both joints were viewed in four positions:
1. Position of primary occlusal contact (POC).
2. Fully occluded position (OP).
3. Contralateral excursion (LP).
4. Maximum opening -- 32mm (MTO).

Both joints present well defined smoothly contoured articular surfaces with interarticular spaces of adequate width which do not decrease in width under biting stress. There is no radiographic evidence of any degenerative joint disease.

There is excellent superimposition of POC and OP in both joints, indicative of no occlusal disharmony gross enough to cause radiographically visible displacement of either condyle when the teeth are firmly occluded.

Translatory movement in LP and MTO is normal in the right joint. In the left, however, both LP and MTO movements are restricted uniformly at a point short of the crest of the articular eminence. This is interpreted as capsular restraint. From the history of painless moderate restriction of opening since a childhood injury, it is presumed to represent capsular fibrosis. The acute painful phase should, therefore, represent capsulitis.

Case No. 11–4,B.—Radiographic tracings of temporomandibular joints.

ARTHRITIC PAIN

Inflammation of the articular surfaces of the joint is termed *inflammatory arthritis*. Normally these surfaces are nonvascularized so that an inflammatory reaction cannot occur. They are also noninnervated so that painful sensation cannot be felt. In order for the joint surfaces to become inflamed, fundamental arthropathic change must occur. Such change may be due to trauma—termed *traumatic arthritis*. It can occur as a result of proliferation of inflamed synovial membrane onto the articular surfaces—termed *rheumatoid arthritis*. It can occur as a result of degeneration of the avascular fibrous tissue that normally constitutes the articular surfaces. When degenerative changes proceed until this tissue no longer is protective, the underlying innervated and vascularized osseous tissue may become exposed to the effects of movement, attrition, and articular pressures, thus becoming inflamed. This is termed *degenerative joint disease* (degenerative arthritis or osteoarthritis).

Inflamed articular surfaces are the source of persistent though variable arthralgia. Although usually felt as a dull aching sensation, sometimes it is described as persistent burning pain. The irritation of occlusal pressure usually increases the discomfort, but sometimes the pressure of clenching the teeth temporarily relieves the pain. Usually pain is increased by chewing food and by all movements that press upon, rub, or irritate the inflamed articular surface.

If the inflammation is acute and widespread, the capsule may become involved so that symptoms of capsulitis are added—pain with movements, swelling of the joint, and palpable tenderness over joint proper. Lesser degrees of inflammation may be accompanied by little or no gross dysfunction other than interference with mandibular movements expressed as discal noise and sensations of altered movements. As acute inflammation occurs and functioning of the joint is decreased due to pain inhibition, inflammatory exudate, or secondary muscle effects, the former noninflammatory dysfunction symptoms may decrease or subside. This effect is presumably due to restraint of condylar movements. If intracapsular edema occurs, some sensation of acute malocclusion may be sensed. This is described as premature occlusion of the teeth on the opposite side. Pain may accompany forceful occlusion of the teeth when such inflammatory edema causes malocclusion. If osseous resorption decreases the vertical height of the mandibular ramus, some occlusal disharmony may be sensed, described as overstressing of the posterior teeth. When this occlusal disharmony is advanced, clinical evidence of progressive anterior open-bite may result (Fig 11–11).

Radiographic evidence of inflammatory arthritis may be variable. Prior to gross structural change, rheumatoid arthritis may present some loss of definition of the osseous articular surfaces suggestive of diffuse surface resorption bilaterally (Fig 11–12). Although not diagnostic, this appearance is sufficient to warrant medical investigation of the possibility of rheumatoid arthritis. Advanced rheumatoid arthritis may present gross bizarre resorption of bone (Fig 11–13). Such changes do not necessarily relate functionally to the clinical symptoms. Fibrous ankylosis may be identified. The inhibitory effect of pain also may be recorded as restriction of mandibular movements.

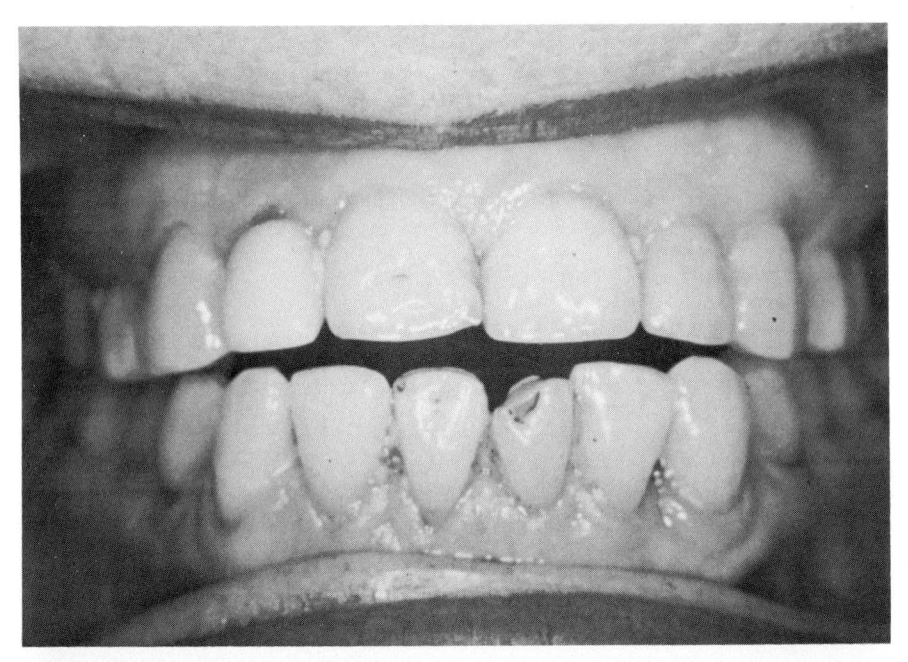

Fig 11-11.—Progressive anterior open-bite due to osseous change in temporomandibular joints as a result of advanced rheumatoid arthritis in a woman aged 49. (From Bell W.E.: Management of temporomandibular joint problems, in Goldman H.M., Gilmore H.W. Royer R.Q., et al. (eds.): *Current Therapy in Dentistry*. St. Louis, C.V. Mosby Co., 1970, vol. 4. Reproduced with permission.)

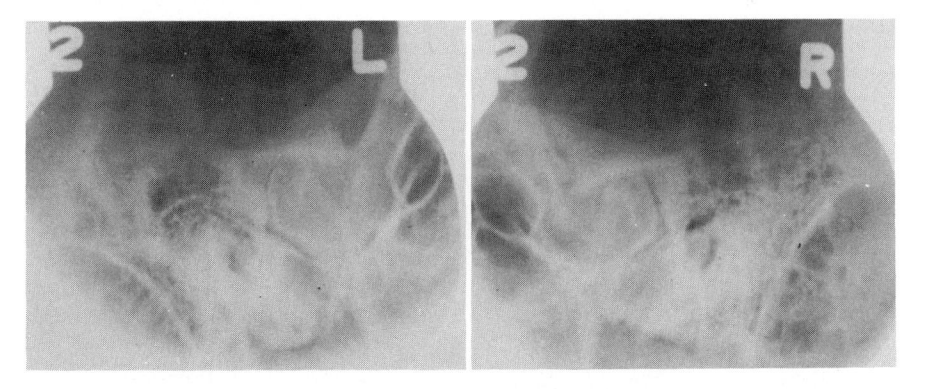

Fig 11-12.—Radiographs of temporomandibular joints of patient with early rheumatoid arthritis. Note lack of definition of osseous surfaces bilaterally.

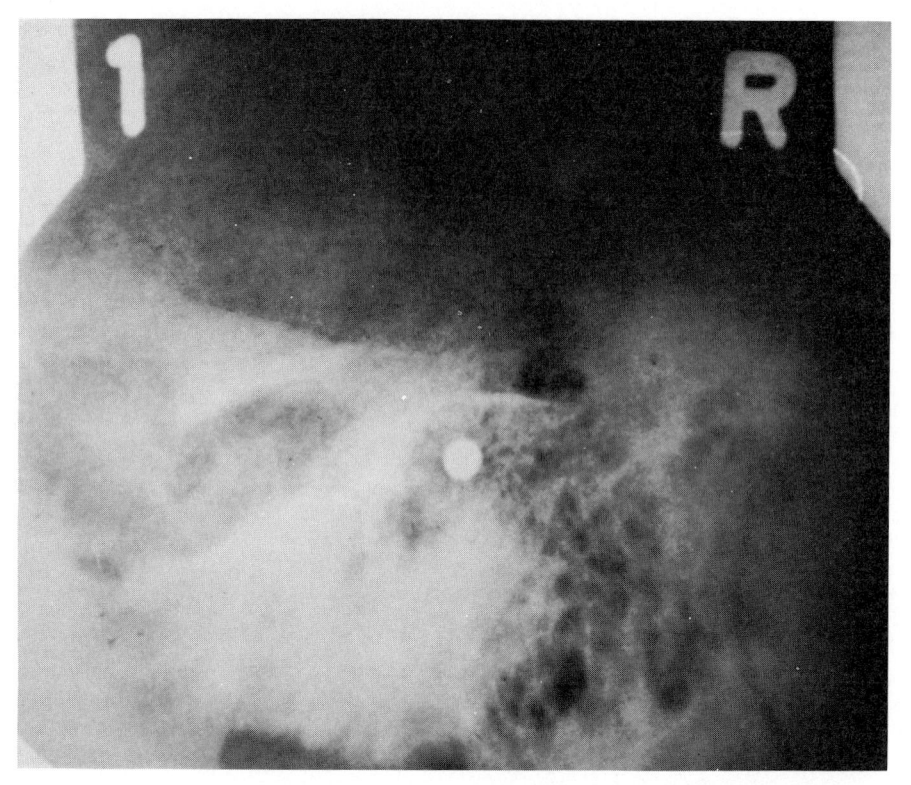

Fig 11–13.—Radiograph of temporomandibular joint with advanced rheumatoid arthritis (see Fig 11–11). Note bizarre osseous resorption that reduces vertical height of mandibular ramus, causing malocclusion, clinically observed as progressive anterior open-bite.

Degenerative joint disease may show little or no radiographic evidence in the early phase. Degenerative changes in the articular disc may sometimes be identified as a decrease in the width of the radiographic interarticular space under biting stress. This is done by comparing the width of the space in primary occlusal contact with the fully occluded position. Degenerative disc changes also may be observed as a significantly narrow interarticular space, especially when the tomographic method is used. As degenerative changes in the osseous surfaces occur, alterations in contour may become evident radiographically. These changes may be identified as flattened paralleled surfaces (Fig 11–14), anterior lipping (Fig 11–15), loss of definition indicative of active osseous resorption (Fig 11–16), or gross change in condylar form (Fig 11–17).

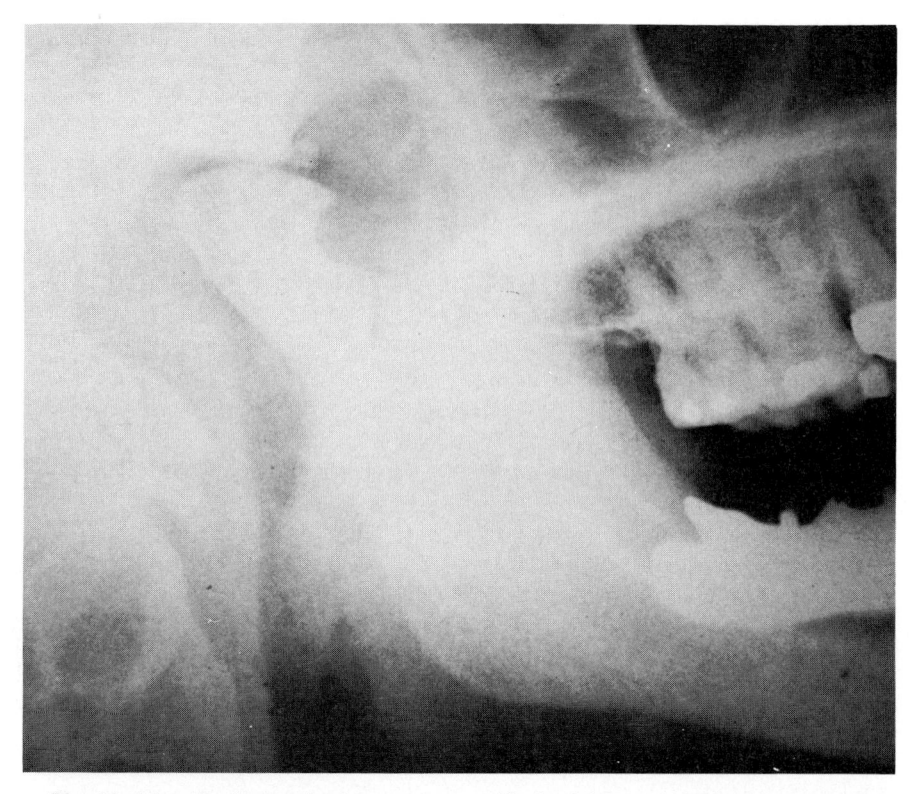

Fig 11-14.—Radiograph of temporomandibular joint undergoing degenerative change expressed as flattening and paralleling of osseous surfaces.

Traumatic arthritis may present similar radiographic changes. In addition, some evidence of former trauma such as malposition due to fracture may be seen (Fig 11-18). Other changes are condylar hyperplasia and malformation (Fig 11-19).

In acute inflammatory arthritis, intracapsular edema sufficient to cause gross occlusal disharmony may be identified as a widened interarticular space in primary occlusal contact position compared with the fully occluded position. If inflammatory swelling immobilizes the joint, restriction of condylar movements will be observed radiographically. Restriction of condylar movement due to disc jamming and the inhibitory influence of pain may also be observed (Case No. 11-5).

Periarticular inflammation that envelops the joint may cause swelling, pain, and immobilization of the joint, the severity of symptoms depending on the degree, extent, location, and phase of the inflammatory reaction. *Both rheumatoid arthritis and hyperuricemia may*

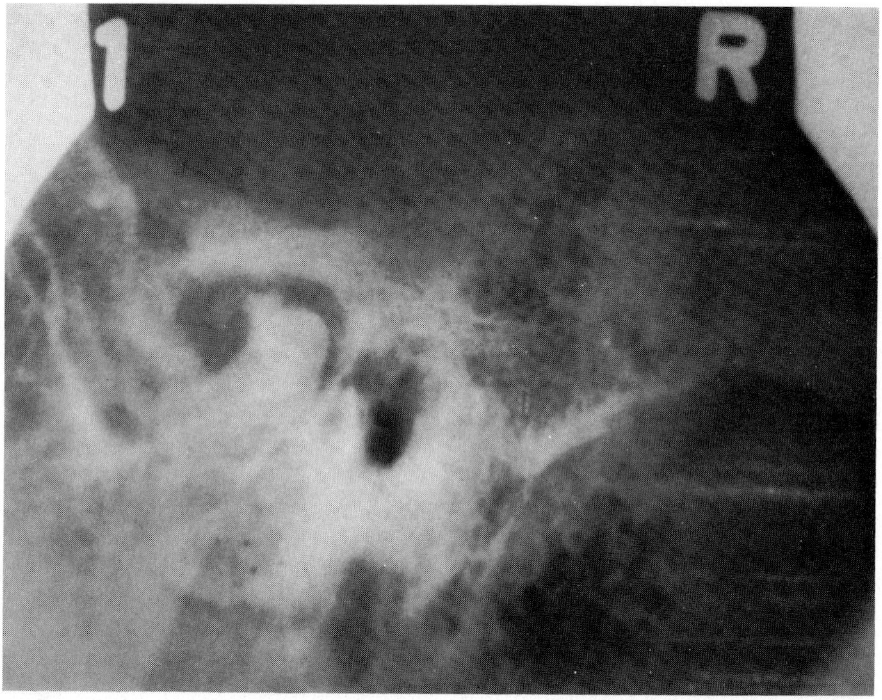
1
R

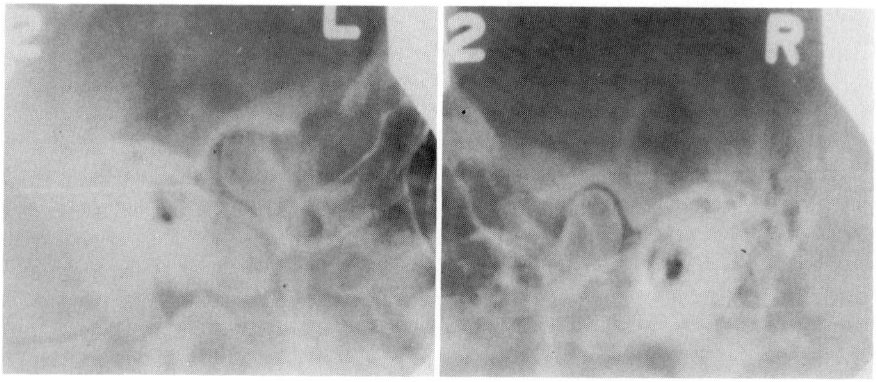
L
2
R

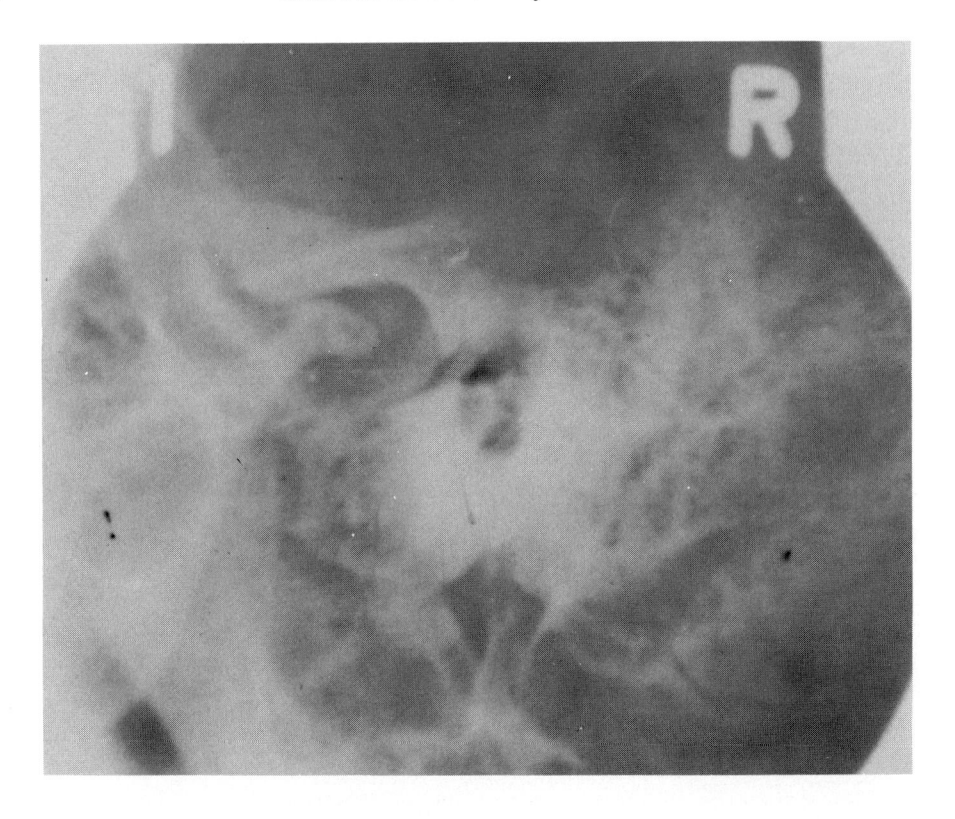

Fig 11–15 (top left page).—Radiograph of a temporomandibular joint with advanced degenerative joint disease. Note irregular articular surfaces and anterior lipping of condylar surface.

Fig 11–16 (bottom left page).—Radiographic appearance of osseous change in left temporomandibular joint due to advanced degenerative joint disease in a woman aged 45. Right joint is not affected. (From Bell W.E.: Management of temporomandibular joint problems, in Goldman H.M., Gilmore H.W., Royer R.Q., et al. (eds.): *Current Therapy in Dentistry.* St. Louis, C.V. Mosby Co., 1970, vol. 4. Reproduced with permission.)

Fig 11–17 (above).—Radiograph of temporomandibular joint exhibiting marked deformation as result of degenerative joint disease.

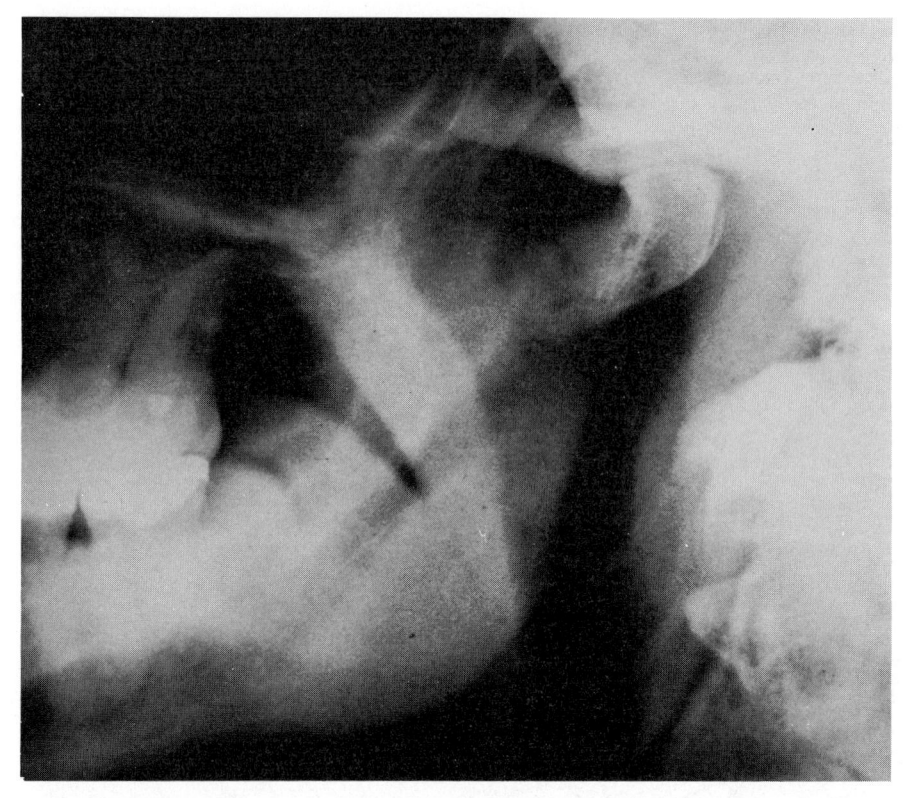

Fig 11–18.—Radiograph of temporomandibular joint with traumatic arthritis due to former injury. Malposition of condyle shows evidence of formerly fractured mandible.

so involve the temporomandibular joints. When periarticular inflammation occurs without other obvious local cause, the examiner should consider the possibility of these causes (Case No. 11–6).

Periarticular inflammation may occur as a result of trauma or by direct extension from another contiguous inflammatory process such as otitis media. Under such circumstances the cause should be so obvious as to present no diagnostic problem. If the injury or infection penetrates the capsule, acute inflammatory or infectious arthritis may follow, and the condition may terminate as a chronic mandibular hypomobility.

In periarticular inflammations, the joints appear normal radiographically except for possible restriction of translatory movement due either

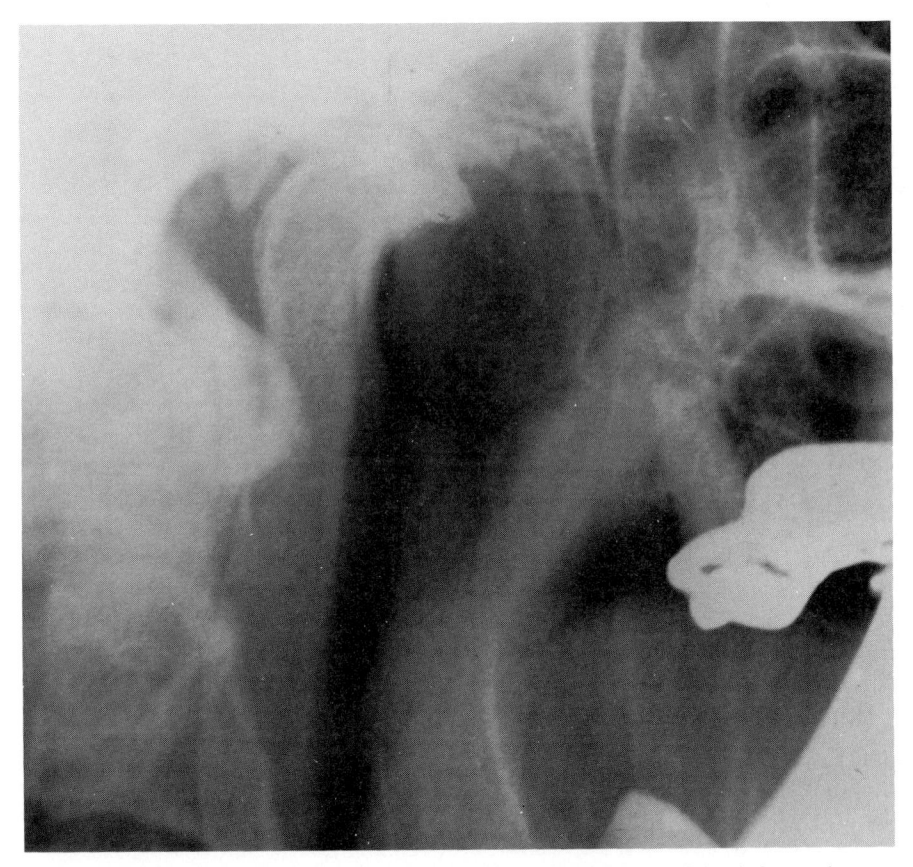

Fig 11–19.—Transfacial radiograph of left mandibular condyle deformed as result of former injury.

to the inflammatory exudate or to the inhibitory influence of inflammatory pain.

As the result of periarticular and articular inflammation, scar tissue may form around the joint, in the fibrous capsule or between the joint surfaces, depending on location of the inflammatory process. Such fibrosis, contracture, or adhesions restrict condylar movements, depending on location and extent of cicatrization. As long as the mandibular movements do not exceed the limitations thus imposed, these conditions usually remain painless. As such, they are classified as chronic mandibular hypomobilities. If the adhesions are injured by straining or applying force to move the mandible beyond such limitations, the adhesions may become inflamed and painful.

Oral and Facial Pain
DR. WELDEN E. BELL
8226 DOUGLAS AVENUE
DALLAS, TEXAS

Name: Male age 61

HISTORY

QUALITY	DURATION	LOCALIZATION	AFFECTED BY	LOCAL EFFECTS
(Mild) Severe	Bright **(Dull)**	**(Continuous)** Intermittent Recurrent	Localized **(Diffuse)**	Face Movement **(Jaw Movement)** Tongue Movement Swallowing Head Position Body Position Activities Tension Fatigue Time of Day	Sensory: Hypesthesia Hyperesthesia Paresthesia Dysesthesia Motor: **(Weakness)** Contraction Spasm	Special Sense: Visual Auditory Olfactory Gustatory Autonomic: Ocular Signs Nasal Signs Cutaneous Signs Gastric Signs
Spontaneous Triggered Induced Paroxysmal **(Steady)**	Pricking Itching Burning **(Aching)** **(Pulsating)**	Momentary Minutes Hours Day long **(Protracted)**	Radiating Spreading Enlarging Migrating Secondary Pain			

Location
Inception
Initial pain
Duration, clinical course
Therapeutic response
Physical and emotional background
Trauma, infection, etc.
Medications in use

Mild to severe continuous protracted steady dull aching and throbbing pain diffusely located in the right preauricular area, accompanied by tenderness and slight swelling over the TM joint and marked restriction of all jaw movements. The pain is aggravated by clenching the teeth, opening, chewing, and talking. Recent malocclusion has been sensed.
The complaint began after an episode of extraordinary chewing about two weeks ago. Prior to that, the right joint was asymptomatic. For a few days, he noticed mild stiffness and vague discomfort in the right TM joint, gradually increasing in severity. After a week, the swelling, localized pain, fixation of the joint, and the sensation of acute malocclusion occurred and these symptoms have remained much the same ever since. Antibiotics prescribed by his physician have not controlled the complaint.
No medications are presently in use other than simple analgesics.

EXAMINATION

B/P 160/90   Neurological Survey   Psychological Survey

Oral

TM joints

Muscle system

Diagnostic blocks

Diagnostic drugs

Trial therapy

Orally: The teeth and mouth are clinically and radiographically negative for cause of pain except that there is subjective occlusal disharmony described as a sensation of premature contact of the right teeth with slight disocclusion of the left. Pain increases when he attempts to fully occlude the teeth. This is reduced by insertion of a tongue blade on either side to prevent intercuspation. There is slight swelling over the right condyle and acute palpable tenderness both directly over the condyle and intraaurally. Pain increases with all joint movements and there is described a feeling of muscular weakness when he moves the mandible. Opening is restricted to about 26mm and deflects to the right. Protrusion is restricted and deflects to the right. Left lateral excursion is almost nil.
TM joints: The left joint appears to be normal. The right joint presents evidence of degenerative changes, preexistent occlusal disharmony, intracapsular edema, and inflammation. (See tracings.)
Muscle system: Essentially negative except for minor tenderness and weakness presumed to represent the inhibitory influence of pain.
Opinion: Radiographic evidence of preexistent degenerative changes in the articular discs, especially the right, with non-symptomatic preexistent occlusal disharmony should represent the predisposing factors present. The acute activating cause was no doubt the extraordinary chewing episode. As a result, acute inflammatory changes of the joint have occurred.

DIAGNOSIS

Degenerative joint disease with acute inflammatory arthritis of the right joint.

Case No. 11–5,A.—Case chart. Temporomandibular arthralgia, expressed as arthritic pain, due to inflammatory degenerative joint disease.

Painful fibrous ankylosis presents clinical symptoms of acute inflammatory arthritis with condylar immobilization. It will be noted that when the acutely painful condition resolves, clinical and radiographic evidence of preexistent fibrous ankylosis remains (Case No. 11–7).

Temporomandibular Examination Radiographic Tracings	Name __Male age 61__	Key to Symbols
DR. WELDEN E. BELL	X-ray File No. _____	POC Primary Occlusal Contact
8226 DOUGLAS AVENUE		OP Occlusal Position
DALLAS, TEXAS	Date _____	RP Rest Position
		LP Contralateral Position
		MTO Maximum Translatory Opening
		PR Protrusive Position

Left T-M Joint	Left LP: 12 MTO: 9	Key	Right LP: 3 MTO: 3	Right T-M Joint
		POC ━━━━		
		OP ┈┈┈┈		
		LP ╌╌╌╌		
		MTO ━ ━ ━		

INTERPRETATION

Each joint was viewed in four transparietal positions:
1. Position of primary occlusal contact (POC).
2. Fully occluded position (OP).
3. Contralateral excursion (LP).
4. Maximum opening - 26mm (MTO).

Both joints present well defined smoothly contoured articular surfaces. The interarticular spaces are moderately thin. In the left joint, this space does not decrease in width under biting stress. In the right, however, it does decrease in width under biting stress, indicative of degenerative changes, presumably due to occlusal disharmony. There is no radiographic evidence of osseous change in either joint. The right articular eminence is slightly more steeply inclined than the left, possibly predisposing to degenerative discal change.

In the left joint, there is excellent superimposition of POC and OP. In the right, this is not so, there being a visible displacement of the condyle anteriorly when the teeth are firmly occluded. This is radiographic evidence of occlusal disharmony. It should be noted that if this disharmony were symptomatic at all, it should be sensed clinically as premature contact of the left-side teeth with slight disocclusion on the right. In this case, however, the premature contact has very recently been sensed on the right with noticeable disocclusion on the left, symptomatic not of preexistent etiologically important occlusal disharmony, but of recent acute malocclusion due presumably to intracapsular edema from joint inflammation. This radiographic finding, therefore, is interpreted not to represent the present symptomatic acute malocclusion of which the patient complains, but rather is indicative of etiologically important preexistent occlusal disharmony. This very likely is the mechanism by which extraordinary chewing initiated the present acute symptoms.

Translatory movement in LP is normal in the left joint but restricted in MTO due presumably to the right-side hypomobility. In the right joint, both LP and MTO movement appears to be arrested at about 3mm, indicative of capsular and intracapsular restraint from acute inflammation, plus the inhibitory effects of pain.

Case No. 11–5,B.—Radiographic tracings of temporomandibular joints.

Most growth problems involving the temporomandibular joints are painless and do not come within the scope of this monograph. However, if lack of structural harmony between the condyle and fossa (Fig 11–20), between the two joints bilaterally (Fig 11–21), or between the joints and the dentition (Figs 11–22 and 11–23) becomes sufficient to interfere seriously with normal functioning, painful conditions may arise.

Oral and Facial Pain
DR. WELDEN E. BELL
8226 DOUGLAS AVENUE
DALLAS, TEXAS

Name Male age 70	Age	Date	
QUALITY	DURATION	LOCALIZATION	AFFECTED BY	LOCAL EFFECTS

HISTORY

QUALITY	DURATION	LOCALIZATION	AFFECTED BY	LOCAL EFFECTS
(Mild) Severe	Bright (Dull)	(Continuous) Intermittent Recurrent	Localized (Diffuse) Radiating Spreading	Face Movement (Jaw Movement) Tongue Movement Swallowing Head Position	Sensory: Hypesthesia Hyperesthesia Paresthesia Dysesthesia	Special Sense: Visual Auditory Olfactory Gustatory
Spontaneous Triggered Induced	Pricking Itching Burning	Momentary Minutes Hours	Body Position Activities Tension	Motor: Weakness	Autonomic: Ocular Signs Nasal Signs
Paroxysmal (Steady)	(Aching) Pulsating	Day long (Protracted)	Fatigue Secondary Pain	Time of Day	Contraction Spasm	Cutaneous Signs Gastric Signs

Location
Inception
Initial pain
Duration, clinical course
Therapeutic response
Physical and emotional background
Trauma, infection, etc.
Medications in use

Mild continuous variable protracted steady dull aching pain diffusely located in the right TM joint area, aggravated by all joint use. There is localized tenderness to touch and pressure directly over the joint proper.
The complaint began about eight weeks ago as very mild tenderness over the right joint and minor discomfort with jaw movements. Some stiffness of the joint was noticed especially in the early mornings. The discomfort has gradually increased until the last two weeks the pain has become great enough to interfere with normal chewing and talking. Increasing restriction of opening and pain with opening has been noticed. He sought aid from his physician who in turn referred him for a temporomandibular joint examination.
He presently is receiving no medications or therapy.

B/P 155/85   Neurological Survey   Psychological Survey

EXAMINATION

Oral
TM joints
Muscle system
Diagnostic blocks
Diagnostic drugs
Trial therapy

Orally: The missing LR4,5,6 and LL6 are replaced with a satisfactory partial denture. The remaining teeth are clinically and radiographically negative for cause of pain. No occlusal disharmony is identified. There is pain with lateral and protrusive movements as well as opening beyond 23mm. Left lateral movement is restricted. Protrusive movement is restricted and deflects to the right. Opening is restricted to about 30mm and deflects to the right.
TM joints: Both joints appear to be within normal limits structurally and the left joint functionally. The right joint presents restricted condylar movement interpreted as being due to periarticular and capsular inflammation plus the effect of pain inhibition. (See tracings.)
Muscle system: There is moderate palpable tenderness in the right masseter muscle.

Serum uric acid: 8.9 mg%.

Opinion: The right joint appears to be acutely inflamed due presumably to hyperuricemia involving the periarticular and capsular structures of the joint. There is moderate secondary muscle pain emanating from the right masseter muscle.

DIAGNOSIS

Periarticular and capsular inflammation of the right TM joint, due presumably to hyperuricemia.

Case No. 11–6,A.—Case chart. Temporomandibular arthralgia, expressed as arthritic pain, due to hyperuricemia.

Temporomandibular Examination Radiographic Tracings DR. WELDEN E. BELL 8226 DOUGLAS AVENUE DALLAS, TEXAS	Name **Male age 70** X-ray File No. Date	**Key to Symbols** POC Primary Occlusal Contact OP Occlusal Position RP Rest Position LP Contralateral Position MTO Maximum Translatory Opening PR Protrusive Position
Left T-M Joint	Left **Key** Right LP: 14 LP: 8 MTO: 18 MTO: 10 POC = OP = LP = - - - - MTO = — · —	Right T-M Joint

INTERPRETATION

Both joints were viewed in four positions:
1. Position of primary occlusal contact (POC).
2. Fully occluded position (OP).
3. Contralateral excursion (LP).
4. Maximum opening - 30mm (MTO).

Both joints present well defined smoothly contoured articular surfaces separated by interarticular spaces of adequate width which do not decrease in width under biting stress. There is no radiographic evidence of degenerative joint disease or other structural arthropathy that involves the osseous structure.

There is satisfactory superimposition of POC and OP indicative of no occlusal disharmony gross enough to cause radiographically evident displacement of either condyle when the teeth are firmly occluded.

Translatory movement in LP and MTO is normal in the left joint. In the right, the condyle appears to be restricted in both LP and MTO but this restriction does not seem to be imposed wholly by capsular or intracapsular causes which would limit condylar movement uniformly in both LP and MTO. Nor does it appear to be due wholly to extracapsular causes which would restrain MTO movement without appreciably affecting LP movement. From the clinical symptoms and history, this is interpreted to represent the effect of both periarticular and capsular inflammation plus the inhibitory effect of pain on joint movement.

Case No. 11–6,B.—Radiographic tracings of temporomandibular joints.

Pain in such instances would probably relate to intrinsic trauma, presenting symptoms of capsulitis, discitis, retrodiscitis, or inflammatory arthritis, depending on what structures are inflamed. Radiographic evidence of malformation may confirm the diagnosis.

Rarely do malignant tumors involve the temporomandibular joints. They have been reported in the literature, and a few have been observed by this writer. The characteristic features have been slow progressive immobilization of the joint without apparent cause and usually painless at first. The early clinical and radiographic features suggest fibrous ankylosis. It is usually the progressiveness of the condition and finally pain with all joint use that lead the examiner to believe that the condition is other than a simple chronic mandibular hypomobility (Case No. 11–8).

218   OROFACIAL PAINS

Oral and Facial Pain
DR. WELDEN E. BELL
8226 DOUGLAS AVENUE
DALLAS, TEXAS

Name: Female age 34

HISTORY

QUALITY	DURATION	LOCALIZATION	AFFECTED BY	LOCAL EFFECTS
(Mild) Bright	(Continuous)	Localized		Sensory: Special Sense:
Severe (Dull)	Intermittent	(Diffuse)	Face Movement	Hy(p)esthesia Vi(s)ual
	Recurrent		(Jaw Movement)	Hyperest(h)esia Au(d)itory
		Radiating	Tongue Movement	Par(e)sthesia Olf(a)ctory
Spontaneous		Spreading	Swallowing	D(y)sesthesia G(u)statory
Triggered Pricking	Momentary		Head Position	
(Induced) Itching	Minutes	Enlarging	Body Position	Autonomic:
Burning	Hours	Migrating	Activities	Motor: Ocul(a)r Sign(s)
Paroxysmal (Aching)	Day long		Tension	W(e)akness Nasa(l) (S)igns
(Steady) Pulsating	(Protracted)	Secondary Pain	Fatigue	Con(t)raction Cu(t)an(e)ous Signs
			Time of Day	S(p)asm Gastric Signs

Location
Inception
Initial pain
Duration, clinical course
Therapeutic response
Physical and emotional background
Trauma, infection, etc.
Medications in use

Mild continuous intermittently severe variable protracted steady dull aching pain diffusely located in the left preauricular area, induced by forceful opening and excursive movements, and accompanied by restricted movement of the left mandibular condyle.
    The complaint followed an automobile accident about 18 months ago in which the patient sustained multiple fractures of the mandible, one through the left condyloid process. Soreness and restricted movement of the left joint persisted after treatment of the fractures and have been present ever since. The pain is related chiefly to efforts to move the jaw for opening. Physiotherapy, muscle relaxants, and corticosteroid injection therapy have failed to give much benefit. Patient was therefore referred for evaluation of the temporomandibular joints.
    No medications are presently being used.

EXAMINATION

B/P 125/80   Neurological Survey   Psychological Survey

Oral
TM joints
Muscle system
Diagnostic blocks
Diagnostic drugs
Trial therapy

Orally: There is no dental or oral cause for the complaint that is evident clinically or radiographically. There is palpable tenderness over the left condyle but no pain described in resting or occlusal positions. No occlusal disharmony is identified. All pain appears to occur with movements that tend to induce translation of the left condyle -- protrusive, contralateral excursion, and opening beyond about 22mm. The severity of pain relates directly to the degree of attempted movement. Protrusion deflects to the left. Right lateral excursion is nil. Opening ceases at about 24mm and deflects to the left.
    TM joints: Both joints appear to be normal structurally. There is restriction of left condylar movement that is interpreted as representing fibrous ankylosis. (See tracings.)
    Muscle system: Essentially negative.

    Opinion: Fibrous ankylosis of the left TM joint appears to have developed as a posttraumatic sequela. As the adhesions matured, continued efforts to execute normal left condylar movements induced inflammation, making them painful.

DIAGNOSIS

Painful adhesions that immobilize the left mandibular condyle. (Ankylosis)

Case No. 11–7,A.—Case chart. Temporomandibular arthralgia, expressed as arthritic pain, due to inflamed fibrous ankylosis.

Temporomandibular Examination Radiographic Tracings DR. WELDEN E. BELL 8226 DOUGLAS AVENUE DALLAS, TEXAS	Name Female age 34 X-ray File No._____ Date_____	Key to Symbols POC Primary Occlusal Contact OP Occlusal Position RP Rest Position LP Contralateral Position MTO Maximum Translatory Opening PR Protrusive Position

Left T-M Joint

Left LP: 2 MTO: 2	Key	Right LP: 10 MTO: 7

Right T-M Joint

POC ▬ ⎱
OP ▬ ⎰ ───────
LP ▬ ─ ─ ─
MTO ▬ ─ ── ─ ──

INTERPRETATION

Both joints were viewed in four transparietal positions:
1. Primary occlusal contact (POC).
2. Fully occluded position (OP).
3. Contralateral excursion (LP).
4. Maximum opening - 24mm (MTO).

Both joints present well defined smoothly contoured articular surfaces with interarticular spaces of adequate width which do not decrease in width under biting stress. There is no radiographic evidence of degenerative joint disease and no osseous change that is interpreted as indicative of former trauma.

There is satisfactory superimposition of POC and OP in both joints, indicative of no occlusal disharmony sufficient to cause radiographically identifiable displacement of either condyle when the teeth are firmly occluded.

Translatory movement in LP is normal in the right joint but restricted in MTO due presumably to the left joint hypomobility.

Translatory movement in the left joint is restricted to about 2mm in both LP and MTO, indicative of intracapsular and capsular fixation of the condyle. This is interpreted to represent fibrous ankylosis of the left TM joint which by history relates to trauma received some 18 months prior.

Case No. 11–7,B.—Radiographic tracings of temporomandibular joints.

Trotter's syndrome,[5] known also as sinus of Morgagni syndrome, consists of the following features:
1. Unilateral deafness
2. Ipsilateral mandibular division pain
3. Ipsilateral defective mobility of the palate
4. Subsequent trismus

The malignant tumor responsible for this syndrome is located in the nasopharynx and infiltrates the pterygoid muscles, thus causing progressive trismus and pain.

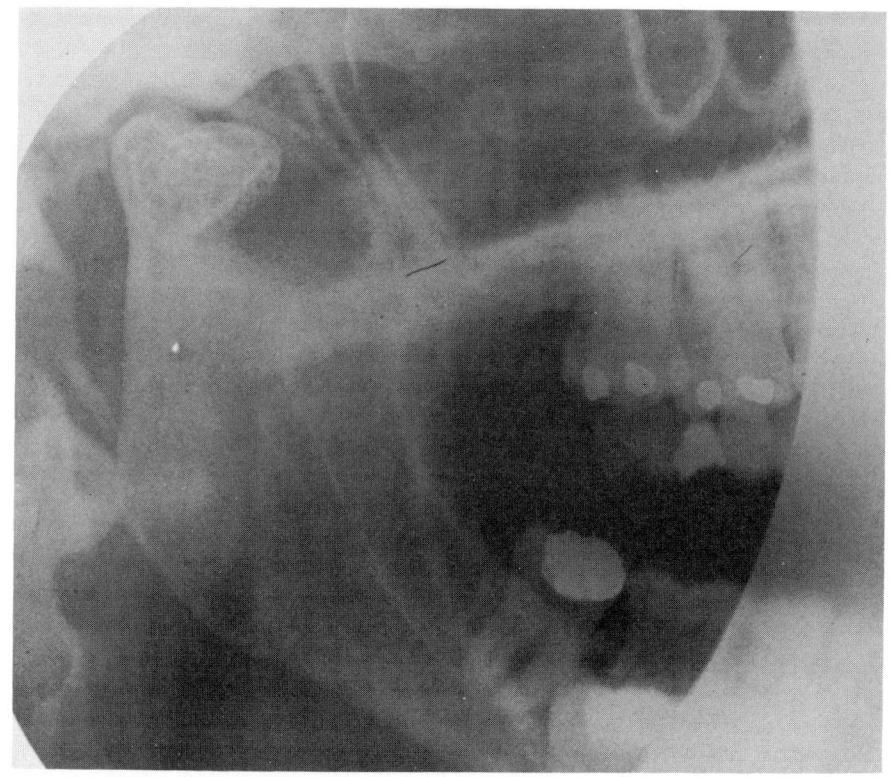

Fig 11-20.—Transfacial projection of mandibular condyle showing massive enlargement that represents obvious structural disharmony between condyle and articular fossa.

The clinical symptoms by which arthritic pain can be recognized are as follows:
1. There is usually some degree of capsular pain as well as other symptoms of synovitis-capsulitis.
2. The pain is accentuated by biting pressure, fast movements, and forced movements.
3. The pain is not decreased by biting against a separator.
4. Dysfunction is expressed as restricted movement, interference during movements, and acute malocclusion. Restricted movement may be due to inflammatory swelling, capsular inflammation, altered synovial fluid function, secondary myospasm, and the inhibitory influence of pain. Interference during movements may be due to disc-condyle complex impairment. Acute malocclusion may be due to increased intracapsular fluid.

Temporomandibular Joint Pains

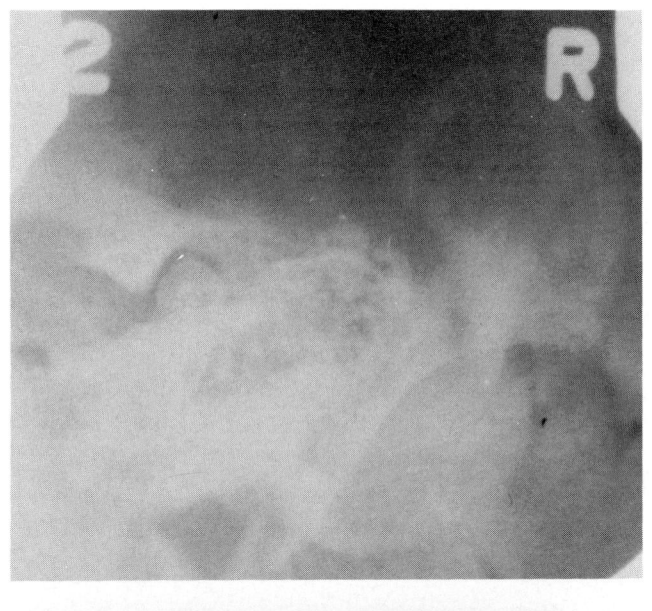

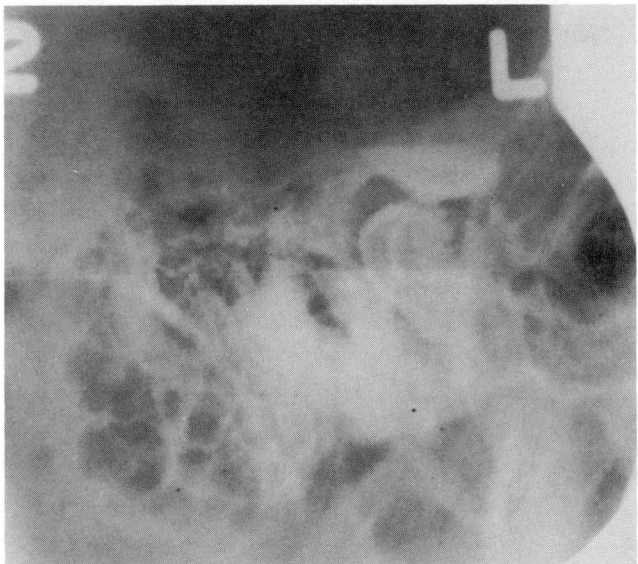

Fig 11-21.—Radiographs of temporomandibular joints illustrating obvious lack of structural harmony between the two joints, the inclination of the left articular eminence being fairly low, whereas that of the right joint is considerably greater.

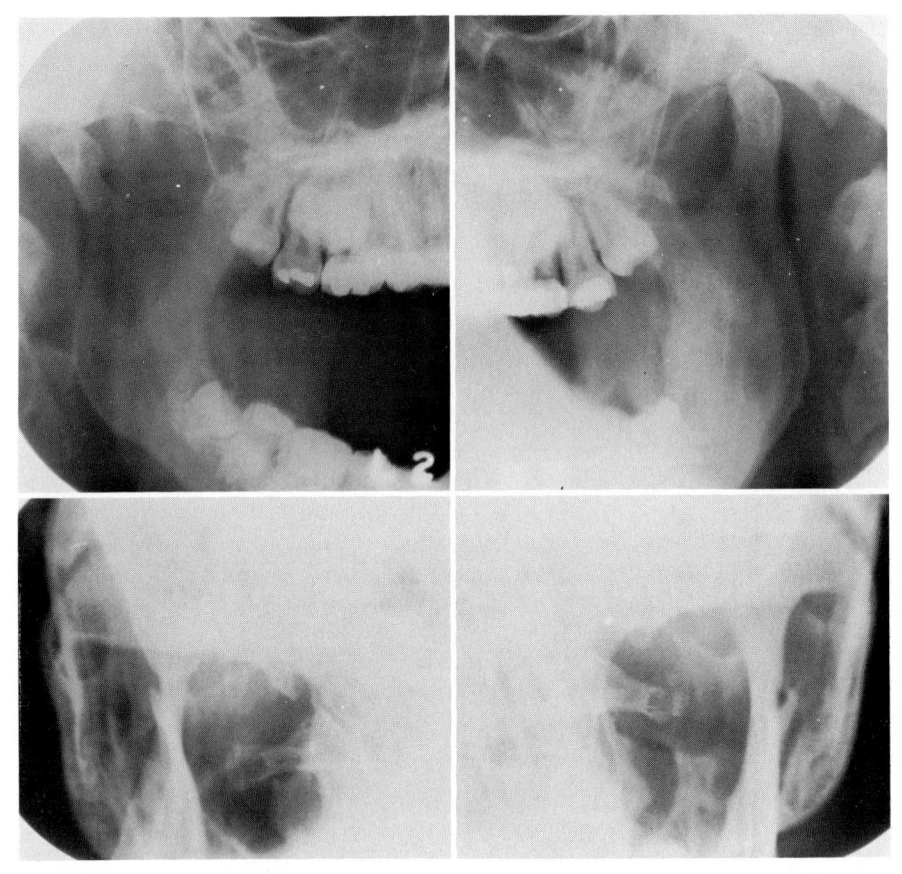

Fig 11–22.—Radiographs illustrating moderate unilateral hyperplasia involving right mandibular condyle. Note that right condyle, neck, and ramus are larger, longer, and thicker than the left, as viewed in transfacial and transorbital projections.

TEMPOROMANDIBULAR JOINT PAINS

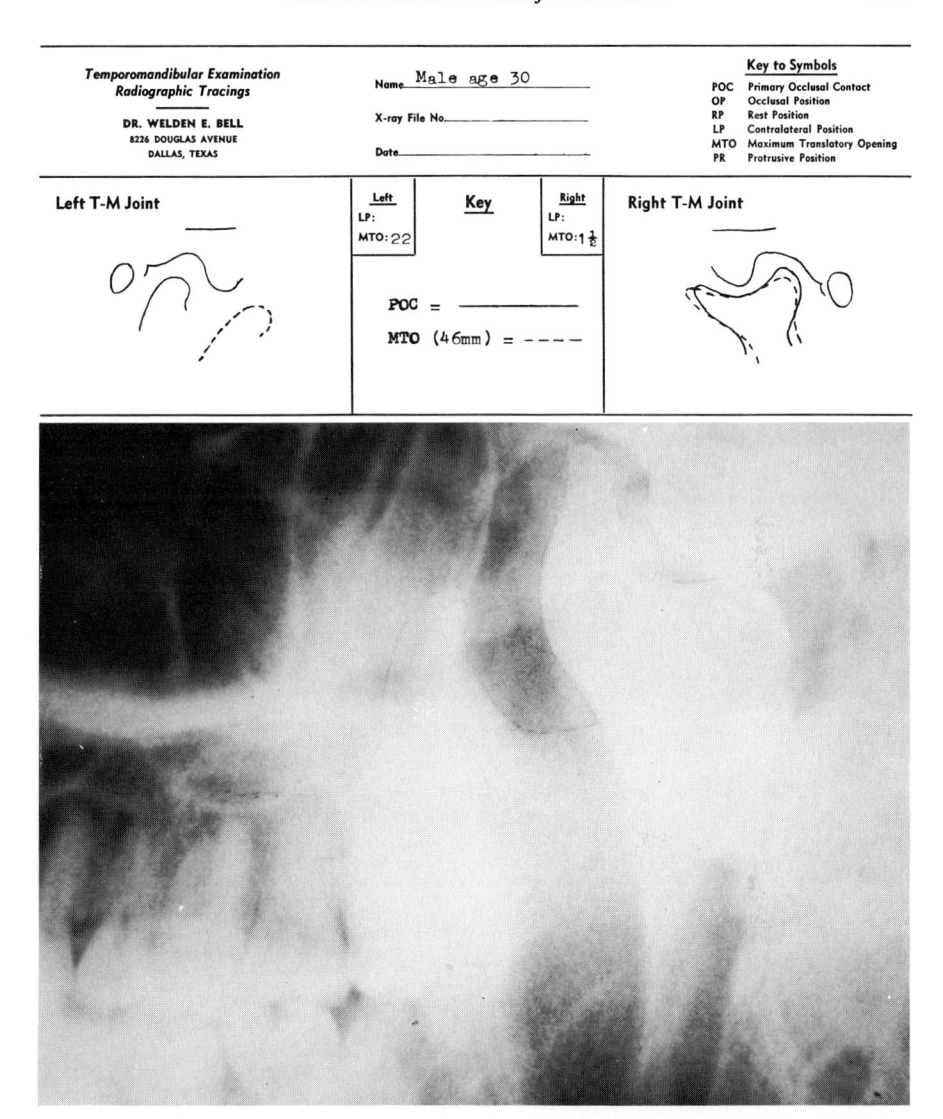

Fig 11-23.—Marked unilateral condylar hyperplasia of right temporomandibular (TM) joint causing cross-bite malocclusion and interference with joint functioning (*top*). Radiographic tracings of the TM joints in POC and MTO showing fixation of malformed massive condyle. *Bottom*, transfacial radiograph of right condyle.

Oral and Facial Pain
DR. WELDEN E. BELL
8226 DOUGLAS AVENUE
DALLAS, TEXAS

Name: Female age 54

QUALITY	DURATION	LOCALIZATION	AFFECTED BY	LOCAL EFFECTS
(Mild) Severe✓	Bright (Dull)	(Continuous) Intermittent Recurrent	Localized (Diffuse)	Face Movement (Jaw Movement) Tongue Movement Swallowing Head Position	Sensory: Hypesthesia Hyperesthesia Paresthesia Dysesthesia	Special Sense: Visual Auditory Olfactory Gustatory
Spontaneous Triggered Induced	Pricking Itching Burning	Momentary Minutes Hours	Body Position Activities Tension		Autonomic: Ocular Signs Nasal Signs
Paroxysmal (Steady)	(Aching) Pulsating	Day long (Protracted)	Enlarging Migrating Fatigue Time of Day Secondary Pain	Motor: Weakness Contraction (Spasm)	Cutaneous Signs Gastric Signs

HISTORY

Location — Mild to severe continuous variable protracted steady dull aching pain diffusely located in the left ear and preauricular area spreading to the temple, face, and submandibular triangle, aggravated by opening 13mm and accompanied by restricted mandibular movements.

Inception
Initial pain
Duration, clinical course — The complaint began about four years ago with no prior history of injury. It began insidiously as left eustachian blockage, followed soon by restriction of opening to about 25mm. ENT therapy was ineffective. Three years ago her dentist made an occlusal splint to "correct the bite". After 2-3 months, mild pain began and has gradually increased ever since. After a year, the splint was discarded. About a year ago, surgery on the opposite ear was followed by an increase in the pain and trismus. Six months ago, she was given a general anesthetic and the "muscles stretched" — without any benefit. Recent muscle relaxant therapy and a corticosteroid injection into the left joint have not been beneficial.

Therapeutic response
Physical and emotional background
Trauma, infection, etc.
Medications in use

B/P 140/80   Neurological Survey   Psychological Survey

EXAMINATION

Oral — Orally: There is no dental or oral cause for her complaint. The left face and ear pain increases with opening beyond 13mm. There is no palpable tenderness over the left condyle. Opening is restricted to 18mm with deflection to the right (suggestive of medial pterygoid spasm). Protrusion deflects to the left. Right lateral excursion is almost nil.

TM joints — TM joints: Both joints appear normal structurally. There is marked restriction of left condylar movement interpreted as being indicative of fibrous ankylosis. (See tracings.)

Muscle system — Muscle system: There is only very slight palpable tenderness in the left temporal and masseter muscles. The medial pterygoid cannot be palpated due to the restricted opening.

Diagnostic blocks — Analgesic blocking of the left medial pterygoid muscle via the sigmoid notch arrested about 75% of the pain but did not alter the dysfunction.

Diagnostic drugs
Trial therapy — Trial therapy for normalization of the medial pterygoid muscle was not effective. Within a few weeks, the pain increased until narcotic analgesics were required at 2-3 hour intervals. Within a year, she was examined at a major medical center and a confirmed diagnosis of carcinoma in the left nasopharynx invading the periarticular structures of the left TM joint was made.

Opinion: In retrospect, no doubt the invasive neoplasm caused the symptoms clinically and radiographically interpreted as fibrous ankylosis complicated by spasm of the left medial pterygoid muscle.

DIAGNOSIS

Immobilization of the left TM joint due to an invasive malignant tumor.

Case No. 11–8,A.—Case chart. Temporomandibular arthralgia, expressed as arthritic pain, due to an invasive malignant tumor.

Temporomandibular Examination Radiographic Tracings DR. WELDEN E. BELL 8226 DOUGLAS AVENUE DALLAS, TEXAS	Name Female age 54 X-ray File No. Date	Key to Symbols POC Primary Occlusal Contact OP Occlusal Position RP Rest Position LP Contralateral Position MTO Maximum Translatory Opening PR Protrusive Position

Left T-M Joint	Left LP: 1½ MTO: 3	Key	Right LP: 9 MTO: 3	Right T-M Joint
		POC = OP = LP = MTO =		

INTERPRETATION

Both joints were viewed in four transparietal positions:
1. Position of primary occlusal contact (POC).
2. Fully occluded position (OP).
3. Contralateral excursion (LP).
4. Maximum opening - 18mm (MTO).

Both joints present well defined smoothly contoured articular surfaces with interarticular spaces of adequate width which do not decrease in width under biting stress. There is no radiographic evidence of degenerative joint disease or other osseous abnormality.

There is excellent superimposition of POC and OP in both joints, indicative of no occlusal disharmony gross enough to cause radiographically apparent displacement of either condyle when the teeth are firmly occluded.

Translatory movement in the right joint is nearly normal in LP. In MTO it is restricted presumably due to the left joint hypomobility. In the left joint, LP is restricted to 1½ and MTO to 3mm, indicative of capsular and intracapsular limitation of condylar movement. Radiographically, this should be suggestive of fibrous ankylosis.

Case No. 11–8,B.—Radiographic tracings of temporomandibular joints.

DIFFERENTIAL DIAGNOSIS

In order to plan effective therapy, accurate identification of pain source is needed. Masticatory pains constitute a major segment of orofacial pain complaints. Frequently, the complaint consists of both myalgic and arthralgic components which should be differentiated. Primary and secondary pains also must be distinguished. This may require considerable diagnostic effort. However, the more accurately it is done, the less complex the management problem and the more predictive the treatment.

Intermittent Arthralgia

Intermittent arthralgic pains relate primarily to the effect of biomechanical abuse. As such, little or no secondary referred pain, secondary hyperalgesia, or myospastic activity results. The pain remains relatively "clean-cut." It is diffusely localizable to the joint region and responds rather faithfully to manual palpation and functional manipulation. Acute intermittent arthralgic pain may induce protective muscle splinting in the masticatory muscles that tends to immobilize the joint in a resting attitude. This may occur bilaterally. It should be noted, however, that protracted muscle splinting may develop into myospasm which, if persistent, may become inflammatory. Thus, it is important to eliminate such pains before complications develop, or else therapy must be instituted for the muscle condition as well.

Chronic intermittent arthralgic pains may cause a change in muscle activity patterns. It is hypothesized that latent memory traces may persist after neural stimulation; thus, repeated stimulation may induce altered habitual patterns of muscle activity. It is presumed that such engram change is responsible for deviations in the midline incisal path during opening-closing movements. (*Deviation* refers to discursive movement that returns again to the centered position; *deflection* refers to discursive movement that terminates eccentricly.) This may account also for such anomalies as avoidance closure movements, slides in centric, and convenience occlusal positions, as well as various habitual jaw movements and mannerisms. Time and repetition are required. Thus, acute and changing conditions do not cause such effects; they induce muscle splinting instead.

Inflammatory Arthralgic Pain

When the condition that induces arthralgic pain becomes inflammatory, continuity of input results, and, with it, the propensity to induce secondary central excitatory effects. Thus, inflammatory arthralgia (retrodiscal pain, capsular pain, and arthritic pain) may be complicated by a variety of secondary effects such as referred pains including headache, secondary hyperalgesia displayed as superficial touchy spots or areas of deep palpable tenderness, or secondary myospasm involving masticatory muscles. Careful differentiation between primary sources of pain input and the secondary effects of deep somatic pain is essential to accurate diagnosis and effective management. It should be noted that while muscle spasm may be induced by deep pain input, it may soon develop as a cycling mechanism. As such, it becomes wholly independent of the initiating cause and requires separate therapeutic effort for resolution.

Arthralgia of Nonmasticatory Origin

From the dental standpoint, it is important to distinguish between arthralgia of masticatory origin, which can reasonably be expected to respond to proper masticatory therapy, and arthralgia of nonmasticatory origin, which may require medical therapy, surgical intervention, or both. Arthralgias from hyperuricemia and rheumatoid arthritis are essentially medical problems in which treatment of the masticatory apparatus would be secondary and supplemental. Infections, traumatic arthritis, and temporomandibular involvement from adjacent pathosis may require considerable interdisciplinary attention. Chronic mandibular hypomobilities and growth disorders are usually surgical problems.

Referred Pain Felt in the Joint Area

True arthralgia that emanates from the temporomandibular joint must be differentiated from heterotopic pain that is felt in the joint area. As discussed in chapter 10, myogenous pain may be referred to the joint. This is especially true of myofascial trigger point pain involving sternocleidomastoid, masseter, medial pterygoid, and lateral pterygoid muscles (Case No. 14–3). But referred pain from any source within the vast trigeminal distribution may also be felt in the joint area. The salivary glands are known sources of such reference (Case No. 14–2).

Eagle's Syndrome

Eagle's syndrome[6,7] may be confused with temporomandibular pain because it typically induces a sensation of persistent raw throat, pain and difficulty with swallowing, pain referred to the auricular area, and limited neck movement.[8] The condition is due to elongation of the styloid process or calcification of the stylohyoid ligament. The elongated styloid process may encroach on the carotid artery, thus causing carotid arteritis. The resulting carotidynia may refer pain through the face to the ophthalmic area. Encroachment on the carotid artery is said to cause faintness or syncope when the head is turned from side to side.[9]

Painful Scar Tissue

Neurogenous pain may emanate from traumatic neuroma formation in scar tissue residual to lacerating injuries or surgery of the joint. Such pain displays the clinical characteristics of neurogenous rather than deep somatic pain. There is no discomfort except when a certain mandibular movement puts the affected scar tissue under stretch. Such pain can be replicated at will by repeating the same jaw movement (Case No. 15–2).

Glossopharyngeal Neuralgia

Another neurogenous pain that may be confused with temporomandibular joint pain is glossopharyngeal neuralgia. This paroxysmal neuralgia is triggered by stimulation of receptors in the pharyngeal mucosa. It is associated therefore with talking as well as with jaw and throat movements incidental to chewing and swallowing. The pain usually is felt deeply in the postmandibular and infra-auricular area. It presents the clinical characteristics of neurogenous rather than deep somatic pain and is temporarily arrested by topical anesthesia of the pharyngeal mucosa (Case No. 15–6).

REFERENCES

1. Bell W.E.: *Clinical Management of Temporomandibular Disorders.* Chicago, Year Book Medical Publishers, 1982.
2. Sicher H.: *Oral Anatomy*, ed. 3. St. Louis, C.V. Mosby Co., 1960.
3. Thilander B.: Innervation of the temporomandibular joint capsule in man. *Trans. R. School Dent.* 7:1, 1961.
4. Bell W.E.: Understanding temporomandibular biomechanics. *J. Craniomand. Pract.* 1(2):27, 1983.
5. Gorlin R.J., Pindborg J.J.: *Syndromes of the Head and Neck.* New York, McGraw-Hill Book Co., 1964.
6. Eagle W.W.: Elongated styloid process: Further observations and a new syndrome. *Arch. Otolaryngol.* 47:630, 1948.
7. Eagle W.W.: Symptomatic elongated styloid process. *Arch. Otolaryngol.* 49:490, 1949.
8. Lawrence F.R., Cornielson E.: Eagle's syndrome. *J. Oral Maxillofac. Surg.* 40:307–309, 1982.
9. Correll R.W., Wescott W.B.: Eagle's syndrome diagnosed after history of headache, dysphagia, otalgia, and limited neck movement. *J.A.D.A.* 104:491–492, 1982.

12

Other Musculoskeletal Pains

FOR PURPOSES OF DESCRIPTION, pains that emanate from musculoskeletal structures of the mouth and face have been divided into separate groups: periodontal odontogenous pains (chapter 9), pains of muscle origin (chapter 10), temporomandibular joint pains (chapter 11), and other musculoskeletal pains of the mouth and face. All such musculoskeletal pains display the clinical characteristics of deep somatic pain, of which they constitute a major subdivision. In addition, they display features that identify them as being of musculoskeletal origin, namely (1) the pain relates reasonably to the demands of function, (2) manual palpation (or functional manipulation) at the site of pain induces a graduated response, and (3) subjective localization of the pain varies in accordance with the need for proprioceptive guidance as demanded by the requirements of function. The *other musculoskeletal pains* of the face and mouth include (1) osseous pains, (2) periosteal pains, and (3) soft connective tissue pains (Fig 12–1). It should be noted that since osseous structures and soft connective tissue are less intimately related to biomechanical function, they are less well innervated proprioceptively and therefore are less localizable subjectively. Also, pains emanating from such structures are less apt to induce muscle effects.

OSSEOUS PAINS

Pains that emanate from the bony structures of the mouth and face exclusive of the periodontal structures and the temporomandibular joints constitute another major subdivision of musculoskeletal pain. Pains from this source are predominantly inflammatory as a result of injury, infection, or surgical procedures.

Osseous pain is more stabile than myogenous pain and follows an inflammatory time frame. It usually differs from cellulitic pain in that initially pain alone dominates the symptom complex, showing less

OROFACIAL PAIN SYNDROMES

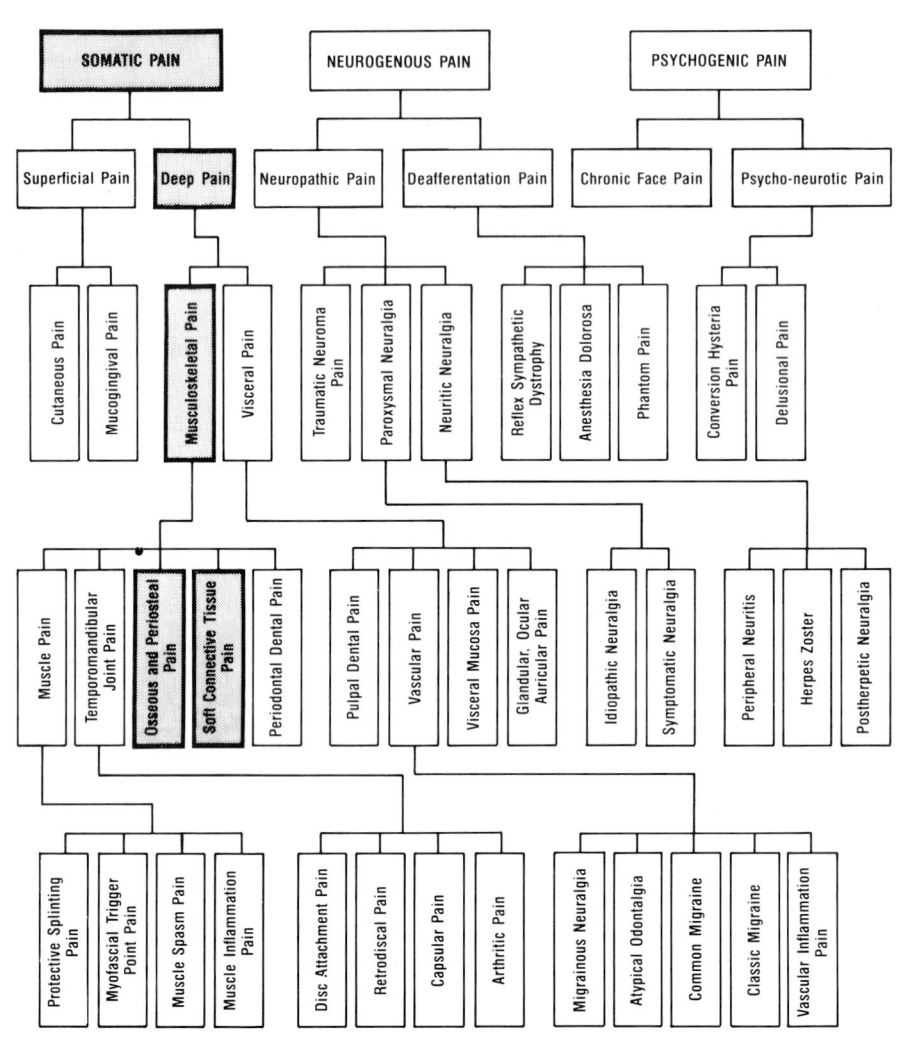

Fig 12–1.—Chart showing classification relationship of osseous, periosteal, and soft connective tissue pains to other orofacial pain syndromes.

evidence of other inflammatory symptoms. Due to the rigid unyielding structure of the tissues involved, inflammatory swelling may not be observed until surrounding structures become involved. During this phase, the pain relates especially to three factors: (1) susceptibility of inflamed osseous tissue to environmental noxious irritation such as mechanical encroachment, movement of fractured or injured parts and contact with saliva; (2) confinement of inflammatory exudate; and (3) type and virulence of the contaminating organism. The pain level usually drops rapidly as these factors are obtunded by natural resolution or therapy. Final relief of pain follows a protracted inflammatory time frame. There is minimal dysfunction other than that due to the inhibitory influence of pain. Secondary factors such as muscle splinting, myospasm, or cellulitis may contribute some dysfunction, however.

By definition, osteitis denotes inflammation of bone involving the haversian spaces, canals, and medullary spaces.[1] Acute septic osteitis is usually designated *osteomyelitis*. The inflammatory reaction occurs in the soft tissues confined within the rigid osseous compartments, a condition that in some ways simulates pulpal inflammation. Congestion within such rigidly confined areas may cause pain out of proportion to that experienced when such confinement is not present. This gives the pain a throbbing quality. It induces necrosis by pressure against the unyielding walls. Thus the inflammatory condition spreads through the bone, following paths of least resistance.

When the cortex is penetrated, the inflammatory process is considerably less confined, and the pain intensity decreases. Subperiosteal spreading occurs with surface swelling and pain, which is readily identifiable by manual palpation. Subperiosteal spreading may proceed until a barrier is reached, such as a muscle attachment. At that point it may rupture through and the inflammation spread to the overlying soft tissues. Confined acute subperiosteal inflammation may be extremely painful due to sensitivity of the periosteum to pain.[2]

When confinement is released by rupture or surgical drainage, the pain intensity drops dramatically, and the throbbing quality disappears. In turn, cellulitic involvement accompanies the osteitis, and further spreading takes place along natural barriers such as the fascial planes. The degree of pain again is determined largely by confinement imposed by the relation of the anatomical features to the quantity of exudate and degree of purulence. Tissues offering little resistance to swelling provide less intense pain, whereas tissues that tightly contain the inflammatory process increase the pain level and incidence of throbbing. Surface rupture and fistulization (or surgical drainage) reduce pain intensity, and the throbbing usually disappears.

It should be evident therefore that the pain behavior is determined by several factors including the type of injury, virulence and behavioral characteristics of the invader, resistance of the host, and anatomical conditions imposed at the site of inflammation. Nonseptic inflammations are less painful. Chronicity may cause pain to disappear entirely

pain. Pains from these structures are predominantly inflammatory and relate to other signs of inflammation by which the source of pain may be identified.

The pain is considerably more stabile than muscle pain and follows an inflammatory time frame. When the inflammatory exudate is confined, the pain develops a pulsatile quality and increases in intensity. When evacuated by penetration, rupture or surgical drainage, pain intensity drops dramatically, and the pulsatile quality disappears. Dysfunction is due chiefly to inflammatory swelling. Response to effective therapy follows resolution of the inflammatory process.

By definition, *cellulitis* denotes inflammation of cellular tissue, especially purulent inflammation of loose connective tissue.[2] Most purulent inflammatory conditions involving the deeper soft tissues of the face and mouth are designated as cellulitis. Specific terms may designate certain types and locations of cellulitic involvement. The intensity of pain depends largely on the acuity, rate of spreading, distension of tissues, and confinement of inflammatory exudate. Manual palpation gives essential information, as do concomitant regional lymphadenitis and systemic effects. Spreading follows the fascial planes. An intimate understanding of these anatomical features is indispensable to the examiner.[3]

Acute cellulitis is usually evident from the swelling and pain, and no diagnostic problem occurs as long as the inflammation is located in accessible regions. When this condition involves the sublingual area, its location relative to the mylohyoid muscle largely determines its clinical features and behavior. Supramylohyoid cellulitis lifts the tongue and interferes with speech and swallowing. Inframylohyoid cellulitis causes external swelling in the submental and submandibular areas and may embarrass respiration if it encroaches on the glottis. Palatal cellulitis causes swelling that interferes with speech and swallowing. In the buccal regions it usually causes external swelling of the face that spreads readily to the eyelids. Confinement, spreading, and location of the swelling relate to the anatomical arrangement of facial muscles and to the anchorage of fascial barriers. Cellulitis in the pterygomandibular space causes trismus due to medial pterygoid muscle involvement. Similar inflammation adjacent to the masseter muscle does likewise. Cellulitis in the infratemporal fossa area causes characteristic facial swelling above the zygoma and trismus due to temporal muscle involvement.

Subacute and chronic cellulitis is less dramatic and may present diagnostic problems of differentiation from cysts and tumors. The history and clinical course plus manual palpation and surgical aspiration are the usual means of establishing the diagnosis.

Pain of cellulitic origin should be differentiated from muscle pain, vascular pain, and glandular pain. Other conditions that may initiate soft connective tissue pain are cysts and tumors, both benign and malignant.

REFERENCES

1. *Dorland's Illustrated Medical Dictionary*, ed. 26. Philadelphia, W.B. Saunders Co., 1981.
2. Wolff H.G., Wolf S.: *Pain*, ed. 2. Springfield, Ill., Charles C Thomas Publishers, 1958.
3. DuBrul E.L.: *Sicher's Oral Anatomy*, ed. 7. St. Louis, C.V. Mosby Co., 1980.

13

Vascular Pains

CLINICALLY, DEEP SOMATIC PAIN occurs either as musculoskeletal or as visceral pain. Musculoskeletal pain derives from the structures that give physical form and stability to the body as well as provide for the biomechanical functions that accomplish posture, locomotion, and other useful working movements. Visceral pain derives from components of the supply and maintenance system that subserve the musculoskeletal structures. The visceral system has to do with oxygen supply, nutrition, metabolism, detoxification, and elimination of waste products. It is composed of organs of many different types, glandular structures, and a network of vessels of different kinds to transport substances throughout the body. Whereas sensation emanating from the musculoskeletal structures relates to more or less conscious volitional biomechanical functions, sensation initiated in visceral structures is largely unconscious and serves to facilitate ongoing automatic metabolic functioning of the body. Pain of musculoskeletal origin therefore relates to biomechanical function as a graduated response, while pain of visceral origin commands attention only to warn that all is not well within. The clinical symptoms displayed by the two kinds of deep somatic pain are sufficiently different to make them identifiable. This is of considerable importance diagnostically.

For purposes of description, the visceral pains have been separated into three groups, namely (1) pulpal odontogenous pains (chapter 9), (2) vascular pains of the mouth and face, and (3) other visceral pains, including those of mucosal, glandular, ocular, and auricular origin (chapter 14). In addition to the clinical characteristics of deep somatic pain, all such visceral pains display certain features by which they may be recognized, namely (1) the pains are of threshold type and do not yield graduated responses, (2) the pains are influenced very little by biomechanical function, and (3) subjective localization of the pain is diffuse, some being nearly nonlocalizable by the subject. Visceral pains are usually not accompanied by distinctive evidence of dysfunction other than that induced by the inhibitory influence of pain.

BEHAVIOR OF VISCERAL PAIN

The mechanism of visceral pain has been described by several authors.[1-5] Ordinarily, sensory information transmitted by afferent neurons of the visceral nervous system remains well below conscious levels. It serves to monitor the involuntary muscle action of vessels, glands, and organs. It reports unusual sensation occurring in the lining membranes of organs and cavities. It helps regulate the automatic functioning of the body by supplying the CNS with a constant inflow of information. When such sensation becomes noxious, pain is felt. Visceral afferent fibers of both the sympathetic and parasympathetic type are known to mediate pain.[4] Visceral pain usually has a distinct stinging or burning quality. It is said that protracted visceral pain tends to provoke vasomotor effects, local edema, and trophic changes.[5]

It appears that conscious visceral sensation is normally of a very low order of intensity, the visceral afferents having high threshold receptors. However, the presence of hyperemia or inflammation may reduce this threshold considerably so that conscious pain becomes evident with little added provocation. For example, the stomach yields minimal sensation other than when it is very empty or very full. But an inflamed gastric mucosa causes the normal stomach contents to excite painful sensation, usually described as "heartburn."

Visceral pain in the maxillofacial region is not rare. Esophagitis and pharyngitis have the dull, diffuse, burning quality of visceral pain. Nasal and ostium maxillare mucosa pain presents a similar burning quality.[3] The major salivary glands, as well as the numerous glands of the lymphatic system, the skin, and the mucous membranes, are other sources of this type of pain.

Some pains arising in the maxillofacial region are mediated by sympathetic afferent fibers that do not enter the CNS via any cranial or cervical nerve sensory root. Rather, these visceral fibers leave the head and pass through the cervical sympathetic chain and finally enter the CNS via the sensory roots of the upper thoracic spinal nerves. *Head and neck pains mediated by this route cannot be arrested by division of any or all cranial and cervical spinal sensory roots.* Such pains are arrested by analgesic blocking of the stellate ganglion through which such afferents pass, even though they undergo no synapse prior to reaching the CNS.[5,6]

Some *vascular pains* arising in the trigeminal area are not arrested by blocking or sectioning the trigeminal sensory root but are arrested by analgesic blocking of the stellate ganglion. This is clinical evidence that such pains are in fact mediated by sympathetic afferent fibers. Occasionally, atypical facial neuralgia is arrested in this way. There appears to be no indication, however, that classic migraine is mediated by this route.[6]

Analgesic blocking of the stellate ganglion does not necessarily arrest some of these vascular pains. This strongly suggests that the cranial parasympathetic constitute the mediating pain pathway, since no parasympathetic afferent fibers pass through the dorsal root of the trigeminal nerve. Rather, they leave this nerve and enter the CNS via the seventh and ninth cranial nerve dorsal roots. Thus division of the trigeminal sensory root will not arrest pains from the trigeminal area that are mediated by parasympathetic afferent fibers.

Visceral pain input tends to provoke central excitatory effects, probably because such pains are frequently continuous and protracted. Referred pains and localized autonomic effects may accompany visceral pains. Sometimes they dominate the symptom picture and constitute the patient's complaint. So-called sinus headache typifies this clinical behavior. Referred pains including toothache are felt throughout the maxillary area, and autonomic symptoms are present.

Manual palpation is useful in locating the site of visceral pain emanating from glandular structures. Confirmation may require further study, use of analgesic blocking techniques, or trial therapy. When the referred pain is felt in and about the ear, it may be mistaken for masticatory pain.

VASCULAR PAINS OF THE MOUTH AND FACE

Of the various pain syndromes that frequently involve the maxillofacial region, the vascular pains until very recently have been the least understood. Wolff[4] and his co-workers explored these pains in depth, and their investigations indicated that pain occurred as a result of dilatation of arteries, which distorted and noxiously stimulated the sensory receptors and afferent fibers in the vascular and perivascular tissues. When a vasoconstricting medication such as ergotamine tartrate reduced the dilatation and amplitude of pulsation of such arteries, the pain decreased or ceased. Also, pressure on the carotid artery diminished the pain. Sensitivity to histamine, certain toxic conditions, fever, posttraumatic syndromes, and certain emotional states also appear to relate to the incidence of vascular pains.

More recently, Wolff indicated that there are several conditions that evoke discomfort in vascular pain syndromes:

1. Dilatation of blood vessels
2. Local edema of the painful site

3. Edema of the vessel wall and perivascular tissue
4. Associated muscle pain, especially in the occipital area

The vascular distension and local edema of the painful site appear to be present in painful episodes of rather short duration such as typical migraine that lasts only a day or less. If it persists, the arterial edema and muscular component almost always become evident. The clinical entity known as temporal arteritis (or cranial arteritis) presents edema and inflammation of the arterial wall as a dominant feature with muscle pains as a secondary component. Persistent episodes of migrainous neuralgia usually present all these features plus central excitatory effects in the form of referred pains and secondary muscle spasms. When there is a component of muscle pain, the patient describes a persistent dull, aching sensation that bridges exacerbations of more severe pain.

The distinctive features of vascular pain is its primary pulsatile or throbbing quality. The pulsations match the heart beat and no doubt stem from the cardiac systoles. The greater the amplitude of vascular dilatation, the more pronounced the throbbing quality of the pain. This quality may be very slight at times and may be masked by coexistent muscle pain. The pulsatile feature of a vascular pain syndrome is not constant but is usually present during exacerbations. Between such peaks of discomfort, the pulsations may diminish in intensity or be imperceptible.

The throbbing quality of true vascular pain must be distinguished from other throbbing pains. Inflammatory pains, especially those confined in such a way that the pulsating vessels in the inflamed area cause noxious stimulation, have a throbbing quality. Examples of such inflammatory pains frequently encountered by the dentist are pulpitis, osteitis, periosteitis, and confined cellulitis. Usually differentiation can be made on the basis of other clinical signs of inflammation and on the basis that the clinical course of the pain complaint follows the usual pattern of other inflammatory processes. Some neoplastic lesions present a pulsatile quality.

It appears that most vascular pains of the maxillofacial region are mediated by somatic afferents and enter the CNS through the sensory roots of cranial nerves. However, there are instances in which vascular pains are arrested by analgesic blocking of the stellate ganglion, indicating that they are mediated by visceral afferents.

Gross[5] has shown that blood vessels are supplied by both visceral and somatic afferents. Nerves at the surface of the media are predominantly sympathetic; those in the more superficial adventitia are predominantly somatic. Hannington-Kiff[7] believes that some vascular pain

dromes that accompany certain illnesses, intoxications, and posttraumatic conditions.

The formulation for vascular pain includes features other than those explicable by the gate control theory of pain mechanisms. The occurrence of cervical muscle pain does not follow the behavior of central excitatory activity as a secondary effect. Rather, it behaves as an accompanying but independent cervical myofascial pain syndrome. It may be presumed that when both the vascular and myogenous components are integral parts of the syndrome and not dependent on each other, they stem from a common cause such as emotional tension. The emotional overlay that so consistently accompanies vascular pain syndromes probably also induces the cervical muscle complaint, which, though less severe, may be the more persistent of the two pain sources. For this reason the muscular component induces mild, nonpulsatile, dull, aching sensations that bridge the periodic throbbing pains that emanate from the vessels.

The formulation for vascular pain includes also another element—that of secondary central excitatory effects. If the pain, either the vascular or the muscle component, is persistent and of sufficient intensity, secondary referred pain and spreading are expected to occur. In the more severe forms of persistent vascular pain, these effects can be clinically identified. *The secondary muscle spasms most frequently involve the masticatory muscles and bring into the symptom complex a component of masticatory pain and sometimes dysfunction as well.* When this occurs, diagnostic differentiation is required; otherwise, unnecessary and futile dental treatment may be instituted. Secondary autonomic effects are commonplace in migrainous neuralgia.

As the role of neurotransmitters, and particularly the discovery of an endogenous antinociceptive system, have modified our understanding of pain mechanisms, the concept that peripheral vasodilatation is the primary factor in vascular pains is no longer valid. Currently, it appears that failure in the endogenous antinociceptive system is largely responsible for vascular pain syndromes.[9] Vasodilatation does not induce headache in normal subjects. Pain and vasodilatation are induced only by such substances as bradykinin, prostaglandins, and histamine. Vascular pain attacks are likely due to the failure of opioid peptides and neurotransmitters of the antinociceptive system which causes supersensitivity to the serotonin precursor 5–hydroxytryptophan and other monoamines (dopamine and norepinephrine).[9]

According to Appenzeller,[10] vascular headaches constitute a central serotonin deficiency together with increased circulatory epinephrine.

During the aura phase, impaired oxygenation of brain tissue has been detected by computed axial tomography (CAT) scans and examination of cerebrospinal fluid (CSF) constituents. During the headache phase, brain blood flow definitely increases. The role of extracranial vessels therefore has been seriously questioned.

There seems to be little doubt that serotonin has a significant role in vascular pains.[11-13] This monoamine is also implicated in emotional states; it is significantly decreased in depressive illness.[14] Histamine also has an important role. It has been shown, however, that the action of histamine in initiating attacks of vascular pain applies only to so-called migraine patients; it does not act in this way with nonmigrainous subjects.[15] It has also been shown that attacks of common migraine display an increase in EMG activity in pericranial muscles.[16,17] Since vascular headache and so-called tension headache have much in common,[9] it is likely that the underlying systemic factors stem from common cause. Currently, it is believed that systemic factors, complex as they are, exercise a dominant role in vascular pain syndromes.

For purposes of description, vascular pain syndromes are classified as (1) migrainous neuralgia, (2) atypical odontalgia, (3) common migraine, (4) classic migraine, and (5) vascular inflammation pains (Fig 13–1). It should be understood, however, that such an arbitrary classification should not be taken to indicate that they constitute specific clinical entities. The most characteristic feature of all vascular pains is their variability. All have a common underlying systemic etiology in which factors of emotional stress and tension play an important role. This classification of vascular pains reflects more the timing and location of symptoms and the predominant features displayed rather than any real difference between them.

MIGRAINOUS NEURALGIA

Migraine variants appear to be less well understood than classic migraine in all its variations. Different investigators have assigned names to some of the more distinctive variants such as migrainous neuralgia, cluster headache, histamine cephalalgia, Horton's headache, sphenopalatine neuralgia, vidian nerve neuralgia, lower-half headache, Sluder's headache, post-traumatic headache, and atypical facial neuralgia. The descriptive difference in these various pain complaints is not impressive since they all have in common the characteristic features of vascular pain, especially the feature of variability. Different vascular sources may alter the location of the pain.

OROFACIAL PAIN SYNDROMES

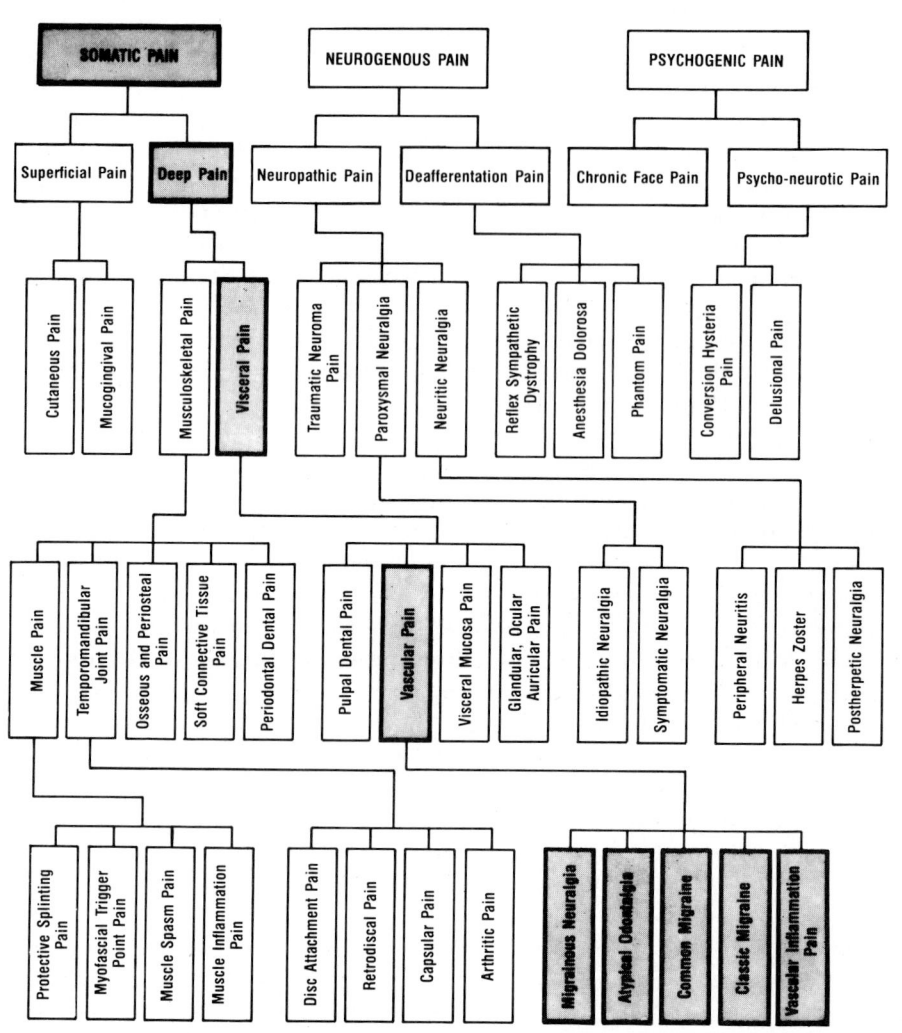

Fig 13–1.—Chart showing classification relationship of vascular pains to other orofacial pain syndromes.

The general term *migrainous neuralgia* may be used to designate all the nonneurogenous neuralgic complaints of the orofacial region. As a group, they should be clearly differentiated from the neuritic and paroxysmal neuralgias that stem from neural causes. The vascular pain

syndromes are deep somatic, not neurogenous. Vascular neuralgias differ from those of neural origin in the following ways[8]:
1. Pain is not limited to the peripheral distribution of a nerve but may spread beyond neurologic boundaries following the vascular arborization.
2. Pain is not precisely controlled by division of the sensory root of a single nerve.
3. Pain is steady, diffuse, aching, and usually throbbing with milder dull, diffuse, nonpulsatile discomfort bridging the more severe exacerbations. It may last for hours, days, or weeks.
4. Summation effects such as triggering from slight stimulation are not observed.
5. The syndrome occurs in younger age groups.
6. Attacks of pain are not induced by stimulation of superficial sensory receptors.
7. Vasoconstriction medications usually decrease the intensity of the throbbing component of pain.

Migrainous neuralgia has some behavioral characteristics that cause it to be confused with other pain syndromes of the face and neck. It initially may be felt as *toothache,* especially in the maxillary canine and biscuspid area (Case No. 13–1). Many teeth have been extracted or treated endodontally for toothache from this cause, and much needless and fruitless dental therapy instituted. Because of its frequency, this pain entity needs to be better understood by all who diagnose and treat pain problems of the teeth, mouth, and face.

Migrainous neuralgia that involves the face is often referred to as *atypical facial neuralgia.*[18] It frequently begins as a "dental pain" involving a maxillary canine or biscuspid. The initiating pain is sufficiently similar to true pulpal toothache to convince the patient, and usually the dentist as well, that a dental cause is present and dental treatment indicated. Unfortunately such dental treatment may be instituted prior to accurate diagnosis and followed by still other forms of therapy. For example, such a tooth may be prepared and filled (when minor caries is identified or the tooth as been previously treated), only to be followed by endodontic treatment, and finally extraction. Then treatment begins on adjacent teeth, and sometimes extensive procedures are attempted. Because of the accompanying nasal symptoms, the patient may be treated for sinusitis, then allergic rhinitis—finally being branded neurotic. As treatment progresses, so does spreading of the complaint. As rapport between patient and doctor breaks down, the patient may blame the initial or subsequent dental treatment for his predicament.

Oral and Facial Pain

DR. WELDEN E. BELL
8226 DOUGLAS AVENUE
DALLAS, TEXAS

Name: Female age 46

HISTORY

QUALITY	DURATION	LOCALIZATION	AFFECTED BY	LOCAL EFFECTS
(Mild) Severe	Bright (Dull)	(Continuous) Intermittent (Recurrent)	Localized (Diffuse)	Sensory: Hypesthesia Hyperesthesia Paresthesia Dysesthesia	Special Sense: Visual Auditory Olfactory Gustatory
Spontaneous Triggered Induced Paroxysmal (Steady)	Pricking Itching Burning (Aching) (Pulsating)	Momentary Minutes Hours Day long (Protracted)	Face Movement Jaw Movement Tongue Movement Swallowing Head Position Body Position Activities (Tension) (Fatigue) Time of Day	Motor: Weakness Contraction Spasm	Autonomic: (Ocular Signs) (Nasal Signs) Cutaneous Signs Gastric Signs
		Radiating Spreading Enlarging Migrating (Secondary Pain)			

Location / Inception / Initial pain / Duration, clinical course / Therapeutic response / Physical and emotional background / Trauma, infection, etc. / Medications in use

Recurrent episodes of mild to severe variable continuous protracted steady dull aching throbbing pain diffusely located in the right teeth and face, aggravated by tension and fatigue, and accompanied by nasal congestion.
The complaint has been recurrently present for 4-5 years, each episode lasting a few weeks, followed by a remission of several months. The present one began about a month ago. There is mild constant aching in the face and some also in the occipital area with severe exacerbations described as throbbing toothache lasting up to an hour occurring once or twice daily, sometimes at night. She has lacrimation and congestion of the nose on the right side that increases when the pain is severe. It was initially treated as sinusitis, then as tic douloureux, and more recently as allergic rhinitis -- without benefit. Dental treatment has included occlusal adjustments, endodontia, extraction of UR6, extraction of LR6, and replacements by dentists of different disciplines. She has been cleared neurologically. The internist wants the dental problem cleared.

EXAMINATION

B/P 135/85   Neurological Survey   Psychological Survey

Oral / TM joints / Muscle system / Diagnostic blocks / Diagnostic drugs / Trial therapy

Orally: There is no clinical or radiographical evidence of any dental, oral, or masticatory cause for the complaint. The quality of dental care reflects expertise technically. Oral hygiene is excellent. There is no occlusal disharmony identified. Masticatory functioning appears to be normal in all respects.
TM joints: Both joints are normal structurally and functionally.
Muscle system: There is no palpable tenderness of any masticatory muscle and no muscular dysfunction. There is vague occipital discomfort that seems to parallel the dental and facial pain.

Trial therapy with ergotamine tartrate gave noticeable relief especially of the spontaneous exacerbations of "toothache". The occipital discomfort and constant mild aching sensation in the face were not affected much.

Opinion: There is no dental, oral, or masticatory cause for the complaint. By history, clinical course, present behavioral characteristics, and trial therapy, the entire pain problem suggests vascular pain clinically classified as atypical facial neuralgia. The dental, nasal, and ocular symptoms are very likely secondary central excitatory effects of the deep vascular pain that presumably involves the right maxillary artery. Management should be on a medical level.

DIAGNOSIS

Toothache secondary to a vascular pain syndrome.

Case No. 13-1.—Heterotopic pain, felt as toothache, due to a vascular pain syndrome (migrainous neuralgia).

The ability of the dentist to recognize and identify this pain syndrome is extremely important—and *only he can do it*. Differential diagnostic criteria are as follows:
 1. The aching tooth is free of reasonable dental cause for the pain.
 2. The toothache has a persistent, episodic, recurrent behavior.

3. Analgesic blocking of the tooth proper may stop the pain in some instances, leading the dentist to assume that the source is of dental origin. At other times its effect is not precise or conclusive and may even aggravate the pain.
4. Definitive therapy such as endodontic treatment or extraction may give temporary, transitory benefit, only to be followed in due time by recurrence of the complaint.
5. Almost invariably there are accompanying ipsilateral autonomic signs involving the eye and nose.
6. With time, the complaint spreads to involve wider areas of the face and neck, even the shoulder. Frequently, occipital muscle effects are observed, with symptoms suggestive of tension headache. Very frequently, chewing pains occur due to secondary painful spasm of the masticatory muscles, and futile efforts to manage a masticatory pain-dysfunction syndrome may follow, sometimes to the point of definitive occlusal treatment measures including reconstruction.
7. Early in the syndrome the pain complaint may be favorably influenced by carotid pressure or administration of ergotamine tartrate, which helps identify it as a vascular pain. This effect diminishes as secondary muscle involvement occurs.

Although atypical facial neuralgia frequently occurs initially as toothache, it may spread to involve the entire maxilla, side of the face, ear, neck, and shoulder. It is episodic and recurrent. Its throbbing quality and muscular component may simulate both odontogenous and masticatory pains. Its extreme variability and sudden exacerbations give it a neuralgic quality that may be mistaken for tic douloureux. The acute pains may occur rather regularly at night. As spreading occurs, the accompanying autonomic effects, i.e., edema of the eyelids and face, lacrimation, and nasal congestion, may be confused with allergic rhinitis and sinusitis. The component of occipital pain that secondarily refers to the frontal region may simulate tension headache.

When expressed as a direct central excitatory effect, the muscle symptoms almost invariably occur in the masticatory muscles because these are innervated by the trigeminal nerve which mediates the pain input. Actual masticatory muscle spasm causing true masticatory pain and representing a masticatory pain-dysfunction syndrome can therefore be a direct secondary effect of persistent vascular pain. When this is true, both the initiating primary vascular pain and the secondary masticatory pain should be identified, and therapy for both pain problems is required for adequate management. This immediately becomes a multidisciplinary effort. If the masticatory component only is treated, prompt relapse occurs when active therapy ceases. If the vascular component only is treated, the secondary masticatory muscle component remains as a complaint. *Proper management depends on diagnostic identification of the dual phenomenon present and simultaneous therapy administered by physician and dentist cooperatively.*

When accompanying muscle discomfort stems from a common cause such as emotional tension, the complaint almost invariably involves the occipital and cervical musculature. It should be recognized that so-called tension headache frequently accompanies persistent vascular pains, and this cervical myofascial pain syndrome may in turn cause referred facial pain or may spread secondarily to cause masticatory muscle spasms. Thus masticatory pain may occur in conjunction with combined vascular and myogenous pain problems of the head and neck. Sometimes, expert diagnostic effort is required to evaluate the condition correctly and point the way to effective management.

Vascular pains have the propensity to cause referred pains about the face, frequently in the preauricular and temporomandibular joint region. Such referred pains require careful diagnostic identification.

Atypical facial neuralgia may be mistaken for true masticatory pain. Although classic migraine tends to produce all these pain effects, usually its duration is too short to become a diagnostic problem. Atypical facial neuralgia, however, is a different matter. Not only may it induce a true masticatory pain-dysfunction syndrome as a central excitatory effect (Case No. 13–2), but the vascular pain syndrome may present a component of nonspastic muscle pain felt in the occipital and sometimes masticatory muscles. When this occurs, discomfort with chewing is experienced even though no actual masticatory dysfunction takes place. This strange manifestation of atypical facial neuralgia may be mistaken for a masticatory pain-dysfunction syndrome and be improperly treated as a masticatory problem (Case No. 13–3).

The dental examiner should be familiar with this behavior of facial vascular pain. Definite similarities exist between atypical facial neuralgia and masticatory pain, since both are representative of deep somatic pain. Both syndromes are variable or recurrent; the pains are steady, not paroxysmal; the pains have a dull, aching quality; the pains are very poorly localized or frankly diffuse; and both syndromes readily induce central excitatory effects. The following points should serve as guidelines to help differentiate them:

1. Vascular pain usually has a characteristic pulsatile, throbbing quality.
2. Atypical facial neuralgia follows the vascular arborization and therefore violates neuroanatomical boundaries. Frequently the

Vascular Pains 249

Oral and Facial Pain
DR. WELDEN E. BELL
8226 DOUGLAS AVENUE
DALLAS, TEXAS

Name: Male age 60

HISTORY

QUALITY	DURATION	LOCALIZATION	AFFECTED BY	LOCAL EFFECTS
(Mild) Severe	Bright (Dull)	(Continuous) Intermittent Recurrent	Localized (Diffuse) Radiating (Spreading)	Face Movement (Jaw Movement) Tongue Movement Swallowing Head Position Body Position Activities Tension Fatigue Time of Day	Sensory: Hypesthesia Hyperesthesia Paresthesia Dysesthesia Motor: Weakness Contraction (Spasm)	Special Sense: Visual Auditory Olfactory Gustatory Autonomic: (Ocular Signs) (Nasal Signs) (Cutaneous Signs) Gastric Signs
Spontaneous Triggered Induced Paroxysmal (Steady)	Pricking Itching Burning (Aching) (Pulsating)	Momentary Minutes Hours Day long (Protracted)	Enlarging Migrating (Secondary Pain)		

Location
Inception
Initial pain
Duration, clinical course
Therapeutic response
Physical and emotional background
Trauma, infection, etc.
Medications in use

Mild to severe continuous protracted steady dull aching pain diffusely located in the left auricular and preauricular area, aggravated by mandibular movement, associated with a continuous but quite variable high and low intensity throbbing pain in the left maxillary teeth, face, orbit, and neck which when intense was accompanied by tearing, swelling, and redness of the left eye, left nasal congestion, and flushing of the left face.

The complaint began about two years ago as a recurrent throbbing pain in the left maxillary teeth, several of which were treated dentally without lasting benefit. He was then unsuccessfully treated for sinusitis and allergic rhinitis. About a year ago, the pain became continuous and soon spread to involve the masticatory system. He has been examined medically, neurologically, and otolaryngologically and the concensus was that he had a temporomandibular joint syndrome. The complaint has remained the same for several months.
No medications are presently being taken.

EXAMINATION

B/P 105/68   Neurological Survey   Psychological Survey

Oral

TM joints

Muscle system

Diagnostic blocks

Diagnostic drugs

Trial therapy

Orally: The teeth and mouth are essentially negative clinically and radiographically. There is pain in the left masseter area with opening beyond 24mm, with chewing eccentrically, and with clenching the teeth. The mandible deflects to the left after about 24-25mm opening. The maximum opening is about 30mm. No occlusal disharmony is identified.

TM joints: Both joints are clinically normal except for left side restriction of opening. Radiographically, the left joint is normal structurally and functionally except for evidence of extracapsular restriction of translatory movement with opening. (See tracings.)

Muscle system: There is palpable tenderness in the left masseter muscle.

Analgesic blocking of the left masseter muscle arrested the masticatory component of the complaint but did not affect the diffuse throbbing pain. Ergotamine tartrate temporarily reduced the throbbing component when used during a period of high intensity pain.

Opinion: It appears that a vascular pain syndrome antedated the masticatory complaint and as such represented the primary pain which secondarily by central excitation induced spasm of the left masseter muscle. Cycling has no doubt occurred. The resulting myofascial pain-dysfunction syndrome involving the masticatory muscle was induced by non-masticatory causes.

DIAGNOSIS

Masticatory pain-dysfunction syndrome expressed as cycling myospasm of the left masseter muscle, secondary to preexistent vascular pain.

Case No. 13–2,A.—Case chart. Masticatory myospasm pain (pain-dysfunction syndrome), secondary to deep vascular pain (migrainous neuralgia).

pain is simultaneously felt in the side of the neck—sometimes in the shoulder. Vessel wall edema may occur, identified as palpable tenderness along the superficial arteries. Occipital muscular discomfort may be present.

Temporomandibular Examination Radiographic Tracings	Name __Male__ age __60__	Key to Symbols
DR. WELDEN E. BELL 8226 DOUGLAS AVENUE DALLAS, TEXAS	X-ray File No. _____ Date _____	POC Primary Occlusal Contact OP Occlusal Position RP Rest Position LP Contralateral Position MTO Maximum Translatory Opening PR Protrusive Position

Left T-M Joint	Left LP: 13 MTO: 9	Key	Right LP: MTO:	Right T-M Joint
	POC = ⎫ OP = ⎬ _____ LP = ---- ---- ---- MTO = --- -- --- --			

INTERPRETATION

The left joint was viewed in four transparietal positions:
1. Position of primary occlusal contact (POC).
2. Fully occluded position (OP).
3. Contralateral excursion (LP).
4. Maximum opening - 30mm (MTO).

This joint presents well defined smoothly contoured articular surfaces with an interarticular space of adequate width which does not decrease in width under biting stress. There is no radiographic evidence of degenerative joint disease or other structural abnormality.

There is excellent superimposition of POC and OP, indicative of no occlusal disharmony that is radiographically evident as gross displacement of the condyle when the teeth are firmly occluded.

Translatory movement of the condyle in contralateral excursion is normal, indicative of freedom of movement within the capsule.

Translatory movement of the condyle with opening is restricted, indicative of the effect of extracapsular causes.

Case No. 13-2,B.—Radiographic tracings of left joint.

3. Atypical facial neuralgia varies in intensity from low to high—low enough almost to go unnoticed, followed by a sudden exacerbation of high-intensity pain. This gives it a neuralgic quality, but the pains are not truly paroxysmal, and the intermissions are not completely pain free. The low-intensity pain is predominantly myalgic and nonpulsatile, whereas the high-intensity exacerbations are usually more characteristically vascular and throbbing. The intense exacerbations may have a temporal regularity unrelated to functioning. These attacks are frequently nocturnal.

4. Atypical facial neuralgia is prone to occur in episodes lasting several weeks and separated by pain-free remissions of several weeks or months. Sometimes it occurs in clusters of short painful episodes followed by long periods of remission. The episodes relate more to emotional tension and fatigue than to functional demands.

Oral and Facial Pain
DR. WELDEN E. BELL
8228 DOUGLAS AVENUE
DALLAS, TEXAS

Name Female age 36		Age	Date		
QUALITY	DURATION	LOCALIZATION	AFFECTED BY	LOCAL EFFECTS	

HISTORY

QUALITY: ~~Mild~~, ~~Severe~~, Spontaneous, Triggered, Induced, Paroxysmal, ~~Steady~~
DURATION: ~~Bright~~, ~~Dull~~, Pricking, Itching, Burning, ~~Aching~~, Pulsating / ~~Continuous~~, Intermittent, ~~Recurrent~~, Momentary, Minutes, Hours, Day long, ~~Protracted~~
LOCALIZATION: Localized, ~~Diffuse~~, Radiating, Spreading, Enlarging, Migrating, ~~Secondary Pain~~
AFFECTED BY: Face Movement, ~~Jaw Movement~~, Tongue Movement, Swallowing, ~~Head Position~~, Body Position, Activities, Tension, Fatigue, Time of Day
LOCAL EFFECTS — Sensory: Hypesthesia, Hyperesthesia, Paresthesia, Dysesthesia; Motor: Weakness, Contraction, Spasm; Special Sense: Visual, Auditory, Olfactory, Gustatory; Autonomic: ~~Ocular Signs~~, ~~Nasal Signs~~, Cutaneous Signs, Gastric Signs

Location
Inception
Initial pain
Duration, clinical course
Therapeutic response
Physical and emotional background
Trauma, infection, etc.
Medications in use

Recurrent episodes of continuous mild protracted steady dull aching pain diffusely located in the left occipital and preauricular areas, apparently aggravated by head movements and hard chewing, punctuated several times daily by spontaneous periods of high-intensity throbbing pain located in the left maxillary teeth and jaw and associated with ipsilateral lacrimation and nasal congestion, sometimes with noticeable nausea. Each episode lasts several weeks separated by irregular intervals of several months.
The complaint began about two years ago and was treated as tension headache. When the chewing discomfort occurred, the physician thought it was due to a "TM joint syndrome" and promptly referred the patient for dental treatment. This has consisted of refilling several left maxillary teeth and adjustments of the occlusion -- without benefit. At times, the remissions were attributed to medical and/or dental therapy. The present episode has lasted five weeks without responding favorably to treatment. No medications presently being taken.

EXAMINATION

B/P 120/80   Neurological Survey   Psychological Survey

Oral

TM joints

Muscle system

Diagnostic blocks

Diagnostic drugs

Trial therapy

Orally: No dental or oral cause for the complaint is found clinically or radiographically. Masticatory function is entirely normal in all respects. No occlusal disharmony is identified clinically or radiographically. There is some minor preauricular and temporal discomfort with hard chewing.
TM joints: Both joints are normal clinically and radiographically.
Muscle system: There is slight palpable tenderness in the left masseter, temporal, occipital and trapezius muscles but no dysfunction of any kind.
Diagnostic drugs: Ergotamine tartrate was administered several times. Each time it arrested the throbbing maxillary component within 30 minutes but it had no noticeable effect on the preauricular and occipital discomfort.
Opinion: The history, clinical course, and present behavioral characteristics of the pain complaint are highly suggestive of a vascular pain syndrome (so-called atypical facial neuralgia) accompanied, as it so frequently is, by muscular, cervical and occipital pain. The left masticatory muscles have become secondarily involved, probably as a central excitatory effect, causing discomfort with hard chewing but no masticatory dysfunction of any kind.

DIAGNOSIS

Vascular pain syndrome with a muscle component mistaken for a masticatory pain-dysfunction syndrome.

Case No. 13-3.—Vascular pain (migrainous neuralgia), mistaken for masticatory pain.

5. Atypical facial neuralgia does not cause appreciable dysfunction unless there is a dominant component of secondarily induced myospasm. Since such effects involve chiefly the masticatory muscles, the symptoms of a masticatory pain-dysfunction syndrome may become evident, and the underlying etiologically

important vascular pain syndrome may go unnoticed. The only indication of its presence may be recurring exacerbations of throbbing pain—a phenomenon wholly inconsistent with true masticatory pain.
6. Atypical facial neuralgia frequently presents characteristic autonomic effects, i.e., nasal congestion, lacrimation, injection of the conjunctiva, edema of the eyelids and face—*on the affected side only.* These central excitatory effects may be confused with allergic rhinitis and sinusitis clinically. It should be noted, however, that allergic rhinitis is always bilateral and sinusitis usually so.
7. When vascular pain is suspected, the throbbing component (but not the muscle component) may be reduced by applying pressure to the carotid artery manually or by administration of ergotamine tartrate.
8. Differentiation between atypical facial neuralgia and true masticatory pain is best made by the accumulation of *positive evidence of the presence of vascular pain on one hand or of masticatory pain on the other.*
9. When the two conditions occur simultaneously, therapeutic trial may be required to confirm the diagnosis.

Atypical facial neuralgia may follow facial trauma, including tooth extraction and other minor oral surgery. As such, it may be confused with other post-traumatic pain problems such as reflex sympathetic dystrophy, atypical neuralgia, and neuritic pain in the trigeminal area.

Because of the extreme versatility of vascular pain and its propensity to simulate other facial pain syndromes, especially those involving dental practice, errors in diagnosis may be made. The dental examiner should be constantly alert to these possibilities because vascular pain is very common.

The dental examiner should have at his command sufficient understanding to be able to identify pains of this type. He should be especially cautious in advising definitive therapy either of the teeth or the masticatory apparatus until a confirmed diagnosis is established.

ATYPICAL ODONTALGIA

In recent years a vascular pain syndrome has been described as atypical odontalgia.[19-21] This condition exhibits all the symptoms of vascular toothache as expressed in migrainous neuralgia, but without the face symptoms. The tooth pain remains the focus of attention.

Without other clinical characteristics of migrainous neuralgia, toothache of this type closely simulates pulpal odontalgia. Several features, however, should lead the examiner to suspect that the pain is of vascular origin, namely (1) lack of adequate local dental cause, (2) persistent and sometimes recurrent toothache without undergoing the usual expected temporal sequence from pulpal to periodontal pain, and (3) the ability of the subject to point out exactly which tooth hurts. This may represent the initial symptom of a beginning vascular pain syndrome.

COMMON MIGRAINE

So-called migraine headache is a vascular pain syndrome of limited duration—usually only a day or so—that recurs periodically. Classic migraine displays a prodromal phase that precedes the headache phase. Common migraine does not prominently display such prodromal symptoms. This complaint has taken on numerous common names such as sick headache, Sunday headache, Monday-morning headache, wash-day headache, examination headache, and menstrual headache. It is frequently associated with stressful life situations. It has been called the most common bodily complaint of civilized man.[22]

Olesen[23] has reported on a large group of patients with migraines. He reported that pain was significantly more right-sided than left. Nausea was present in 86% of his subjects, with nearly half of them actually vomiting. Pain was described by 68% as "severe." Pulsatile quality was reported by nearly half of the subjects. Interictal pain was reported by nearly half. Some muscle tenderness was reported by about 70% of the subjects, it being felt especially in the cervical and masticatory areas.

Dental and masticatory pains occur frequently with migraine headache. They usually do not constitute a clinical complaint, however, because of the limited duration. Most migraine sufferers know that such is part of the headache problem and give it no thought. Mistakes in this regard are usually those of the doctor who mistakenly thinks the headaches are due to a dental or masticatory cause.

CLASSIC MIGRAINE

Classic migraine is a well-known vascular pain syndrome. It is described[8] as periodic headache, usually unilateral in onset but which later may become generalized; it is associated with irritability, nausea, photophobia, constipation, or diarrhea. Frequently the attack has a prodromic phase, with visual disturbance affecting half the visual field, paresthesias, and speech difficulties. Usually it affects only the upper head, but it may spread to include the face and neck. At times it induces rather typical toothache. Widespread autonomic effects that induce strange symptoms throughout the body are commonplace. The complaint may vary from trifling symptoms that go almost unnoticed to severe, disabling illness. It may last from a few hours to several weeks. The longer it lasts, the more pronounced the autonomic effects and accompanying muscle pains. Severe attacks may induce secondary muscle spasms in segmentally related areas. Many variations of typical migraine occur, and perhaps its most typical feature is its variability. It may occur at any age but is especially common among adolescents and young adults.

Blau and Dexter[24] have used the following criteria to decide if the pain emanates from intracranial or extracranial sources. Intracranial pain is said to be increased by head jolt, coughing, or holding the breath for 30 seconds. Extracranial pain is said to be relieved by digital compression of superficial scalp arteries or by inflation of a cuff around the head. Of 50 subjects studied during migraine attacks, all but one, by these criteria, had intracranial pain, while 28 had extracranial pain also.

VASCULAR INFLAMMATION PAIN

While most vascular pains are noninflammatory, sometimes the vessels become inflamed, and the pain that results takes on the clinical characteristics of inflammatory pain. According to Dalessio,[2] cranial or temporal arteritis is a rare, febrile, inflammatory disease of variable duration. It afflicts the aged of both sexes and appears to be related to inflammation and distension of cranial arteries. It becomes particularly evident in the superficial temporal arteries because of their accessibility. The distended arteries are extremely tender on palpation. Frequently headache, scalp hyperalgesias and painful mastication accompany the arteritis. Vision may be affected. Many arteries usually are involved, and the localized pain is accompanied by systemic symptoms suggestive of subacute or chronic infection.

The natural history is that of a self-limiting disease of many months' duration with a tendency to relapse. It is nonfatal, and recovery may be complete except for specific conditions such as impaired vision due to vascular changes. Although the cause of arteritis is unknown, there is some evidence that it is a type of immunologic vasculitis.[2]

This condition differs from other vascular pains that have such characteristics as periodic and intermittent timing; variability; recurrence; noninflammatory pulsatile pain, especially with exacerbations; intensity unrelated to function or provocation; more obvious emotional overlay; and response to vasoconstricting medications. Cranial arteritis in contrast has an inflammatory time frame, is localizable subjectively and objectively, can be provoked by manual palpation, and displays characteristic local and systemic symptoms. The diagnosis may be confirmed by biopsy.[25]

Cranial arteritis seems to occur more frequently in females. It may arise as a nonspecific pain that induces heterotopic pain, headaches, and burning sensations. Discomfort in the throat is common. The masticatory muscles may display heterotopic pain as areas of palpable tenderness due to secondary hyperalgesia. The affected blood vessels are tender to manual palpation, and manipulation accentuates the symptoms.[26]

Carotodynia is a rare vascular pain syndrome that causes pain in the neck and face. Some of these conditions are noninflammatory and appear to be migraine variants.[27] Others are definitely inflammatory and are identified as cranial arteritis.[28] Carotodynia causes episodic throbbing pain in the carotid region. It occurs in females four to one. The head cannot be hyperextended away from the affected side. There is pain with swallowing and some difficulty with mastication. A variety of secondary central excitatory effects may be displayed. Carotodynia may be a complication of Eagle's syndrome when the styloid process is elongated enough to encroach on the carotid vessels.

REFERENCES

1. Bonica J.J.: *The Management of Pain.* Philadelphia, Lea & Febiger, 1953.
2. Dalessio D.J.: *Wolff's Headache and Other Head Pain,* ed. 3. New York, Oxford University Press, 1972.
3. Wolff H.G., Wolf S.: *Pain,* ed. 2. Springfield, Ill., Charles C Thomas, Publishers, 1958.
4. Finneson B.E.: *Diagnosis and Management of Pain Syndromes,* ed. 2. Phildelphia, W.B. Saunders Co., 1969.
5. Gross D.: Pain and autonomic nervous system, in Bonica J.J. (ed.): *Advances in Neurology.* New York, Raven Press, 1974, vol. 4, pp. 99–103.
6. Moore D.C.: *Stellate Ganglion Block.* Springfield, Ill., Charles C Thomas, Publisher, 1954.
7. Hannington-Kiff J.G.: *Pain Relief.* Philadelphia, J.B. Lippincott Co., 1974.
8. Wolff H.G.: *Headache and Other Head Pain,* ed. 2. New York, Oxford University Press, 1963.
9. Sicuteri F.: Headache as the most common disease of the antinociceptive system: Analogues with morphine abstinance, in Bonica J.J., Liebeskind J.C., Albe-Fessard D.G. (eds.): *Advances in Pain Research and Therapy.* New York, Raven Press, 1979, vol. 3, pp. 359–365.

10. Appenzeller O.: Headache: Clinical and pathogenetic aspects, in Bonica J.J., Liebeskind J.C., Albe-Fessard D.G. (eds.): *Advances in Pain Research and Therapy.* New York, Raven Press, 1979, vol. 3, pp. 345–358.
11. Dvilansky A., Rishpon S., Nathan I., et al.: Release of platelet 5–hydroxytryptamine by plasma taken from patients during and between migraine attacks. *Pain* 2:315–318, 1976.
12. Anthony M., Hinterberger H., Lance J.W.: Plasma serotonin in migraine and stress. *Arch. Neurol.* 16:544–552, 1967.
13. Anthony M., Hinterberger H., Lance J.W.: The possible relationship of serotonin to the migraine syndrome. *Arch. Clin. Stud. Headache* 2:29, 1969.
14. Seltzer S., Marcus R., Stoch R.: Perspectives in the control of chronic pain by nutritional manipulation. *Pain* 11:141–148, 1981.
15. Krabbe A.A., Olesen J.: Headache provocation by continuous intravenous infusion of histamine: Clinical results and receptor mechanisms. *Pain* 8:253–259, 1980.
16. Clifford T., Lauritzen M., Bakke M., et al.: Electromyography of pericranial muscles during treatment of spontaneous common migraine attacks. *Pain* 14:137–147, 1982.
17. Bakke M., Tfelt-Hansen P., Olesen J., et al.: Action of some pericranial muscles during provoked attacks of common migraine. *Pain* 14:121–135, 1982.
18. McArdle M.J.: Atypical facial neuralgia, in Hassler R., Walker A.E. (eds.): *Trigeminal Neuralgia.* Stuttgart, Georg Thieme Verlag, 1970, pp. 35–42.
19. Rees R.T., Harris M.: Atypical odontalgia. *Br. J. Oral Surg.* 16:212–218, 1979.
20. Brooke R.I.: Atypical odontalgia. *J. Oral Surg.* 49:196–199, 1980.
21. Kreisberg M.K.: Atypical odontalgia: Differential diagnosis and treatment. *J.A.D.A.* 104:852–854, 1982.
22. Bassoe P.: Migraine. *J.A.M.A.* 101:599, 1933.
23. Olesen J.: Some clinical features of the acute migraine attack: An analysis of 750 patients. *Headache* 18:268–271, 1978.
24. Blau J.N., Dexter S.L.: The site of pain origin during migraine attacks. *Cephalgia* 1:143, 1981.
25. Paine R.: Vascular facial pain, in Alling C.C., Mahan P.E. (eds.): *Facial Pain,* ed. 2. Philadelphia, Lea & Febiger, 1977, pp. 57–70.
26. Trolano M.F., Gaston G.W.: Carotid system arteritis: An overlooked and misdiagnosed syndrome. *J.A.D.A.* 91:589, 1975.
27. Murray T.J.: Carotidynia: A cause of neck and face pain. *Can. Med. Assoc. J.* 120:441–443, 1979.
28. Scheitler L.E., Balciunas B.A.: Carotidynia. *J. Oral Maxillofac. Surg.* 40:121–122, 1982.

14

Other Visceral Pains

DEEP SOMATIC PAIN OF VISCERAL TYPE may arise from other structures of the mouth and face besides the pulps of teeth (chapter 9) and the vascular tissues (chapter 13). For descriptive purposes, such pains can be divided into (1) pains emanating from the mucosa of the pharynx, nose, and paranasal sinuses, (2) pains arising from glandular structures of the face, (3) ocular pains, and (4) auricular pains (Fig 14–1).

PRIMARY PAINS OF VISCERAL MUCOSA

While pain emanating from the oral mucogingival tissues is exteroceptive in character and therefore displays clinical characteristics of superficial somatic type, pain from other mucosal structures of the face is definitely interoceptive in character and exhibits the clinical characteristics of deep pain of visceral type. This refers particularly to the mucosal linings of the pharynx, the nasal cavity, and the paranasal sinuses.

Being of the deep somatic category, pain from these structures usually displays the following symptoms:
1. The pain has a dull, depressing quality.
2. Subjective localization of the pain is variable and somewhat diffuse.
3. The site of pain may or may not identify the correct location of its true source.
4. Response to provocation at the site of pain is fairly faithful in incidence and intensity, but not in location.
5. Accompanying secondary central excitatory effects are frequently displayed.

In addition, visceral pain is of threshold type and does not give a graduated response to stimulation. It has little or no relationship to biomechanical function, and is nearly nonlocalizable by the subject. These clinical characteristics clearly differentiate the mucosal pains

OROFACIAL PAIN SYNDROMES

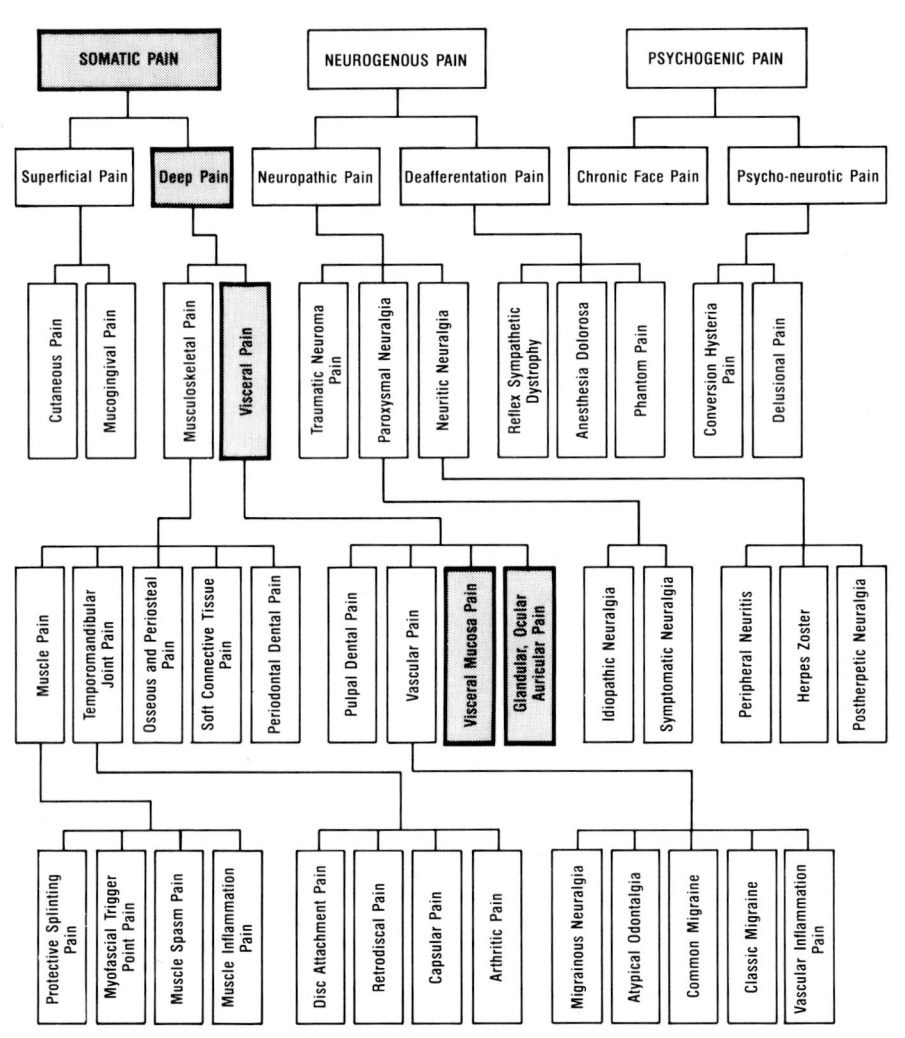

Fig 14–1.—Chart showing classification relationship of visceral mucosal, glandular, ocular, and auricular pains to other orofacial pain syndromes.

from those of the superficial somatic category that emanate from the oral mucogingival tissues as previously described.

Ordinarily, sensory perception of visceral mucosa linings remains below conscious levels. This rule applies especially to the more deeply situated structures. The closer such tissues are located to external environmental sources of stimulation, however, the more responsive they are to all stimuli, and the more conscious such sensation becomes. For example, the nasal mucosa is more sensitive to low-level stimulation than the pharyngeal mucosa, while that of the esophagus is less reactive. The fine sensibility of nasal mucosa applies also to the ostium maxillare, but the lining membrane of the maxillary sinus remains resistant to all stimuli. The external portion of esophageal mucosa is highly responsive to stimuli of threshold intensity, but the more deeply situated portion is nearly insensible to all noxious stimuli. It should be noted that there is a transitional zone where the oral mucogingival tissue joins the pharyngeal mucosa in which symptoms of both superficial somatic and deep visceral pain categories may be displayed.

An appreciation of the different types and degrees of sensibility of the lining membranes of the oral, nasal, and pharyngeal structures is needed to understand the nociceptive sensations that emanate from these tissues.

The normal inflow of sensation from visceral mucosa serves to regulate automatic functioning. Several reflex mechanisms are recognized. Irritation of the nasal mucosa excites the sneeze reflex; the pharyngeal mucosa initiates the swallowing and gag reflexes; upper esophageal mucosa may induce esophageal spasm; upper tracheal and laryngeal irritation stimulates the cough reflex. When mucosal stimulation becomes noxious, burning pain is felt.[1-4] It is said that continuing visceral pain tends to provoke vasomotor effects, local edema, and trophic changes.[5] The normally high-threshold level of sensibility is lowered in the presence of hyperemia and inflammation so that nociceptive impulses may be generated by otherwise nonnociceptive stimuli.

Nociceptive pathways from orofacial mucosal structures likely involve afferent elements of both the somatic and the visceral nervous systems. Somatic afferents are mediated by the fifth, seventh, and ninth cranial nerves. Parasympathetic visceral afferents are mediated by the seventh and ninth cranial nerves only. Sympathetic visceral afferents escape entry into the CNS by way of cranial nerves. Instead, they leave the head and travel the cervical sympathetic chain to enter through the upper thoracic spinal nerves. Pain mediated by sympathetic visceral afferents can be arrested by analgesic blocking of the stellate ganglion, through which such pathways pass even though they undergo no synapse prior to reaching the CNS.[6]

Like other forms of deep pain, visceral mucosa pain tends to initiate central excitatory effects. Many times, the secondary symptoms predominate while the primary pain input remains silent or goes unnoticed. Some orofacial pain syndromes are almost exclusively expressed as secondary central excitatory effects. Caution should be exercised in differentiating such effects from the true source of primary input.

PHARYNGEAL MUCOSA PAIN

Inflammatory conditions of the pharyngeal mucosa expressed as "sore throat" point up the marked difference between nociceptive conditions involving the oral mucogingival tissues and the visceral mucosa of the pharynx. While the pharyngeal mucosa is quite susceptible, the oral lining membranes are resistant.

Nonspecific pharyngitis is usually viral in origin and occurs in conjunction with nasal and laryngeal symptoms. Pain on swallowing is characteristic. Central excitatory effects include referred pain especially with swallowing. The reference zone is usually deep in the ear, and the pain is sensed as sharp and lancinating. Secondary hyperalgesia may be felt as deep palpable tenderness in the throat, larynx, neck, or face, or as superficial touchiness of the facial skin or scalp. Secondary autonomic symptoms may include puffy swelling of the eyelids, lacrimation, and nasal secretion. Sneeze and cough reflexes are active. Referred headache is common. Several clinical entities are recognized such as so-called strep throat and tonsillitis.

STREPTOCOCCAL PHARYNGITIS.—Streptococcal pharyngitis is typified by sore throat, fever, acutely inflamed pharyngeal mucosa, and referred pains including headache. Cervical and submandibular lymphadenitis is present. Laryngitis, coughing, and nasal congestion are not due to streptococcal infection. When present, other etiologic agents coexist. Definitive diagnosis rests on laboratory examination to identify the Group A beta-hemolytic organism.

TONSILLITIS.—Tonsillitis is an acute inflammation of the palatine tonsils, due usually to viral and/or streptococcal infection. Severe pain on swallowing, fever, malaise, headache, and regional lymphadenopathy are common. Differential diagnosis includes diphtheria, Vincent's angina, and infectious mononucleosis, each of which requires laboratory examination for identification.

Differential Diagnosis

Pharyngeal mucosa pain should be differentiated from Eagle's syndrome, glossopharyngeal neuralgia, geniculate neuralgia, and Ramsay

Hunt syndrome. *Eagle's syndrome* is due to an elongated styloid process or calcification of the stylohyoid ligament. The symptoms are persistent raw throat, ear pain, pain and difficulty with swallowing, and limited jaw movement.[7,8] *Glossopharyngeal neuralgia* is typical neurogenous pain of the paroxysmal neuralgia type that is triggered by throat movement incidental to swallowing, talking, and chewing food. *Geniculate neuralgia* is an extremely rare neurogenous pain of the paroxysmal neuralgia type that is felt as sharp lancinating pain within the depths of the ear. It is triggered by touching the external ear canal or by movement of the auricle.[3] *Ramsay Hunt syndrome* is herpes zoster of the nervus intermedius portion of the seventh cranial nerve. It is felt as ongoing burning pain deep in the ear and is accompanied by herpetic lesions in the external auditory canal and sometimes on the soft palate as well.

NASAL MUCOSA PAIN

Pain that emanates from the nasal mucosa is typically a dull, burning sensation that exhibits the clinical characteristics of visceral mucosa pain. Pain arising from the external lining of the nasal ala exhibit features of the superficial somatic category. When the deeper nasal mucosa is irritated as a result of viral or bacterial infection or as an expression of allergic rhinitis, typical deep visceral pain along with a variety of central excitatory effects may occur spontaneously or with the normal passage of air through the nose. The primary pain may go unnoticed because of the predominance of secondary effects such as referred pain, secondary hyperalgesia, and autonomic symptoms.

Primary pain in the inferior turbinate area has secondary reference zones that include all the ipsilateral maxillary teeth and areas of the face (Fig 14–2). Pain from the region of the ostium maxillare induces referred pain in the upper molar teeth and on the face (Fig 14–3).[4] The referred pain may be sensed as spontaneous toothache (Case No. 14–1). Secondary hyperalgesia may be felt as tender teeth or areas of touchy gingiva. Pain emanating from the nasal mucosa may induce referred pain throughout the entire upper face. It may be sensed as headache. Secondary hyperalgesia may be felt as areas of deep palpable tenderness in the upper face or as superficial touchy areas of skin, scalp, or mucogingival tissue.

Central excitatory effects are frequently expressed as autonomic symptoms. This includes puffy swelling of the eyelids and other loose facial tissue, injection of the conjunctiva, lacrimation, nasal secretion, and nasal congestion. When such symptoms occur in conjunction with

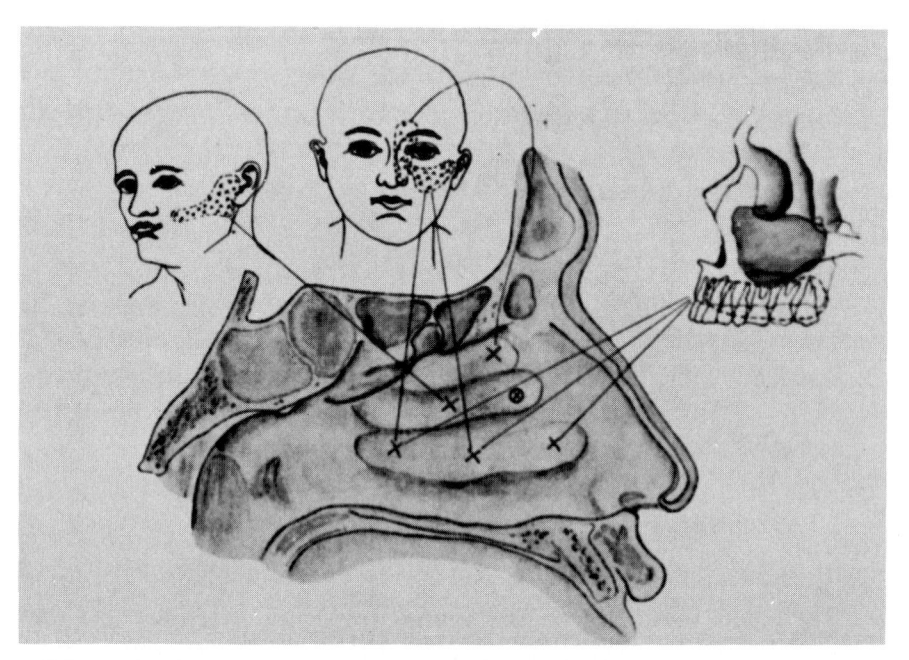

Fig 14–2.—Points stimulated on turbinates, indicated by *large crosses*, causes referred pain to be felt in all maxillary teeth as well as in the face. (From Wolff H.G.: *Headache and Other Head Pain*, ed. 2. © 1963 by Oxford University Press, New York. Reproduced with permission.)

diffuse maxillary pain, the condition is usually thought to be due to maxillary sinusitis. When complicated by spontaneous maxillary toothache or tender teeth, the condition may cause doctor and patient alike to think that it constitutes a dental problem—or a sinus problem—or both. Not finding adequate dental cause, the dentist may refer the patient for ear, nose, and throat evaluation—or vice versa.

When the referred pain is sensed as headache, the condition is popularly known as "sinus headache." This is especially so when allergic rhinitis is the precipitating cause. Several proprietary remedies are offered the public for this common ailment. The condition illustrates the behavior of visceral mucosa pain when secondary effects mask the primary pain input.

Upper respiratory infections frequently involve the nasal and pharyngeal mucosa as well as that of the larynx and upper trachea. The inflammatory reaction is of the serous type which produces serous exudate on the surface. When the nasal mucosa is inflamed, the secondary effects of referred pain, secondary hyperalgesia, or autonomic

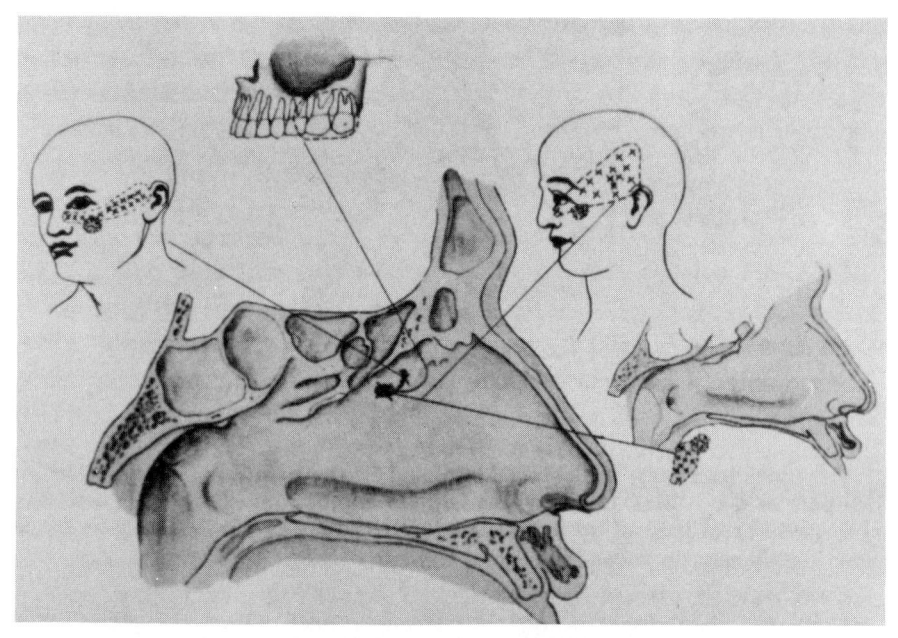

Fig 14-3.—Stimulation of ostium maxillare causes referred pain to be felt in the maxillary molar teeth and in the face. (From Wolff H.G.: *Headache and Other Head Pain* ed. 2. © 1963 by Oxford University Press, New York. Reproduced with permission.)

symptoms may be displayed throughout the maxillary region and upper face. Such symptoms frequently include aching or tender teeth. The differential diagnosis depends on distinguishing between the primary pain and its secondary effects. A topical anesthetic applied to the nasal mucosa will arrest spontaneous referred toothache but will not arrest stimulus-evoked tenderness of the teeth, which is a heterotopic expression of secondary hyperalgesia. Analgesic blocking of the tooth may reduce, but does not arrest, the symptoms of secondary hyperalgesia. (Note: If the tooth were the primary source of pain, analgesic blocking would arrest it.)

With such conditions, the question may arise as to whether it represents a complication of maxillary sinusitis. The symptoms as described do not emanate from maxillary sinusitis except in so far as the ostium maxillare, nasal mucosa, or both are involved by direct extension from the antrum. The lining membrane of the maxillary sinus does not initiate appreciable secondary excitatory effects of any kind. Whether the antrum is truly involved in such conditions requires radiography and other specific examining techniques.

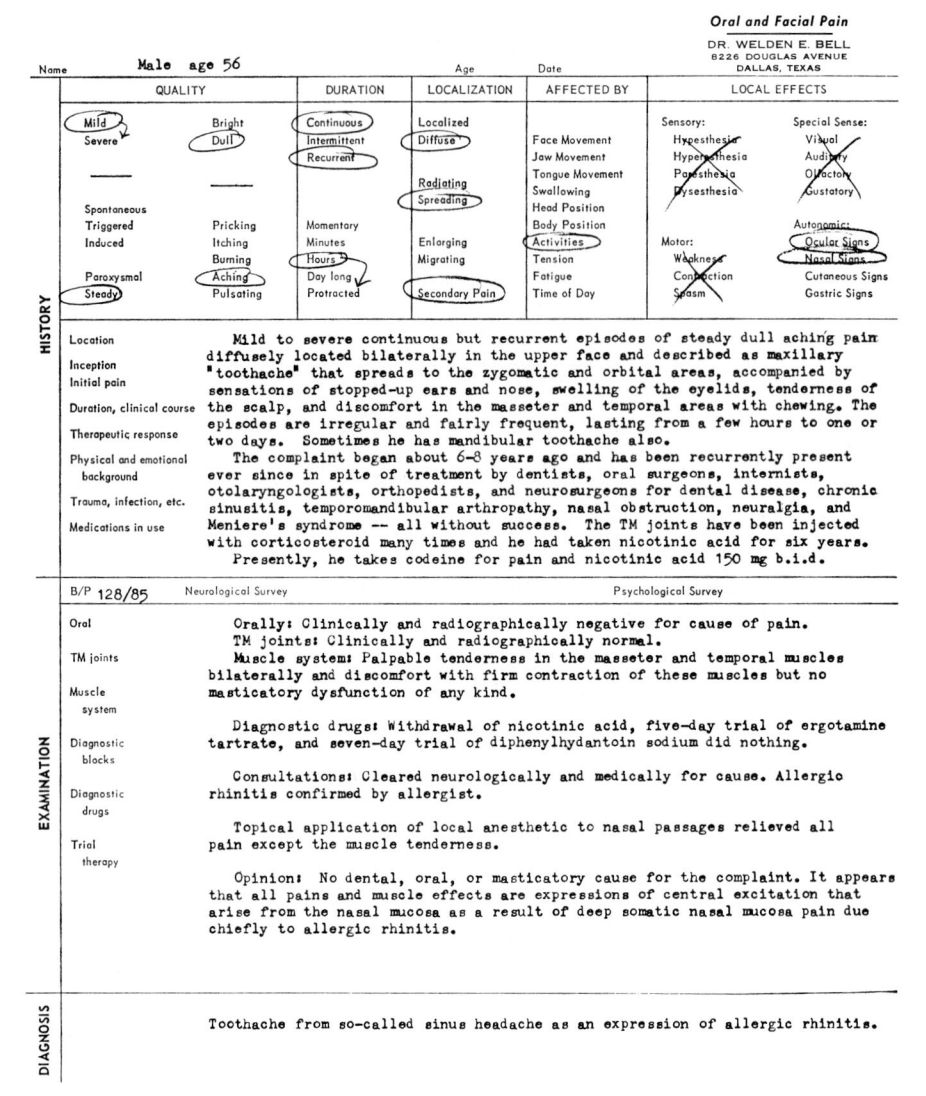

Oral and Facial Pain
DR. WELDEN E. BELL
8226 DOUGLAS AVENUE
DALLAS, TEXAS

Name: Male age 56

QUALITY	DURATION	LOCALIZATION	AFFECTED BY	LOCAL EFFECTS
(Mild) / Severe	Bright / (Dull)	(Continuous) / Intermittent / Recurrent	Localized / (Diffuse)		Sensory: (Hypesthesia) / Hyperesthesia / (Paresthesia) / (Dysesthesia)	Special Sense: Visual / Auditory / Olfactory / Gustatory
			Radiating / (Spreading)	Face Movement / Jaw Movement / Tongue Movement / Swallowing / Head Position		
Spontaneous / Triggered / Induced	Pricking / Itching / Burning	Momentary / Minutes / (Hours)	Enlarging / Migrating	Body Position / (Activities) / Tension / Fatigue / Time of Day	Motor: Weakness / Contraction / Spasm	Autonomic: (Ocular Signs) / (Nasal Signs) / Cutaneous Signs / Gastric Signs
Paroxysmal / (Steady)	(Aching) / Pulsating	Day long / Protracted	(Secondary Pain)			

HISTORY

Location
Inception
Initial pain
Duration, clinical course
Therapeutic response
Physical and emotional background
Trauma, infection, etc.
Medications in use

Mild to severe continuous but recurrent episodes of steady dull aching pain diffusely located bilaterally in the upper face and described as maxillary "toothache" that spreads to the zygomatic and orbital areas, accompanied by sensations of stopped-up ears and nose, swelling of the eyelids, tenderness of the scalp, and discomfort in the masseter and temporal areas with chewing. The episodes are irregular and fairly frequent, lasting from a few hours to one or two days. Sometimes he has mandibular toothache also.

The complaint began about 6-8 years ago and has been recurrently present ever since in spite of treatment by dentists, oral surgeons, internists, otolaryngologists, orthopedists, and neurosurgeons for dental disease, chronic sinusitis, temporomandibular arthropathy, nasal obstruction, neuralgia, and Meniere's syndrome -- all without success. The TM joints have been injected with corticosteroid many times and he had taken nicotinic acid for six years. Presently, he takes codeine for pain and nicotinic acid 150 mg b.i.d.

B/P 128/85   Neurological Survey   Psychological Survey

EXAMINATION

Oral
TM joints
Muscle system
Diagnostic blocks
Diagnostic drugs
Trial therapy

Orally: Clinically and radiographically negative for cause of pain.
TM joints: Clinically and radiographically normal.
Muscle system: Palpable tenderness in the masseter and temporal muscles bilaterally and discomfort with firm contraction of these muscles but no masticatory dysfunction of any kind.

Diagnostic drugs: Withdrawal of nicotinic acid, five-day trial of ergotamine tartrate, and seven-day trial of diphenylhydantoin sodium did nothing.

Consultations: Cleared neurologically and medically for cause. Allergic rhinitis confirmed by allergist.

Topical application of local anesthetic to nasal passages relieved all pain except the muscle tenderness.

Opinion: No dental, oral, or masticatory cause for the complaint. It appears that all pains and muscle effects are expressions of central excitation that arise from the nasal mucosa as a result of deep somatic nasal mucosa pain due chiefly to allergic rhinitis.

DIAGNOSIS

Toothache from so-called sinus headache as an expression of allergic rhinitis.

Case No. 14–1.—Heterotopic pain, felt as toothache, referred from inflamed nasal mucosa (so-called sinus headache).

PARANASAL SINUS PAIN

Inflammatory conditions of the maxillary antrum and other paranasal sinuses are generally misunderstood. The syndrome of symptoms usually thought to be clinically indicative of "sinusitis" are chiefly secondary autonomic and sensory effects induced by primary pain emanating from the nasal mucosa as previously described. Whether such symptoms occur in conjunction with antral disease depends chiefly on patency of the ostium maxillare. Inflammatory exudate that accumulates in the antral cavity remains below the opening of the antrum into the middle meatus of the nose as long as the head is erect. Bending forward, however, permits the fluid to wash over the pain-sensitive tissue around the ostium, thus eliciting pain. If the ostium is open, antral inflammation can spread to the nasal mucosa and thereby initiate the symptoms as described previously. If the ostium is closed by swollen membrane or mucous polyps, the maxillary sinus may remain essentially nonsymptomatic. This is because the lining membrane is nearly insensible to pain. This is altered very little even when the sinus is inflamed.[4] Contrary to popular belief, pain is not a highly characteristic symptom of paranasal sinusitis, and chronic sinusitis seldom gives rise to facial pain or headache.[9] Waltner[10] stated that in his experience no more than 20% of patients treated for "sinus disease" had any disease of the sinus at all. Chronic obstructive sinusitis exhibits symptoms of fullness or pressure, but not pain or headache, unless the nasal mucosa is conjointly affected.

The question may arise whether the teeth and the maxillary sinus are affected in a common disease process. Sinusitis, of course, can result from dental sepsis just as antral disease can spread to involve teeth. A determination, however, of which is the primary source cannot be made from the clinical symptoms alone. If the cause of the sinusitis is dental, adequate clinical and radiographic evidence of the dental sepsis should be forthcoming. If the teeth are secondarily involved by direct extension of prior antral disease, the dental pain will be sensed initially as periodontal in type, with pulpal pain coming later. This, it should be noted, is the reverse of what takes place in the usual temporal sequence of pain of odontogenous origin.

Referred spontaneous toothache and secondary hyperalgesia involving the teeth and mouth do not arise as a result of antral inflammation. There is, however, a condition that does cause tooth pain. This is neuritic neuralgia that occurs as a result of inflammation of elements of the superior alveolar plexus by direct extension of antral inflammation. The neuritic symptoms occur in the peripheral distribution of the affected nerve. Thus, any ipsilateral maxillary tooth can be painful. The quality and character of the pain, however, is that of the neuritic type of neurogenous pain. It is also accompanied by other sensory symptoms that may go unnoticed. These include hyperesthesia, hypoesthesia, paresthesia, and anesthesia of other maxillary teeth, the adjacent gingiva, or the tissues around the infraorbital foramen. To confirm the diagnosis, clinical or radiographic evidence of preexistent antral disease is needed. Positive confirmation can be had by surgical aspiration of the maxillary sinus (Case No. 15–7).

GLANDULAR PAINS OF THE MOUTH AND FACE

Primary visceral pain that emanates from glandular structures of the mouth and face is not uncommon. A diagnostic problem may occur especially when heterotopic pains, secondary myospasms, autonomic symptoms, or a combination are displayed. The source of such pain includes the major salivary glands, mucous and sebaceous glands, lacrimal and oil glands, and especially the lymph glands.[11]

Most glandular pain is inflammatory and therefore relates to infection, trauma, or sialolithiasis. Cystic degeneration or tumor formation may be present. Lymphadenitis results from infection primarily. Infectious mononucleosis and neoplasia may be other causes. The major salivary glands are subject to the irritating effects of mineral deposits and retrograde infection through the ducts that communicate with the oral cavity. Distension and compression may accentuate the pain. Salivary gland pain usually increases at mealtime and therefore may be associated with mastication. Submandibular salivary gland pain is frequently accentuated by chewing and swallowing movements. It may be mistaken for masticatory pain (Case No. 14–2).

Because most painful glands are inflammatory, the pain can be localized quite well by manual palpation and by the presence of other signs of inflammation. Secondary central excitatory effects may complicate the symptom picture. Occasionally, heterotopic pains constitute the entire complaint. Careful diagnostic identification of pain source is important. Lymphadenopathy, especially of low-grade or chronic type, may be mistaken for a cyst or tumor.

OCULAR PAINS

Primary pains emanating from the nonmuscular structures of the orbit are mediated by the trigeminal nerve. Ocular muscle pain displays the clinical characteristics of musculoskeletal pain, while pain from the eye proper is chiefly visceral in type. All such pains should be diagnosed and managed by a competent ophthalmologist.

Heterotopic pain felt in the eye is frequently of muscle origin. Eye pain is usually accompanied by headache. Retro-orbital pain has some-

OTHER VISCERAL PAINS

Oral and Facial Pain
DR. WELDEN E. BELL
8226 DOUGLAS AVENUE
DALLAS, TEXAS

Name: Male age 38

QUALITY	DURATION	LOCALIZATION	AFFECTED BY	LOCAL EFFECTS
(Mild) / Severe	Bright / (Dull)	(Continuous) / Intermittent / Recurrent	Localized / (Diffuse)	Face Movement / (Jaw Movement) / Tongue Movement / Swallowing / Head Position / Body Position / Activities / Tension / Fatigue / Time of Day	Sensory: Hypesthesia / Hyperesthesia / Paresthesia / Dysesthesia — Special Sense: Visual / Auditory / Olfactory / Gustatory
Spontaneous / Triggered / Induced / Paroxysmal / (Steady)	—	Pricking / Itching / Burning / (Aching) / Pulsating	Momentary / Minutes / Hours / Day long / (Protracted)	Radiating / Spreading — Secondary Pain	Motor: Weakness / Contraction / Spasm — Autonomic: Ocular Signs / Nasal Signs / Cutaneous Signs / Gastric Signs

HISTORY

Location
Inception
Initial pain
Duration, clinical course
Therapeutic response
Physical and emotional background
Trauma, infection, etc.
Medications in use

Mild continuous protracted steady dull aching pain located diffusely in the left preauricular and facial area, aggravated by chewing and opening widely but without any accompanying masticatory dysfunction.
   The complaint began about a year ago as intermittent pain in the left face. It continued to increase in frequency and severity until about six months ago; it was constant but variable. During the last six weeks it has become severe enough to seek medical aid. His ENT physician found nothing wrong with the ear and advised a dental examination. His dentist removed the LL8 tooth, injected the left TM joint with corticosteroid, and then prescribed nicotinic acid, all without benefit. He then referred him to another dentist who made a temporary occlusal splint which seemed to aggravate the complaint. He was then referred for a temporomandibular joint examination.
   No medications are presently being taken.

B/P 125/80   Neurological Survey   Psychological Survey

EXAMINATION

Oral
TM joints
Muscle system
Diagnostic blocks
Diagnostic drugs
Trial therapy

Orally: Although the dentition is mutilated by three missing first molar teeth, the remaining ones are clinically and radiographically negative for cause of pain. No occlusal disharmony is identified. All jaw movements are adequate in amplitude and symmetric. Tongue movements are normal. There is no palpable tenderness except in the left submandibular triangle where an indurated mass is felt and acute pain is elicited on firm palpation. An occlusal radiograph revealed a large irregular calcific mass in the region of the left submandibular salivary gland and this was seen also in the left lateral oblique film of the mandible. This mass was interpreted to represent massive sialolithiasis. Manipulation of the left submandibular gland seemed to increase the left facial and preauricular pain.
   TM joints: Normal structurally and functionally. (See tracings.)
   Muscle system: Negative for pain and dysfunction.

   Opinion: The patient's masticatory discomfort appears to be a secondary manifestation of primary pain arising from the left submandibular gland presumably from the sialolith radiographically observed. The primary pain apparently is largely inhibited except when stimulated by firm manual palpation. Normal mandibular movements seem sufficient to induce impulses that are felt as referred pain in the left preauricular area and face.

DIAGNOSIS

Masticatory pain referred from primary sources in the submandibular gland.

Case No. 14–2,A.—Case chart. Heterotopic pain, felt as preauricular pain, referred from inflamed submandibular gland.

times been attributed to masticatory causes. It usually is referred from nonmasticatory muscles, however. The occipital portion of the occipitofrontalis, the splenius cervicis, and the sternocleidomastoid muscles are the chief sources of such pain. It occurs frequently in con-

Temporomandibular Examination
Radiographic Tracings

DR. WELDEN E. BELL
8226 DOUGLAS AVENUE
DALLAS, TEXAS

Name: Male age 38
X-ray File No.
Date

Key to Symbols
POC Primary Occlusal Contact
OP   Occlusal Position
RP   Rest Position
LP   Contralateral Position
MTO Maximum Translatory Opening
PR   Protrusive Position

Left T-M Joint

Left
LP: 11
MTO: 20

Key

Right
LP: 11
MTO 21

Right T-M Joint

POC ▬
OP   ▬
LP   ▬ ▬ ▬ ▬
MTO ▬ · ▬ · ▬

INTERPRETATION

Both joints were viewed in four transparietal positions:
1. Position of primary occlusal contact (POC).
2. Fully occluded position (OP).
3. Contralateral excursion (LP).
4. Maximum opening - 44mm (MTO).

Both joints present well defined smoothly contoured articular surfaces with interarticular spaces of adequate width which do not decrease in width under biting stress. There is no radiographic evidence of degenerative joint disease or other structural arthropathy.

There is excellent superimposition of POC and OP in both joints indicative of no occlusal disharmony gross enough to cause radiographically discernible displacement of either condyle when the teeth are firmly occluded.

Translatory movement in LP and MTO is normal and symmetrical in both joints.

Case No. 14–2,B.—Radiographic tracings of temporomandibular joints.

junction with tension headache. Careful diagnostic identification of the pain source is needed to avoid therapeutic errors.

AURICULAR PAINS

Since the ear is innervated by several different cranial and cervical nerves, the symptom "earache" is nearly meaningless. Primary pain emanating from the ear may arise from different causes and be mediated by different nociceptive pathways. All such complaints should be diagnosed and managed by a competent otologist.

External auditory canal pain is of considerable interest to the dentist. Such pain is usually inflammatory and causes heterotopic symptoms in the face as well as deeply in the ear and throat. Since it usually is accentuated by swallowing, it may be mistaken for masticatory pain or glossopharyngeal neuralgia. Otitis externa may be mistaken for temporomandibular arthralgia. One point of difference, however, is that the ear pain is accentuated by movement of the auricle.

Since it is common practice to palpate the mandibular condyle through the external auditory canal, consideration should be given to the condition of the ear prior to inserting the finger. It should be inspected visually using a speculum and direct light if an otoscope is not available.

Earache, like headache and retro-orbital pain, is frequently a heterotopic manifestation of deep somatic pain located elsewhere. Frequent sources of such pain are the deep masseter and the clavicular portion of the sternocleidomastoid muscle (Case No. 14–3). Earache

Oral and Facial Pain
DR. WELDEN E. BELL
8226 DOUGLAS AVENUE
DALLAS, TEXAS

Name	Male age 46		Age	Date		
	QUALITY	DURATION	LOCALIZATION	AFFECTED BY		LOCAL EFFECTS
HISTORY	Mild ✓ Severe ――― Spontaneous Triggered Induced ✓ Paroxysmal Steady ✓	Bright Dull ✓ ――― Pricking Itching Burning Aching ✓ Pulsating	Continuous Intermittent ✓ Recurrent Radiating Spreading Momentary Minutes ✓ Hours Day long Protracted	Localized Diffuse ✓ ――― ――― ――― Enlarging Migrating Secondary Pain	Face Movement Jaw Movement ? Tongue Movement Swallowing Head Position ? Body Position Activities Tension Fatigue Time of Day	Sensory: Hypesthesia Hyperesthesia Paresthesia Dysesthesia ― Motor: Weakness Contraction Spasm	Special Sense: Visual Auditory Olfactory Gustatory ― Autonomic: Ocular Signs Nasal Signs Cutaneous Signs Gastric Signs

	Location	Intermittent short periods of mild to severe steady dull aching pain diffusely located in the left auricular and preauricular area, lasting a few minutes each time, and vaguely related to head and jaw movements.
	Inception Initial pain	
	Duration, clinical course	The complaint began about two years ago following a severe upper respiratory infection and was initially diagnosed as otitis media. The periods of increased discomfort had been such that he sought only medical attention for his "bad ear". Recently, he went to an ENT physician who found the ear to be normal and suggested it to be a "bite problem". His dentist was unable to find any cause, so returned him to the physician who then prescribed therapy for "neuralgia" without benefit. He was then returned to his dentist to "take care of this dental problem" and was promptly referred for a TM joint examination.
	Therapeutic response	
	Physical and emotional background	
	Trauma, infection, etc.	
	Medications in use	Presently, he is taking no medications.

	B/P 130/80	Neurological Survey		Psychological Survey	
EXAMINATION	Oral	Orally: Dentally and orally negative for cause of pain. No occlusal disharmony is identified either clinically or radiographically. All mandibular functioning is well within normal limits. No discomfort of any kind is elicited by mandibular movements.
	TM joints	
	Muscle system	TM joints: Both joints are clinically and radiographically normal. Muscle system: The masticatory muscles are entirely negative for cause of pain or dysfunction. There is palpable tenderness in the midbody of the left sternomastoid muscle which when squeezed causes acute pain to be felt in the left ear and preauricular area.
	Diagnostic blocks	
	Diagnostic drugs	Analgesic blocking of the left sternomastoid muscle trigger site arrested all local tenderness as well as the induced ear and preauricular pain.
	Trial therapy	Opinion: The present pain complaint does not stem from masticatory, dental, or oral causes. It appears to be referred pain arising from stimulation of a painful myofascial trigger site in the left sternomastoid muscle.

DIAGNOSIS	Preauricular nonmasticatory pain referred from the sternomastoid muscle.

Case No. 14–3.—Heterotopic pain, felt as preauricular pain, due to trigger point pain affecting the sternocleidomastoid muscle.

may be referred from inflamed dental pulps and from the pharyngeal mucosa. Such ear pain is a dominant symptom of "sore throat." Preauricular pain is frequently referred from the medial and lateral pterygoid muscles.

Ear pain such as that of otitis media has the propensity to induce a variety of central excitatory effects including myospasm of masticatory muscles, thus producing a masticatory pain-dysfunction syndrome. The cycling nature of muscle spasm may perpetuate the condition long after the initiating deep pain input has disappeared. Although such a complaint constitutes a true masticatory disorder, requiring treatment by the dentist, the condition is not of masticatory origin. Careful diagnosis as to etiology is therefore essential for effective management of the condition.

Since ear pains and masticatory pains have an intimate interrelationship, it is important that the pain source be accurately identified prior to definitive therapy by either dentist or otologist.

REFERENCES

1. Bonica J.J.: *The Management of Pain*. Philadelpha, Lea & Febiger, 1953.
2. Wolff H.G., Wolf S.: *Pain*, ed. 2. Springfield, Ill., Charles C Thomas, Publisher, 1958.
3. Finneson B.E.: *Diagnosis and Management of Pain Syndromes*, ed. 2. Philadelphia, W.B. Saunders Co., 1969.
4. Dalessio D.J.: *Wolff's Headache and Other Head Pain*, ed. 3. New York, Oxford University Press, 1972.
5. Gross D.: Pain and autonomic nervous system, in Bonica J.J. (ed.): *Advances in Neurology*. New York, Raven Press, 1974, vol. 4, pp. 93–103.
6. Moore D.C.: *Stellate Ganglion Block*. Springfield, Ill., Charles C Thomas, Publisher, 1954.
7. Lawrence F.R., Cornielson E.: Eagle's syndrome. *J. Oral Maxillofac. Surg.* 40:307–309, 1982.
8. Correll R.W., Wescott W.B.: Eagle's syndrome diagnosed after history of headache, dysphagia, otalgia, and limited neck movement. *J.A.D.A.* 104:491–492, 1982.
9. Boles R.: Paranasal sinuses and facial pain, in Alling C.C., Mahan P.E. (eds.): *Facial Pain*, ed. 2. Philadelphia, Lea & Febiger, 1977, pp. 115–133.
10. Waltner J.G.: Otolaryngeal sources of pain. *J.A.D.A.* 51:417, 1955.
11. Procacci P., Zoppi M.: Pathophysiology and clinical aspects of visceral and referred pain, in Bonica J.J., Lindblom U., Iggo A. (eds.): *Advances in Pain Research and Therapy*. New York, Raven Press, 1983, vol. 5, pp. 643–658.

15

Neurogenous Pains

NEUROGENOUS PAIN IS DUE TO ABNORMALITY in the nervous system itself rather than to noxious stimulation of otherwise normal neural structures, as with superficial and deep somatic pain syndromes. The cause of neurogenous pain lies within the nerves, and its clinical significance relates to such abnormality. Whereas somatic pains are predominantly a warning system that noxious stimulation is present, neurogenous pain is symptomatic of structural abnormality in the peripheral sensory nerves.

Neurogenous pains of the mouth and face may be classified as (1) neuropathic pains and (2) deafferentation pains. The neuropathic pains may be subdivided into traumatic neuroma pains, paroxysmal neuralgias, and neuritic neuralgias (Fig 15–1).

NEUROPATHIC PAINS OF THE MOUTH AND FACE

Pains of neuropathic origin present distinctive clinical characteristics. It is by recognizing these characteristics that pains of this category can be identified.
1. The pain has a bright, *stimulating* quality that provokes some degree of alarm reaction in the subject.
2. The site of pain is accurately localizable by the subject.
3. The site of pain (where it is felt) is not due to lowered pain threshold at that point. It may mislead the patient as to the location of the neuropathy that causes it. Traumatic neuromas are exceptions to this rule.
4. The pain is disproportionate in intensity to the exciting stimulus, usually being considerably greater than if no neuropathy were present. Sometimes the pain does not relate accurately to the stimulus in temporal behavior—duration and timing.
5. If accompanying effects are present, they are anatomically related to the neuropathy and not due to central excitation.

OROFACIAL PAIN SYNDROMES

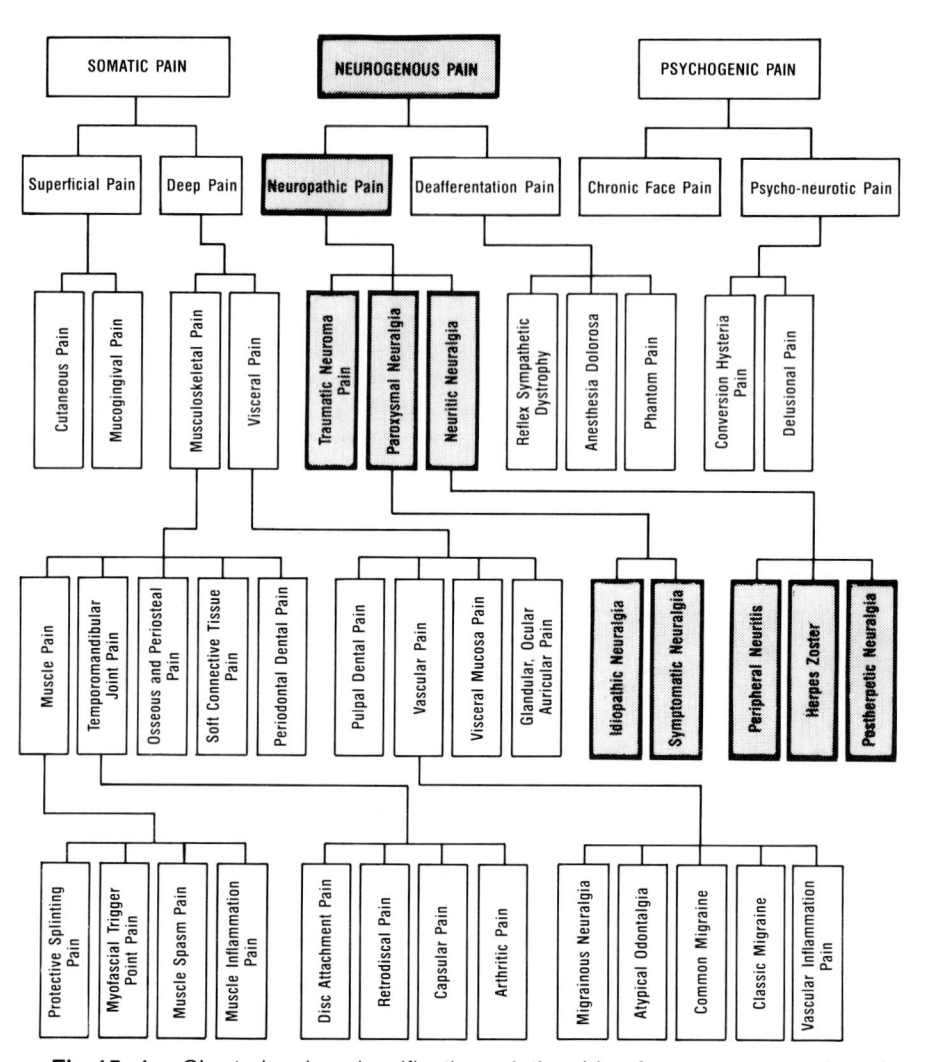

Fig 15–1.—Chart showing classification relationship of neurogenous pains of neuropathic origin to other orofacial pain syndromes.

6. Topical anesthesia of the site of pain does not arrest it except for mucosa-triggered neuralgia.

Neuropathy alters neural behavior due to changes in receptivity, the transmission of impulses, or the peripheral inhibitory system so that neural impulses initiated by ordinary peripheral stimulation are markedly modulated prior to reaching the higher centers. Neuropathic pain results largely from neural deficits.

Traumatic neuromas are not true neoplasms. Rather, they consist of a random overgrowth of intertwined extraneural and intraneural tissues and Schwann's cells that develops as part of the regeneration process after a nerve is cut. It is a disorganized mass of nerve tissue that is painless in itself but that elicits a neurogenous type of pain when stimulated by pressure, impingement, or stretching. This is due not so much to neural deficit as to neural overabundance, and pain is an accident of location where adequate stimulation can be brought to bear on it. Since the resultant pain has the essential qualities of other neurogenous pains, it is included among the neuropathies.

Neuritic pain occurs as a result of alteration of sensory fibers that mediate pain and is felt in the peripheral distribution of the affected fibers. The inflammatory process alters the relative activity of fibers that mediate pricking and burning pain, elevating the threshold for pricking pain but lowering it for burning pain.[1] This gives the pain a characteristic burning quality along with the other characteristics of neurogenous pain, i.e., bright, stimulating, precisely localizable pain that is accurately related in location to the site of inflammation as far as the anatomical distribution of those fibers is concerned. It is inaccurately related, however, to the intensity of the stimulus. In fact, the pain persists regardless of added stimulation, only increasing when stimulated. No secondary excitatory effects are seen.

In light of the gate control theory of pain mechanisms, it appears that the neuritic process alters the peripheral large/small-fiber activity ratio, depressing the larger myelinated fast-conducting fibers that mediate pricking pain.[2] The decreased large-fiber activity opens the synaptic gate in the brain stem widely enough for otherwise normal ongoing sensation mediated by the small fibers to pass through as pain—burning pain. This gives the neuropathy its characteristic persistent unremitting burning quality irrespective of added stimulation. Additional stimulation only increases the pain. Although variable in degree, neuritic pain has a strange constancy that relates to the incidence and resolution of the inflammatory process. Its temporal behavior is less dramatic than that of other neurogenous pains.

Paroxysmal neuralgia refers to paroxysmal pain that extends along the course of a nerve. It is sometimes referred to as typical neuralgia. *Idiopathic neuralgia* includes the neuralgic pain syndromes induced by neuropathic change in the fibers of the ganglion and dorsal root, the cause of which is not known.[3] This is sometimes referred to as primary or major neuralgia. *Symptomatic neuralgia* designates the neuralgic pain syndromes that result from identifiable pathologic conditions such as multiple sclerosis, neoplasms and aneurysms. This is sometimes referred to as secondary or minor neuralgia.

Until recently, the mechanism of idiopathic neuralgia was not known. Kerr [4,5] has shown that significant pathologic change occurs in the myelin sheath of fibers in the ganglion, dorsal root, or both. This change, recognizable by both light and electron microscopy, consists of disintegration of the myelin sheath—demyelination (Figs 6–1 and 6–2), the cause of which is not known.[6] Demyelination affects the large fibers, which alters their ability to transmit impulses. According to the gate control theory, this depresses the peripheral inhibitory mechanism and allows impulses initiated by light touch and superficial movement to be felt as pain. There is no significant change in the receptors, no lowering of pain threshold, no primary hyperalgesia. The receptors are stimulated normally, but the impulses are modulated to painful proportions.

According to the gate control theory, reduced large-fiber activity (presumably due to demyelination) elevates the critical firing level in the gating mechanism so that impulses reaching the synapse must first summate until a higher firing level is reached. This not only causes a momentary delay, it also permits the summated impulses to burst across explosively as an intense volley of paroxysmal pain.[7] A refractory period usually follows a severe barrage of painful impulses.

There is some evidence that demyelination results from a progressive degenerative process that permits ephaptic transfer of neural impulses.[8] It has been established that the pathogenesis of trigeminal neuralgia is not related to deficiency of opioid peptides.[9] Whatever the mechanism, it seems quite certain that it is peripheral and not central.[8,10]

What may be a very significant breakthrough in understanding pain mechanisms is the recent report by Wall and Devor[11] that afferent impulses originate in the dorsal root ganglia as well as from normal peripheral nerves, and that this phenomenon is accentuated by nerve injury. These impulses contribute a tonic, low-level, spontaneous background discharge that is propagated orthodromically into the root and antidromically into the peripheral neurons. Since this newly discovered source of spontaneous afferent activity is increased when a nerve is injured, it likely has an important role in deafferentation syndromes. It has also been reported that heretofore unidentified synapses are to be found in the dorsal root ganglia.[11] This may have bearing on mechanisms responsible for idiopathic neuralgia.

TRAUMATIC NEUROMA PAIN

Large traumatic neuromas are not reported in the oral structures, presumably due to the size of the nerve trunks that may be sectioned.

Most such sensory nerves are situated within bony canals where they are protected against injury, and, if sectioning should occur and a neuroma develop, it is unlikely that pain would occur due to the protection of overlying osseous tissue. Following fracture of facial bones and deep lacerations, one should be alert to the inherent possibility of neuroma formation as a cause of post-traumatic pain. The oral surgeon especially should know the characteristic features of this source of neurogenous pain.

Of considerably greater importance is the formation of minute neuromas in scar tissue, as these may be a cause of painful scars.[12] Microscopic examination of painful scar tissue excised from the mouth is not remarkable, and the pathologist should not expect to find typical end-bulb neuromas. Usually, considerable fibrous tissue is seen with small nerve fibers, which appear thicker than normal, nodular, and terminating in little whorls. The time lapse between wound healing and development of painful scar varies considerably. Once a painful neuroma becomes clinically evident, the complaint will continue until the mass is surgically excised.

The actual cause of neuroma pain is not clear. The ephaptic transfer of signals is very likely. Scar tissue that elicits pain only when stretched indicates that traction may be the adequate stimulus for pain. Compression of a neuroma may represent adequate stimulus for pain, as indicated by the success that attends burying the nerve stump in bone and shielding with tantalum. A recent tubulation technique to prevent end-bulb neuroma formation has been described.[13]

Mucogingival scars following minor oral surgical procedures, such as extraction of teeth and alveoloplasty, when compressed by a denture base, can elicit typical neurogenous pain. Such minute painful spots can easily be overlooked by the examiner (Case No. 15–1).

The diagnostic features of mucogingival scars with neuroma formation are as follows:
1. History of prior surgery or *lacerating* injury at the site of pain.
2. Usually no visible or palpable mass.
3. No complaint of pain except when the site is aggravated by pressure or stretching.
4. Decisive arrestment of pain for duration of anesthesia by injection of a drop of anesthetic at pain site.

Traumatic neuromas may form in temporomandibular joint adhesions and contractures that result from operation or lacerating trauma (Case No. 15–2). Pain from this source must be differentiated from arthralgia due to inflammatory conditions of the joint. Such pains also may be confused with neuralgic pains of the trigeminal and glosso-

Oral and Facial Pain

DR. WELDEN E. BELL
8226 DOUGLAS AVENUE
DALLAS, TEXAS

Name: Female age 65

	QUALITY	DURATION	LOCALIZATION	AFFECTED BY	LOCAL EFFECTS	
HISTORY	~~Mild~~ **(Severe)** Spontaneous Triggered **(Induced)** Paroxysmal **(Steady)**	Bright Dull — Pricking Itching **(Burning)** Aching Pulsating	Continuous **(Intermittent)** Recurrent — **(Momentary)** Minutes Hours Day long Protracted	**(Localized)** Diffuse Radiating Spreading — Enlarging Migrating Secondary Pain	Face Movement Jaw Movement Tongue Movement Swallowing Head Position Body Position **(Activities)** Tension Fatigue Time of Day	Sensory: Hypesthesia Hyperesthesia Paresthesia Dysesthesia Motor: Weakness Contraction Spasm	Special Sense: Visual Auditory Olfactory Gustatory Autonomic: Ocular Signs Nasal Signs Cutaneous Signs Gastric Signs

Location
Inception
Initial pain
Duration, clinical course
Therapeutic response
Physical and emotional background
Trauma, infection, etc.
Medications in use

Mild to severe bright steady burning pain induced momentarily by denture or finger pressure at a point in the edentulous UR1 area about halfway between the crest of the ridge and the mucobuccal fold. The pain is proportionate to the pressure. There is no spontaneous or triggered pain. Location is precise and the pain predictable.
Complaint began about 30 years ago following the extraction of the anterior maxillary teeth and has remained the same ever since. Many doctors have been consulted and therapy of different types unsuccessfully tried, including all types of topical applications, systemic medications, denture adjustments, and surgically smoothing the underlying alveolar bone.
No medications are presently being taken.

B/P 155/90   Neurological Survey   Psychological Survey

Oral
TM joints
Muscle system
Diagnostic blocks
Diagnostic drugs
Trial therapy

Orally: The mouth is edentulous with no evidence of hyperemia, ulceration, or palpable tenderness other than precisely at the "spot" in question. That site appears normal radiographically and there is no abnormal prominence of the bone beneath. Pain is readily elicited when this site is pressed with the finger.
TM joints and muscle system: Negative.
Application of a topical anesthetic to the painful site did not prevent pain when pressed. Injection of a drop of local anesthetic directly into the painful site immediately arrested all pain from pressure for the duration of anesthesia.
Opinion: The complaint is typical of that elicited by pressing upon a painful neuroma located in the mucoperiosteum. Full-thickness excision of the painful site was done and the pathological diagnosis obtained by biopsy of the excised tissue was: "Neuromatous formation, benign, involving skeletal muscle tissue." The pain did not return following excision.

DIAGNOSIS

Painful neuroma located in the mucoperiosteum of edentulous right maxillary alveolar ridge.

Case No. 15–1.—Traumatic neuroma pain, located in edentulous mucogingival tissue (postsurgical).

Oral and Facial Pain
DR. WELDEN E. BELL
8226 DOUGLAS AVENUE
DALLAS, TEXAS

Name: Male age 27

HISTORY

QUALITY	DURATION	LOCALIZATION	AFFECTED BY	LOCAL EFFECTS
Mild ✓ Severe	**Bright** ✓ Dull	**Continuous** **Intermittent** ✓ Recurrent	**Localized** ✓ Diffuse	Face Movement **Jaw Movement** ✓ Tongue Movement Swallowing Head Position Body Position Activities Tension Fatigue Time of Day	Sensory: Hypesthesia Hyperesthesia Paresthesia Dysesthesia Motor: Weakness Contraction Spasm	Special Sense: Visual Auditory Olfactory Gustatory Autonomic: Ocular Signs Nasal Signs Cutaneous Signs Gastric Signs
Spontaneous Triggered **Induced** ✓ Paroxysmal **Steady** ✓	Pricking Itching **Burning** ✓ Aching Pulsating	**Momentary** ✓ Minutes Hours Day long Protracted	Radiating Spreading Enlarging Migrating Secondary Pain		

Location
Inception
Initial pain
Duration, clinical course
Therapeutic response
Physical and emotional background
Trauma, infection, etc.
Medications in use

Mild to severe momentary intermittent steady bright burning pain located in the left temporomandibular joint area, induced by mandibular movements, and accompanied by some restriction of jaw movements.
The complaint began about six months ago and has remained much the same ever since. Some 12 months prior, patient sustained bilateral mandibular condyle fractures in an automobile accident. Reduction was closed via intermaxillary fixation for six weeks. When released, his opening was said to have been about 15mm. This increased to about 32mm during the ensuing year with little or no change since. Although he has some restriction of mandibular movements and definite malocclusion, his chief complaint during the last six months has been the acute burning pain that occurs almost every time he tries to open the mouth to chew. Presently, he is wearing an occlusal splint that seems to have improved his occlusion but it has not altered the sharp pains.

EXAMINATION

B/P 120/80   Neurological Survey   Psychological Survey

Oral
TM joints
Muscle system
Diagnostic blocks
Diagnostic drugs
Trial therapy

Orally: There is malocclusion which seems to have been very well corrected with an occlusal splint. All mandibular movements are restricted, lateral and protrusive movements being almost nil. He has some mild dull constant discomfort in the left masseter and joint area but this does not seem to constitute his chief complaint. There is sharp burning pain when he opens 32mm and with extended protrusive and lateral excursions. This pain does not occur in occlusal position, with eccentric biting, or with actual chewing.
TM joints: Both joints show evidence of malposition presumed to be due to trauma and cicatrization. (See tracings.)
Muscle system: There is palpable tenderness in the left masseter muscle.

Analgesic blocking of the left masseter muscle reduced the discomfort only partially.
Trial therapy consisting of one corticosteroid injection into the left TM joint did nothing to reduce the pain complaint.

Opinion: Since the sharp burning pain does not stem from the muscles or inflamed adhesions and since the behavioral characteristics are those of neurogenous pain, it is presumed that the pain arises from painful neuroma formation associated with the cicatrization sequential to trauma. Surgical management is suggested.

DIAGNOSIS

Painful neuroma formation in cicatricial tissue due to a traumatized TM joint.

Case No. 15–2,A.—Case chart. Traumatic neuroma pain, located in the temporomandibular joint (post-traumatic).

Temporomandibular Examination Radiographic Tracings

DR. WELDEN E. BELL
8226 DOUGLAS AVENUE
DALLAS, TEXAS

Name: Male age 27
X-ray File No.
Date

Key to Symbols
POC Primary Occlusal Contact
OP   Occlusal Position
RP   Rest Position
LP   Contralateral Position
MTO Maximum Translatory Opening
PR   Protrusive Position

Left T-M Joint	Left LP: 1 MTO: −4	Key	Right LP: 5 MTO: 3	Right T-M Joint
		POC = ——— Splinted OP = ——— LP = − − − MTO = −·−·−		

INTERPRETATION

Both joints were viewed in four transparietal positions:
1. Position of primary occlusal contact (POC).
2. Splinted occlusal position.
3. Contralateral excursion (LP).
4. Maximum opening − 32 mm (MTO).

Both condyles appear to be situated in a forward position relative to the articular fossae. The left is estimated to be about 15mm forward, the right about 5mm. This is interpreted as malposition sequential to the former trauma.

The splinted occlusal position appears to coincide quite well with POC, indicative of reasonably satisfactory artificial correction of the occlusal disharmony.

Translatory movements in the right joint are limited to 5mm in LP and about 3mm in MTO. Presuming the condyle to be malposed anteriorly, the LP movement may not be as restricted as it appears and MTO movement may well reflect the left joint hypomobility.

Translatory movement in the left joint is nil in LP and a negative 4mm in MTO. Considering the forward displacement of the condyle, this restriction suggests more capsular restraint than intracapsular ankylosis.

Both joints show evidence of trauma and cicatrization.

Case No. 15–2,B.—Radiographic tracings of temporomandibular joint.

pharyngeal nerves. True paroxysms of the spontaneous type do not occur, and triggering from slight stimulation of the peripheral sensory receptors does not take place.

The diagnostic features that differentiate the pain of traumatic neuromas in joint adhesions from inflammatory arthralgia are as follows:
1. Prior history of surgery or lacerating trauma.
2. Clinical characteristics of neurogenous rather than deep somatic pain.
3. Evidence that adhesions restrain joint movements.
4. No complaint of pain except at the moment that such adhesion is stretched.

Traumatic neuroma pain can be differentiated from other neurogenous pain syndromes by the following criteria:

1. The pain is neither spontaneous nor triggered. The condition is painless except when stimulated by compression or stretching. Although the evoked pain is greater in intensity than would be expected from the applied stimulus, the nociceptive response is quite faithful in incidence and duration.
2. There are no accompanying sensory or motor symptoms indicative of a neural deficit.
3. The pain is arrested by injecting a drop or two of local anesthetic at the site of pain.

PAROXYSMAL NEURALGIA

The paroxysmal neuralgias are forms of neurogenous pain. They are characterized by sudden, brief, recurrent volleys of stabbing, electriclike, burning pain that is felt heterotopically in the exact peripheral distribution of the affected nerve. The pain occurs spontaneously or is triggered in response to nonnoxious stimulation of the peripheral receptors by light touch, currents of air, or movements. The paroxysmal neuralgias may be idiopathic or symptomatic, depending on etiology. The cause of idiopathic neuralgia is unknown; symptomatic neuralgia results from pathologic lesions such as tumors, aneurysms, and multiple sclerosis.

Idiopathic Neuralgia

Most paroxysmal neuralgias occur without known cause. They are characterized by several features[14]:
1. Severe paroxysmal pain.
2. Unilateral location.
3. Initiation of pains by minor superficial stimulation in the peripheral distribution of sensory fibers of the affected nerve—so-called triggering of pain.
4. Freedom from neurologic deficits in either sensory or motor functions of the structures involved.

The behavioral characteristics of the pain are neurogenous. The pains are bright and *stimulating*. They are usually described as burning, hot, shocking, or electriclike and can be accurately located by the patient. The relationship between the initiating stimulus and location of the pain is anatomically accurate so that analgesic blocking is decisive. The relationship between the initiating stimulus and intensity of the pain is inaccurate in that the pains are extremely intense compared to the degree of stimulation. In fact, the pains occur spontaneously from the normal stimulation induced by ordinary functioning, and frequently the patient will refrain from actions that excite the pains. Such activities as eating, talking, washing the face, and shaving may become too painful to bear. The impulses from surface stimulation or movement received by the sensory receptors of the nerve are painless until they summate to threshold level—then burst through as excruciating pain. There may be delays of up to half a minute between stimulation and pain response. Frequently after a period of severe pain, there may be an interval during which pain cannot be induced, a so-called refractory period.

There are no central excitatory effects—no referred pains or secondary hyperalgesias, no autonomic effects, and no secondary painful muscle spasms. There are no other sensory changes, as seen in neuritis, or muscle effects other than the hard contractions induced by the paroxysms of pain and perhaps some slight local muscular soreness incidental to such contractions. Both the pain and the triggering are promptly arrested by analgesic blocking of the sensory pathways that conduct impulses from the peripheral receptors of the affected nerve. If such impulses arise in the oral mucosa, application of a topical anesthetic at that site likewise will arrest the pain and triggering.[15]

The pains of typical neuralgia occur as momentary, extended, or rapidly repeated volleys of jabs, separated by pain-free intermissions. This feature is characteristic. However, it should be noted that all neuralgias do not necessarily present this pain-free intermittent behavior. In addition to the paroxysms, some patients with true trigeminal neuralgia may have a mild steady background aching sensation that usually is bearable.[16]

Idiopathic neuralgia occurs in other than the trigeminal nerve, but in no other nerve does it present itself in such a dramatic manner. Besides trigeminal neuralgia, glossopharyngeal and geniculate neuralgias are encountered in the maxillofacial region.

Tic Douloureux

Trigeminal neuralgia[1, 6, 12, 14, 17, 18] has been known for centuries and is one of the most painful afflictions of mankind. Only recently has it been identified as a true neuropathy. Although the cause of idiopathic tic douloureux is still unknown, clinical evidence suggests it may relate to other degenerative conditions that accompnay the aging process. It occurs predominantly during middle and old age, the incidence increasing with age. It occurs more frequently in women.

The clinical behavior of tic douloureux has lost much of its mystery with the introduction of the gate control theory of pain mechanisms.[7] A single nerve branch may be affected without involving other branches, the entire division, or other divisions of the nerve. The pains and triggering occur in the receptor area of the affected nerve so precisely that analgesic blocking to interrupt the passage of impulses from the superficial peripheral receptors accurately arrests both pain and triggering. This effect is diagnostic. Yet the peripheral receptors are not hyperalgesic. The stimulus for pain is the normal sensation induced by surface stimulation due to such factors as movement, contact, and thermal change, giving the paroxysms a spontaneous character. Triggering may occur from light touch or movement of the same receptor areas.

The pain usually is unilateral and remains in the anatomical distribution of the affected nerve regardless of intermissions or remissions. Sometimes it may slowly spread to involve more extensive portions of the nerve—even to affect all divisions of the nerve simultaneously. There have been reports of pain occurring bilaterally but not at the same time. Rapid-spreading, bilateral involvement or simultaneous involvement with other nerve trunks should suggest *symptomatic* neuralgia, indicating the need for a thorough neurologic search for pathologic cause. Examples of simultaneous involvement with other major nerve trunks are tic convulsif,[18] which afflicts both the fifth and seventh cranial nerves, and occurrence of symptoms in both the trigeminal and glossopharyngeal areas, a condition that is not rare. Spontaneous pain-free remissions are characteristic of idiopathic neuralgia, but not so with the symptomatic type.

Typically, the individual pains are paroxysms of hot, shocking, burning, or electriclike volleys of jabs that last from a few seconds to several minutes. They may be repeated so frequently that the pains are nearly continuous. The quality of the jabbing pain differs from the steady flowing pain of other syndromes. Following severe pains, there may be refractory periods during which no pain can be elicited. There may be noticeable delays of several seconds between stimulation and pain reaction, indicating temporal summation. Although muscular contractions accompany severe pains, and some dysfunction may result from the inhibitory influence of fear of the pains, referred pains and secondary myospasms as true central excitatory effects do not occur. The pains are promptly and completely arrested by analgesic blocking of the pain pathway from the peripheral sensory receptors of the nerve involved. Such interruption arrests both the triggering and the paroxysms. Spontaneous periods of remission, followed in due time by recurrence, are fairly common. Paresthesia and motor symptoms are generally absent. Between attacks, there is usually no discomfort other than some slight muscular soreness due to the hard contractions that may accompany the paroxysms. It should be noted that some cases of idiopathic tic douloureux have a mild steady background sensation between paroxysms of intense pain. When this is encountered, adequate neurologic examination is advised to search for a pathologic cause such as multiple sclerosis or malignancy.

Usually, the longer the condition lasts, the more typical it becomes. Sometimes incipient neuralgia has rather atypical features and is difficult to diagnose accurately. It should be noted that drug therapy also may change the typical features of true neuralgia because drugs appear to act primarily on the paroxysmal behavior of the syndrome.

Occasionally only the auriculotemporal branch may be involved. The pains and triggering are located in the auricle as well as in the temple region. This entity may be confused with geniculate and glossopharyngeal neuralgias. Analgesic blocking clearly differentiates them (Case No. 15–3).

Since triggering frequently relates to facial and tongue movements incidental to chewing and swallowing, tic douloureux must be differentiated from masticatory pain which has the clinical characteristics of deep somatic rather than neurogenous pain. It may be induced by jaw movements, and the pain may be intense, but true triggering by light superficial touch and slight movement does not occur. Masticatory pain is not arrested by a conventional mandibular local anesthetic block because the nerves mediating pain either from the joint or the masticatory muscles are not so anesthetized (Case No. 15–4).

Neuropathies such as neuralgia cause tooth pains of nondental origin that at times may be difficult to identify properly. In the past it has not been unusual to examine a patient with obvious tic douloureux who had lost some or all teeth to the midline on the side of pain. Such cases bear witness that true neuralgia of the maxillary or mandibular divisions of the trigeminal nerve causes pain that may be felt as toothache of sufficient intensity to induce the patient to demand removal of the painful tooth (Case No. 15–5). Unfortunately, the following characteristics of true neuralgia contribute to this situation:

1. Stimulation of a tooth by percussion or other means may trigger the neuralgic paroxysm, or a spontaneous paroxysm may be felt in the tooth. This is because the teeth are part of the sensory receptor system of the affected nerve trunk.
2. The pain is immediately and completely arrested by analgesic blocking of the tooth that hurts, leading the dentist and patient to believe that the "proper offending tooth" has been identified.

Neurogenous Pains

Oral and Facial Pain
DR. WELDEN E. BELL
8226 DOUGLAS AVENUE
DALLAS, TEXAS

Name: Female **age** 75

HISTORY

QUALITY	DURATION	LOCALIZATION	AFFECTED BY	LOCAL EFFECTS
(Mild) Severe ✓ Spontaneous Triggered ✓ Induced Paroxysmal Steady ✓	Bright ✓ Dull ——— Pricking Itching Burning ✓ Aching Pulsating	Continuous ✓ Intermittent Recurrent ✓ Momentary Minutes Hours Day long Protracted ✓	Localized ✓ Diffuse Radiating Spreading Enlarging Migrating Secondary Pain	Face Movement ✓ Jaw Movement ✓ Tongue Movement Swallowing Head Position Body Position Activities Tension Fatigue Time of Day	Sensory: Hypesthesia Hyperesthesia ✓ Paresthesia Dysesthesia Motor: Weakness Contraction Spasm	Special Sense: Visual Auditory Olfactory Gustatory Autonomic: Ocular Signs Nasal Signs Cutaneous Signs Gastric Signs

Location
Inception
Initial pain

Recurrent episodes of mild to severe continuous protracted steady bright burning pain localized in the left auricular, periauricular, and temporal areas, aggravated by jaw movements as well as by superficial touch and movement of the painful structures. Exacerbations are nearly paroxysmal.

Duration, clinical course
Therapeutic response
Physical and emotional background
Trauma, infection, etc.
Medications in use

The complaint has been recurrent for several years in irregular episodes of several weeks or months separated by painfree remissions of several months' duration. The discomfort is of low intensity except when stimulated by opening, chewing, or touching the left ear, periauricular structures, and temple. Such stimulation causes nearly paroxysmal pain. She has been treated with vitamins, B-12, iron, and liver extract. She has been cleared medically for sinusitis, allergies, nutritional deficiency, anemia, and diabetes. Her complaint was presumed to be of masticatory origin. Her dentist has adjusted the occlusion, altered her partial dentures, and extracted several teeth without benefit. He referred patient for a TM joint examination. Present episode began 6 months ago.

EXAMINATION

B/P 150/90 **Neurological Survey** **Psychological Survey**

Oral
TM joints
Muscle system
Diagnostic blocks
Diagnostic drugs
Trial therapy

Orally: There is no dental or oral cause for the complaint. The masticatory system functions normally and no pain results from any mandibular movement except when the speed and amplitude causes movement of the temporal and auricular structures.

TM joints: Both joints are structurally and functionally normal.

Muscle system: There is no palpable tenderness in any masticatory muscle and no muscular dysfunction of any kind.

Analgesic blocking of the left inferior alveolar nerve intraorally did not affect the pain. Blocking of the left auriculotemporal nerve where it crosses the zygomatic arch anterior to the tragus promptly and completely arrested all pain and triggering for the duration of anesthesia.

Opinion: There is no dental, oral, or masticatory cause for the pain complaint. The history, clinical course, behavioral characteristics, and effect of analgesic blocking are indicative of neural pain involving the auriculotemporal branches of the left trigeminal nerve. The complaint probably should be classified clinically as atypical idiopathic trigeminal neuralgia.

DIAGNOSIS

Auriculotemporal pain mistaken for masticatory pain.

Case No. 15-3.—Paroxysmal neuralgia of the auriculotemporal nerve, mistaken for masticatory pain.

3. Extraction of the tooth, or for that matter any surgery or even the analgesic block itself, may interrupt the neuralgic paroxysms for days or weeks, convincing both patient and dentist that the offending cause has been found and removed.

Name	Female age 33			Age	Date	Oral and Facial Pain DR. WELDEN E. BELL 8226 DOUGLAS AVENUE DALLAS, TEXAS
	QUALITY		DURATION	LOCALIZATION	AFFECTED BY	LOCAL EFFECTS
HISTORY	Mild (Severe) (Spontaneous) Triggered Induced (Paroxysmal) Steady	(Bright) Dull Pricking Itching (Burning) Aching Pulsating	Continuous Intermittent Recurrent Momentary Minutes Hours Day long Protracted	(Localized) Diffuse Radiating Spreading Enlarging Migrating Secondary Pain	Face Movement Jaw Movement Tongue Movement Swallowing Head Position Body Position Activities Tension Fatigue Time of Day	Sensory: Hypesthesia Hyperesthesia Paresthesia Dysesthesia Motor: Weakness (Contraction) Spasm	Special Sense: Visual Auditory Olfactory Gustatory Autonomic: Ocular Signs Nasal Signs Cutaneous Signs Gastric Signs

HISTORY	Location Inception Initial pain Duration, clinical course Therapeutic response Physical and emotional background Trauma, infection, etc. Medications in use	Recurrent episodes of frequent intermittent short paroxysms of severe bright burning pain located in the left face, upper lip, nose, and lower eyelid, occurring both spontaneously and triggered by light touch to the upper lip and nose and by movement of the face and jaw, especially opening widely, chewing food, and touching the palate with the tongue. The complaint began about two years ago. It was diagnosed as a left TM joint syndrome and treated by injections with corticosteroids. During the painfree remissions, it was thought that the injections had been beneficial. The present episode began about two months ago and has continued despite joint therapy. Another dentist has given her muscle relaxants without benefit. Her physician thought the complaint consisted largely of "nerves" and prescribed phenothiazine therapy. Since the complaint has persisted, she was referred for a TM joint examination.
	B/P 140/85 Neurological Survey	Psychological Survey
EXAMINATION	Oral TM joints Muscle system Diagnostic blocks Diagnostic drugs Trial therapy	Orally: The mouth is completely edentulous and patient is wearing artificial dentures that appear to be satisfactory. There is no hyperemia or palpable tenderness. Masticatory function is entirely normal in all respects. At times severe face pain accompanied by contraction of facial muscles is triggered by light touch, face and lip movement, and extended mandibular movements. The pain continues even though the mandible is stabilized by biting against a bite block. TM joints: Both joints are structurally and functionally normal. Muscle system: There is no palpable tenderness in any masticatory muscle and no muscular dysfunction. Analgesic blocking of the left infraorbital and anterior palatine nerves promptly and completely arrested both the pain and the triggering for the duration of anesthesia. Opinion: By the history, clinical course, behavioral characteristics, and effect of analgesic blocking, it is concluded that no masticatory pain is present. Rather, the complaint is that of neurogenous pain typical of idiopathic neuralgia of the maxillary division of the left trigeminal nerve.
DIAGNOSIS		Tic douloureux mistaken for masticatory pain.

Case No. 15–4.—Paroxysmal neuralgia of the maxillary nerve, mistaken for masticatory pain.

These characteristics of the usual behavior of neuralgia should be well known to the dentist so that he may guard against being deceived by them and be able to convince the patient that such dental treatment is unnecessary and futile. The differential diagnostic criteria for identifying toothache caused by tic douloureux are as follows:

Oral and Facial Pain
DR. WELDEN E. BELL
8226 DOUGLAS AVENUE
DALLAS, TEXAS

Name Female age 65		Age Date			
QUALITY	DURATION	LOCALIZATION	AFFECTED BY	LOCAL EFFECTS	
Mild	*(Bright)*	Continuous	*(Localized)*	Face Movement	Sensory:	Special Sense:
(Severe)	Dull	*(Intermittent)*	Diffuse	Jaw Movement	Hypesthesia	Visual
		Recurrent		Tongue Movement	Hyperesthesia	Auditory
			Radiating	Swallowing	Paresthesia	Olfactory
(Spontaneous)			Spreading	Head Position	Dysesthesia	Gustatory
(Triggered)	Pricking	*(Momentary)*		Body Position		Autonomic:
Induced	Itching	Minutes	Enlarging	Activities	Motor:	Ocular Signs
	(Burning)	Hours	Migrating	Tension	Weakness	Nasal Signs
(Paroxysmal)	Aching	Day long		Fatigue	*(Contraction)*	Cutaneous Signs
Steady	Pulsating	Protracted	Secondary Pain	*(Time of Day)*	Spasm	Gastric Signs

HISTORY

Location
Inception
Initial pain
Duration, clinical course
Therapeutic response
Physical and emotional background
Trauma, infection, etc.
Medications in use

Severe intermittent momentary paroxysms of bright burning pain localized to the left mandibular teeth, jaw, tongue, and lower lip. The paroxysms sometimes occur so frequently as to cause nearly continuous pain for up to five minutes. It is spontaneous and triggered by light touch and movement of the lower lip, sometimes also the tongue. The pains are accompanied by muscular contractions of the face that leave minor discomfort between attacks. Otherwise, the intermissions are entirely painfree.
The pains began about three weeks ago and have increased slightly in frequency and severity. She has on the average about five severe paroxysms daily, none at night. She promptly went to her dentist because of the dental pain but he has not been able to decide which tooth is causing it. He has referred her for more complete diagnostic evaluation.
No medications are presently in use since analgesics seem to do no good.

B/P 170/90   Neurological Survey   Psychological Survey

EXAMINATION

Oral
TM joints
Muscle system
Diagnostic blocks
Diagnostic drugs
Trial therapy

Orally: There is no clinical or radiographic evidence that the pain stems from the teeth or mouth. All the teeth are asymptomatic and no occlusal disharmony is identified. The pain may sometimes be triggered by very light touch or minor movement of the lower lip. Manual palpation, pressure, and gross movement do nothing. There is no hyperesthesia, hyperalgesia, or paresthesia.
TM joints: Both joints are clinically within normal limits.
Muscle system: There is no palpable tenderness in any masticatory muscle and no discernible muscular dysfunction.
Analgesic blocking of the left mandibular nerve promptly and completely arrested all pain and triggering for the duration of anesthesia.
Trial therapy with diphenylhydantoin sodium, 100 mg., t.i.d. reduced the pain to limits readily controllable with simple analgesics in about three days.
Opinion: No dental, oral, or masticatory cause is present for the pain complaint. The behavioral characteristics and results of trial therapy are indicative of typical neurogenous neuralgia of the mandibular division of the left trigeminal nerve (tic douloureux).

DIAGNOSIS

Dental pain from trigeminal neuralgia.

Case No. 15-5.—Paroxysmal neuralgia of the mandibular nerve, mistaken for dental pain.

1. There is lack of reasonable dental cause for the pain.
2. The toothache has a recurrent, paroxysmal, burning character of fairly short duration with intermissions that may be pain free.

3. Symptoms that are clinically evident should alert the dentist to the presence of a neuropathic pain entity in which the teeth are only incidentally involved.

Ninth Nerve Neuralgia

Neuralgia of the glossopharyngeal nerve[1, 12, 14, 15, 19, 20] occurs frequently enough to be considered in orofacial pain differential diagnosis. The pain is felt diffusely in the pharynx, ear, infra-auricular area, and postmandibular area. It is triggered by swallowing, talking, and chewing—functional movements associated with mastication that stimulate the pharyngeal mucosa, the site of triggering. Since the pains relate to jaw use, they usually are confused with those emanating from the temporomandibular joint and masticatory muscles (Case No. 15–6).

Glossopharyngeal neuralgia usually is not as dramatic as tic douloureux and for this reason may be confused with neuritic pain. It can be distinguished from glossopharyngeal neuritis by application of a topical anesthetic to the mucosa of the pharynx. Such anesthesia does not arrest neuritic pains.

It occurs fairly frequently in conjunction with trigeminal neuralgia. Unless they are separate entities, a neurologic search should be made to determine if a common lesion could be responsible for both conditions.

Sometimes the pain is felt deeply in the ear only, and when this occurs it is usually designated as *tympanic plexus neuralgia.* The ear pain may be excruciating. Such neuralgia may be indistinguishable from geniculate neuralgia when that syndrome occurs only in the ear. Precise differentiation may at times require surgical exposure of these nerves under local anesthesia and direct stimulation to determine which nerve is involved.[14, 20]

Glossopharyngeal neuralgia may be accompanied by vagal symptoms, and the examiner should be watchful for such signs. Syncope, arrhythmia, and even cardiac arrest may accompany the paroxysms of glossopharyngeal neuralgia.[20]

Clinical differentiation of glossopharyngeal neuralgia from masticatory pain may be made as follows:
1. Masticatory pain has the clinical features of deep somatic pain, whereas the neuralgia is neurogenous.
2. Masticatory pain is arrested or decreased by immobilization of the mandible with a bite-block. This does not prevent triggering of neuralgia by tongue movement and swallowing.

Oral and Facial Pain
DR. WELDEN E. BELL
8226 DOUGLAS AVENUE
DALLAS, TEXAS

Name: Female age 61

QUALITY	DURATION	LOCALIZATION	AFFECTED BY	LOCAL EFFECTS
(Mild) Severe✓	(Bright) Dull	Continuous (Intermittent) (Recurrent)	(Localized) Diffuse	Face Movement / Jaw Movement / Tongue Movement / (Swallowing) / Head Position	Sensory: Hypesthesia / Hyperesthesia / Paresthesia / Dysesthesia	Special Sense: Visual / Auditory / Olfactory / Gustatory
Spontaneous (Triggered) Induced	—	Pricking Itching (Burning) Aching Pulsating	Momentary Minutes Hours Day long Protracted	Body Position Activities Tension Fatigue Time of Day	Motor: Weakness Contraction Spasm	Autonomic: Ocular Signs Nasal Signs Cutaneous Signs Gastric Signs
(Paroxysmal) Steady			Enlarging Migrating Secondary Pain			

HISTORY

Location
Inception
Initial pain

Recurrent episodes of mild to severe intermittent short paroxysms of bright burning pain located in the right ear, postmandibular area, throat, and tongue, occurring both spontaneously and triggered by jaw movements, talking, and swallowing.

Duration, clinical course
Therapeutic response
Physical and emotional background
Trauma, infection, etc.
Medications in use

The complaint began 5 years ago as sharp pains in the right ear, throat, and tongue induced by jaw use. Her ENT physician found no aural cause and thought it was neuralgia. Her neurologist thought the pain was TM arthralgia. So her dentist remade her dentures to "correct the bite". Soon a painfree remission occurred and lasted 3 years with only minor breakthroughs. Two years ago, it recurred as before. The neurologist treated with B-12, nicotinamide, alcohol injection of the right mandibular nerve, corticosteroids, and various injections. An oral surgeon was called. He did several TM joint injections, used ethyl chloride spray, physiotherapy, and finally did a right condylectomy. After 3 months another remission of 7 months occurred; then the present episode began. Another oral surgeon blocked again with alcohol, then referred her for TM exam.

B/P 155/90   (Neurological Survey)   Psychological Survey

EXAMINATION

Oral
TM joints
Muscle system
Diagnostic blocks
Diagnostic drugs
Trial therapy

Orally: The mouth has been edentulous for 8 years with satisfactory dentures. There is no oral cause for the pain. She has right TM hypomobility and localized tenderness due presumably to the surgery. This is not her chief complaint. There is mandibular anesthesia from the alcohol block. Normal function.
TM joints: Radiographically, a surgical defect in the right condyle is seen and there is condylar fixation due presumably to cicatrization. Left is normal.
Muscle system: There is palpable tenderness over the right condyle and in the right masseter muscle presumably secondary to the arthralgia.
Neurologic consultation was requested to differentiate between very likely neurogenous neuralgia and TM arthralgia which was presumed to reflect only the surgical interference, numerous injections, and cicatrization. His diagnosis based chiefly on cocainization of the throat was glossopharyngeal neuralgia. Complete relief followed 9th nerve rhizotomy.
Opinion: No doubt the recurrent glossopharyngeal neuralgia was the chief complaint during the five years. Unfortunately, triggering from jaw movements misled all concerned and was diagnosed repeatedly as masticatory pain. Only with failure of TM therapy was neurogenous neuralgia considered. Then it was diagnosed as trigeminal instead of glossopharyngeal.

DIAGNOSIS

Glossopharyngeal neuralgia mistaken for masticatory pain.

Case No. 15–6.—Paroxysmal neuralgia of the glossopharyngeal nerve, mistaken for masticatory pain.

3. Masticatory pain is not arrested by application of a topical anesthetic to the pharyngeal mucosa.

Glossopharyngeal neuralgia has pain characteristics similar to those of trigeminal neuralgia, but the location of the initiating stimulus for both spontaneous and triggered pain is different. This distinction can be made by immobilizing the mandible and face by having the patient bite on a bite-block, which minimizes stimulation of the trigeminal structures, and by noting if pain still occurs from tongue movement and swallowing. A more positive means of distinguishing between the two neuralgias is by application of a topical anesthetic to the pharyngeal mucosa. This arrests glossopharyngeal neuralgia triggering but does not affect that of trigeminal neuralgia.

Geniculate Neuralgia

Geniculate neuralgia is a rare paroxysmal neuralgia of the intermediate nerve of Wrisberg,[1,12,14,15,20] the sensory component of the facial nerve. In 1937, Ramsay Hunt produced evidence that this somatic sensory nerve innervates the external ear, part of the external auditory canal, and a small area on the posterior surface of the cleft between the ear and the mastoid process. This illustrates vestigial overlapping innervation of the ear by sensory fibers from the fifth, seventh, ninth, and tenth cranial nerves plus cervical spinal nerve afferents contained in the great auricular and small occipital nerves.

In the neuralgic process one part of the afferent distribution may be involved without implication of the whole nerve, and the site of pain varies accordingly. Since some vestigial fibers of the facial nerve innervate the anterior two thirds of the tongue and part of the soft palate, the actual propensity for numerous sites of pain and triggering is great indeed.

The pain may be felt in front of and deeply in the ear with occasions of pain in the palate and tongue and deeply in the facial musculature. When the triggering is caused by touching the ear, topical anesthesia of the external auditory canal may arrest it. The pains, although typically those of neuralgia, are not especially dramatic, and the diagnosis may not be evident. Neurosurgical exposure of the cerebellopontine angle under local anesthesia makes possible accurate identification of the affected nerve prior to sectioning. The nervus intermedius can be isolated so that no facial paralysis results from rhizotomy to control geniculate neuralgia.

Geniculate neuralgia may be confused with migrainous neuralgia. It may be differentiated as follows:
1. The vascular pain has deep somatic category characteristics, usually with a component of throbbing. The pain distribution follows the vascular arborization. The neuralgia is neurogenous and has precise though widespread distribution that makes anatomical sense to a knowledgeable examiner.

2. The vascular pain is accompanied by central excitatory effects not evident with the neuralgia.
3. If a surgical approach is contemplated and positive identification of the affected nerve is required, this can be done by a neurosurgical suboccipital exposure under local anesthesia for direct stimulation of the nervus intermedius.[14, 20]

Differential Diagnosis

Neurogenous pains in the orofacial region that are influenced by jaw movement may be mistaken for masticatory pain. It is necessary that they be clearly differentiated. The examiner can distinguish between paroxysmal neuralgic pains of all types and true masticatory pain by observing the following points:
  1. Neuralgia is precisely localized, bright, *stimulating*, burning pain occurring in spontaneous or triggered paroxysms induced by *normal* functioning, light touch, superficial stimulation, or movement, the pain being wholly disproportionate to the stimulus and exhibiting characterstics of temporal and spatial summation.
  Masticatory pain, in contrast, is poorly localized, dull, *depressing*, aching pain, sometimes punctuated by sharper lancinating pain or having a minor burning component. It is more consistently related to functional demands and is not so clearly intermittent or triggered by insignificant stimulation. The pain is more proportional to the stimulus and does not exhibit characteristics of summation.
  2. Neuralgia is not accompanied by dysfunction other than muscular contractions with severe paroxysms or the inhibitory influence of fear of the pain. Masticatory pain is usually related to symptoms of masticatory dysfunction and commonly induces secondary referred pains and spreading myospasm activity.
  3. Neuralgia is promptly and completely arrested by interrupting the input from the sensory receptors of the affected nerve. This can be done by analgesic blocking. Mucosal triggering can be arrested by application of a topical anesthetic. Masticatory pain is arrested by analgesic blocking of the source only—the joint proper or the masticatory muscles.
  4. In differentiating glossopharyngeal neuralgia from masticatory pain, both of which are stimulated by mastication, it is well to insert a small bite-block between the teeth to restrain movements of the masticatory muscles and joints. With the mandible

thus stabilized, if throat stimulation and tongue movements continue to trigger the pain, it is probably of glossopharyngeal origin. Analgesic blocking of the joint, masticatory muscles, or both does not arrest glossopharyngeal pain. Topical anesthesia of the throat does.
5. The best differentiation between masticatory pain and the paroxysmal neuralgias is by identification of positive evidence of masticatory pain by completing an adequate examination and applying trial palliative therapy to arrive at a confirmed working diagnosis.

Symptomatic Neuralgia

About 2% of the paroxysmal neuralgias of the orofacial region result from pathologic lesions. Although such symptomatic neuralgias are only rarely encountered, they must be considered in the differential diagnosis of neurogenous pains about the face and mouth. When symptomatic neuralgias simulate the idiopathic type, differentiation may be difficult if not impossible. They usually present features that will indicate that some pathologic lesion is present. When one or more of the following features are observed by the dental examiner, referral for a neurologic consultation is indicated, i.e.:
1. Atypical manifestations such as prolonged or nearly continuous paroxysms of pain.
2. Definite bridging of paroxysms with a more continuous aching or burning pain.
3. Bilateral neuralgic pains.
4. Neuralgic involvement of two or more cranial nerves simultaneously.
5. Neuralgia accompanied by other sensory manifestations such as hypoesthesia, paresthesia, dysesthesia, or anesthesia.
6. Neuralgia accompanied by muscular weakness or paralysis or by unusual autonomic signs.
7. Rapid or significant change in behavior of the symptom complex.
8. Failure of complaint to respond to reasonable therapy.
9. Typical paroxysmal neuralgia in young persons.

Multiple sclerosis[1, 6, 14, 18] may present pain as the initial symptom, which, once established, may continue throughout the course of the disease. Occasionally the pain may be paroxysmal trigeminal pain that may simulate tic douloureux. At autopsy, sclerotic plaques have been found at the entrance zone of the trigeminal root when trigeminal neuralgia had been present. Such plaques in the descending root and sensory nucleus have been observed without associated paroxysmal pains.

When trigeminal neuralgia occurs in a patient with known multiple sclerosis, little difficulty should be encountered in making the proper diagnosis. If it is the initiating symptom, the patient's age may be important, since multiple sclerosis is most likely to develop between the ages of 20 and 40. Neuralgia from this cause may be bilateral.

Trigeminal neuralgia is said to be caused by compression of the nerve root by an aberrant branch of the superior cerebellar artery or by angulation over the petrous apex. When aneurysms are present in trigeminal neuralgia, they are always extramedullary. Such lesions have been reported in the middle posterior fossa and in the cerebellopontine angle.[18]

Meningioma of Meckel's cavity, epidermoid cyst, and arteriovenous aneurysm of the cerebellopontine angle are the more common causes of symptomatic neuralgia. It is established that malignant tumors that initiate pain are extramedullary.[14, 18] Destructive lesions of the nerve located within the brain tissue from the entrance of the trigeminal nerve into the pons throughout the numerous sensory circuits to the cortex do not cause neuralgia.[21]

Post-traumatic trigeminal neuralgia presents features that identify it as neurogenous. It combines the characteristics of both painful neuritis and paroxysmal neuralgia so that the examiner may be unable to clearly call it one or the other. The syndrome has the persistent unremitting though variable, bright, burning pain that suggests painful neuritis, and it may be accompanied by other sensory, motor and/or autonomic effects that characterize a neuritic manifestation. These effects are anatomically direct and do not behave as central excitatory effects. *This basic background neuritic pain is interrupted by paroxysms of typical neuralgic pain.* The term *atypical trigeminal neuralgia* has been used to designate this syndrome.

Neuralgic pains of this type frequently constitute part of what has been referred to as the *post-traumatic pain syndrome,* a more or less all-inclusive term that includes also post-traumatic headaches, atypical facial neuralgias, and minor reflex sympathetic dystrophies. This implies a variety of underlying causes, namely, mentation, deafferentation, and organic neuropathies. Some painful neuritic conditions and symptomatic neuralgias are also to be included in this classification.

It has recently been demonstrated that deeply located, *permanent,* degenerative change may take place following peripheral nerve trauma.[22] It is likely that atypical trigeminal neuralgia represents such degenerative change in fibers located in the ganglion or dorsal root areas. By history it usually follows trauma of some type.

NEURITIC NEURALGIA

Neuritic pains[1,23,24] occur as a result of inflammatory influence on pain-conducting fibers. The location of the pain relates anatomically to the peripheral distribution of the affected nerve. All effects are direct and anatomically related to the particular nerve. Central hyperexcitability seldom if ever occurs. The symptoms therefore closely follow dermatome geography. It is by this feature that the responsible nerve may be identified.

The symptoms relate to which fibers are affected and to what degree. This gives neuritis important identifying characteristics, i.e., other sensory effects such as hyperesthesia, hypoesthesia, paresthesia, dysesthesia, and anesthesia. If motor efferent fibers are present in the nerve trunk and also affected, then muscular signs become evident such as muscular tic, weakness, or paralysis. If autonomic fibers are present, various autonomic effects become clinically evident. The symptom complex therefore depends on the types of fibers affected, the degree of change, the peripheral distribution of the affected fibers, and the state of the inflammatory process. A knowledgeable examiner can utilize these clinical symptoms to locate the site of inflammation. When the inflammatory process occurs within a bony canal, compression effects from the inflammatory exudate may occur. The relationship between the clinical symptoms and inflammatory process is strictly anatomical. *The effects are directly the result of peripheral fiber involvement and do not represent central excitatory phenomena.*

Neuritic pains of the mouth and face may be classified as follows:
1. Peripheral neuritis (designating the entire peripheral nerve trunk, not just nerve endings and terminal branches)
2. Herpes zoster
3. Postherpetic neuralgia

Peripheral Neuritis

Peripheral neuritis occurs as the result of inflammatory influence along the course of a nerve trunk. Sensory, motor, and autonomic symptoms may be present, depending on the fiber content of the affected nerve. Analgesic blocking peripheral to the site of neuropathy may reduce discomfort by shutting off the input of noxious impulses received by the sensory receptors, but it does not arrest the ongoing burning pain that characterizes neuritis. Analgesic blocking central to the site of neuropathy arrests the neuritic pain.

Several clinical types of neuritis occur about the mouth and face, and names have been assigned to some of them. The clinical features of each depend on the factors previously discussed.

Inferior alveolar neuritis involves the mandibular dental nerve within the mandibular canal. It usually results from trauma or direct extension of inflammation from dental sepsis or surgery. The pain may be felt in any or all the structures innervated by these fibers. Other sensory effects including hyperesthesia, hypoesthesia, paresthesia, or anesthesia may accompany the persistent burning neuritic pain. No muscle symptoms are present.

Superior alveolar neuritis involves the maxillary dental plexus and usually occurs by direct extension of inflammation of the antral mucosa. The pain may be felt in any or all of the structures innervated by these fibers, including the maxillary teeth to the midline. Other sensory effects may accompany the persistent burning neuritic pain. No muscle symptoms are present.

Trigeminal Neuritis

Inflammation of the peripheral branches of the trigeminal nerve most frequently involves the inferior and superior alveolar branches. More centrally located inflammatory lesions may induce pain that is more widely located peripherally. With the mandibular division, it may be accompanied by weakness or paralysis of masticatory muscles. Some salivary gland and taste effects may occur, depending on the location of the inflammation. Auriculotemporal neuritis deserves special attention since it can be mistaken for masticatory pain.

Toothache and other pains felt in and around the teeth, periodontal structures, and oral mucogingival tissues may be due to neuritis. The pain is a direct neurologic manifestation of a nerve trunk, and the symptoms relate to the types of nerve fibers thus inflamed and to the precise anatomical distribution of those fibers. Referred pains and other central excitatory effects do not occur. Therefore a direct organic relationship exists between the toothache and its neuritic cause, and the symptoms presented identify this relationship. For example, if dental pain is the only symptom, the location of the neuritis should be sought in the terminal dental branches of the maxillary or mandibular nerves, i.e., the superior alveolar plexus above and the inferior alveolar nerve below. If the neuritis is more centrally located, sensory symptoms in other areas would be expected along with muscular and autonomic signs when such fibers are present in the nerve trunk at the site of inflammation.

Neuritic pain has a persistent, unremitting, nonvariable, burning quality that is fairly characteristic. Thus, toothache from this cause would be expressed as discomfort that differs considerably from typical odontogenous toothache. Perhaps more important is that neuritis almost invariably causes sensory symptoms other than hyperalgesia—especially paresthesia or anesthesia. Such symptoms occur in the peripheral distribution of the affected nerve so that other teeth may feel strange or "dead" and may thus respond to electric pulp testing. Either pain, dysesthesia, paresthesia, or anesthesia may occur in the superficial soft tissues supplied by the affected nerve. This would include not only the cutaneous distribution of the infraorbital and mental nerves above and below, respectively, but also the areas of mucogingiva supplied by the affected nerves. A good understanding of the local neuroanatomy therefore is essential in the diagnosis of neuritic symptoms.

The cause of neuritic toothache arising from the dental branches of the maxillary and mandibular nerves should be well understood. Neuritis of the superior dental plexus occurs most frequently as a result of contiguous inflammation in the maxillary sinus. The dental nerves frequently lie just below the lining mucosa or are separated by very thin osseous structure. They are vulnerable to involvement by direct extension. It should be noted that this is not a tooth-root relationship but a neural relationship. When antral disease causes inflammation of the dental nerve plexus, neuritic toothache may occur in *any maxillary tooth* on that side. The symptoms may be pain, hypoesthesia, paresthesia, and/or anesthesia of a tooth, several teeth, mucogingiva, or the cutaneous area supplied by the infraorbital nerve. When anterior teeth are thus affected, and they frequently are, especially when the antral symptoms are silent due to the relative insensibility of the antral mucosa, a very real diagnostic problem confronts the dentist. Many teeth so affected have been treated endodontally and even extracted, only to find continuance of the pain. For example, such a tooth endodontally treated may not only continue to ache, the pain may actually be excited by electric stimulation—a condition anatomically impossible from pulpal sources. *Therefore, diffuse maxillary toothache occurring as a direct result of maxillary sinusitis may be neuritic if its behavior follows the rules that apply to neuritis.* This should be well understood by all dentists and otolaryngologists (Case No. 15–7).

Neuritic toothache arising from inflammation of the inferior dental nerve occurs most frequently from contiguous inflammation in the mandibular canal, usually from trauma or infection. The most common source is surgery involving deeply embedded mandibular third molars. However, spreading of dental sepsis to the mandibular canal is also a cause of this condition (Fig 15–2). Sometimes such neuritic pain

	QUALITY	DURATION	LOCALIZATION	AFFECTED BY	LOCAL EFFECTS	
Name: Female age 65					Sensory:	Special Sense:
	(Mild) Severe	(Bright) Dull	(Continuous) Intermittent Recurrent	(Localized) Diffuse	Face Movement Jaw Movement Tongue Movement Swallowing Head Position Body Position Activities Tension Fatigue Time of Day	(Hypesthesia) (Hyperesthesia) (Paresthesia) Dysesthesia	Visual Auditory Olfactory Gustatory
	Spontaneous Triggered Induced Paroxysmal (Steady)	Pricking Itching (Burning) Aching Pulsating	Momentary Minutes Hours Day long (Protracted)	Radiating Spreading Enlarging Migrating Secondary Pain		Motor: Weakness Contraction Spasm	Autonomic: Ocular Signs Nasal Signs Cutaneous Signs Gastric Signs

HISTORY

Location
Inception
Initial pain
Duration, clinical course
Therapeutic response
Physical and emotional background
Trauma, infection, etc.
Medications in use

Mild to severe variable but protracted continuous steady bright burning pain located in the right maxillary teeth and gingiva, accompanied by some sensations of hypesthesia, hyperesthesia, and paresthesia. The pain is located in the UR1-3 region where the teeth have recently been extracted.
The complaint began three months ago as intermittent burning pain in the UR2-3 teeth which were treated endodontically without benefit. After about thirty days, she had some burning pain and sensations of swelling of the right labial and buccal maxillary mucogingival tissues. This has persisted as a variable tingling and numb sensation. About six weeks ago, the dental pain became severe and more constant. A few days ago the UR1,2,3 were extracted in a futile attempt to control the patient's pain.

EXAMINATION

B/P 140/85 Neurological Survey   Psychological Survey

Oral
TM joints
Muscle system
Diagnostic blocks
Diagnostic drugs
Trial therapy

Orally: The UR1-3 area shows evidence of recent operation for removal of the UR1,2,3 teeth. No surgical complications are evident. The remaining right maxillary teeth appear to be normal clinically and radiographically except for decreased pulp tester response of the UR4 and UR6 teeth.
TM joints and muscle system: Entirely negative.
Local anesthetic infiltration of the UR1-4 area failed to arrest the pain. Right second division analgesic block nearly completely arrested the pain for the duration of anesthesia.
Opinion: The persistent bright burning pain accompanied by other definite sensations, especially in the absence of central excitatory effects such as referred pain and secondary myospasms, is highly suggestive of neuritic pain rather than true odontalgia. A presumptive diagnosis, therefore, of superior alveolar neuritis probably secondary to antral disease was made. Subsequent consultation with an otolaryngologist confirmed the diagnosis.

DIAGNOSIS

Superior alveolar neuritis due to maxillary sinusitis, felt as "toothache".

Case No. 15–7.—Neuritic neuralgia of the superior alveolar nerve, due to maxillary sinusitis, expressed as maxillary toothache.

involves all mandibular teeth to the midline. Frequently, paresthesia or anesthesia of the lower lip is encountered. Paresthesia sensed as tightness of dental contacts and various "dead" feelings may be described. Mucogingival pain and sensations of swelling in the peripheral distribution of the inferior alveolar nerve are common. All such

Fig 15-2.—Radiograph of mandibular third molar showing extensive radiolucency indicative of interradicular abscess that communicated with the mandibular canal. The patient's clinical symptoms were those of localized periodontal odontogenous pain in third molar region accompanied by neuritic pain in other mandibular teeth, with paresthesia and hypoesthesia of structures supplied by mental nerve.

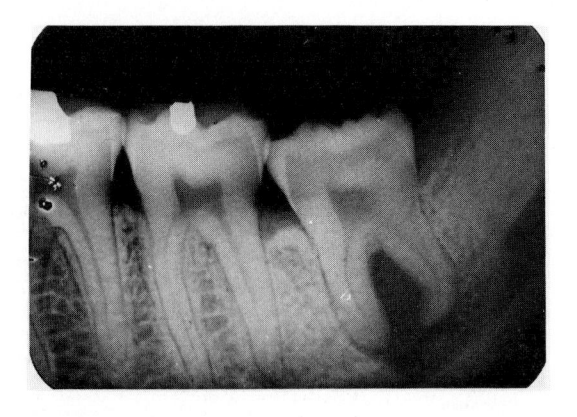

mandibular toothache complaints due to inferior alveolar neuritis follow the rules that apply to neuritis (Case No. 15–8).

The differential diagnostic criteria for identifying toothache of neuritic origin are as follows:

1. The pain is less variable, is more persistent, has more of a burning quality, and is less likely to be accompanied by central excitatory effects than is true odontogenous pain.
2. The pain is likely to be accompanied by other sensory effects such as hypoesthesia, dysesthesia, paresthesia, or anesthesia in other teeth or in the superficial mucogingival and cutaneous tissues innervated by fibers of the affected nerve.
3. More centrally located inflammation involving a nerve trunk may cause motor or autonomic symptoms if efferent somatic and visceral fibers are present in the nerve trunk at the site of inflammation.
4. Electric pulp testing may give results indicative of the varied sensory responses characteristic of neuritis.
5. Analgesic blocking stops the pain if placed central to the site of inflammation.
6. Neuritis of the superior dental plexus may be confirmed by evidence of antral disease. In the absence of clinical or radiographic evidence of maxillary sinusitis, direct surgical aspiration of the antrum may be done. This is a simple intraoral procedure accomplished by infiltrating a small amount of local anesthetic in the canine fossa area superior to the bicuspid teeth and drilling a small hole through the facial wall of the antrum superior to the root ends of the bicuspid teeth (as guided by the dental radiograph). A No. 1 round bur may be used. An

Oral and Facial Pain
DR. WELDEN E. BELL
8226 DOUGLAS AVENUE
DALLAS, TEXAS

Name Female age 45		Age	Date		
QUALITY	DURATION	LOCALIZATION	AFFECTED BY	LOCAL EFFECTS	
(Mild)	(Bright)	(Continuous)	(Localized)	Sensory:	Special Sense:
Severe	Dull	Intermittent	Diffuse	Hypesthesia	Visual
		Recurrent	Face Movement	Hyperesthesia	Auditory
			Jaw Movement	(Paresthesia)	Olfactory
		Radiating	Tongue Movement	Dysesthesia	Gustatory
Spontaneous		Spreading	Swallowing		
Triggered	Pricking	Momentary	Head Position		Autonomic:
Induced	Itching	Minutes	Body Position	Motor:	Ocular Signs
	(Burning)	Hours	Activities	Weakness	Nasal Signs
Paroxysmal	Aching	Day long	(Tension)	Contraction	Cutaneous Signs
(Steady)	Pulsating	(Protracted)	(Fatigue)	Spasm	Gastric Signs
			Secondary Pain	Time of Day		

HISTORY

Location
Inception
Initial pain
Duration, clinical course
Therapeutic response
Physical and emotional background
Trauma, infection, etc.
Medications in use

Mild continuous but variable protracted steady bright burning pain located in the left mandibular teeth, accompanied by some paresthesia described as a tingling sensation. The discomfort increases with firm biting pressure on the teeth and when she is tired and nervous.
The complaint began about four months ago following the extraction of the lower left third molar tooth about two months before. The immediate postoperative pain was intense for several days. This was followed by a period of numbness that lasted several weeks and then subsided. As the numbness decreased, the present mild burning pain was felt in several left mandibular teeth, especially the LL7. The "toothache" has been more annoying than actually painful. It worries her and makes her nervous. The last few weeks the complaint seems to be decreasing gradually.
Medically negative for cause. No medications presently being taken.

B/P 140/80 Neurological Survey   Psychological Survey

EXAMINATION

Oral
TM joints
Muscle system
Diagnostic blocks
Diagnostic drugs
Trial therapy

Orally: The left mandibular teeth are clinically and radiographically free of obvious cause for the complaint. The LL8 alveolus appears to be healing satisfactorily. The root ends appear to have been in close proximity to the mandibular canal. There is no palpable tenderness. All the teeth respond within normal limits to electric pulp testing.
TM joints and muscle system: Entirely negative for cause.

Opinion: The descriptive behavior of the complaint from its inception is highly suggestive of neurogenous pain of neuritic type rather than any form of true odontogenous pain. It appears that the inflammatory process incidental to the surgery and the healing process enveloped the mandibular neurovascular bundle causing first severe pain, then anesthesia, and subsequently neuritis. The dental pain and tingling sensation seem to be subsiding as the inflammatory process resolves naturally.

DIAGNOSIS

Mandibular toothache due to postoperative neuritis of the left inferior alveolar nerve.

Case No. 15–8.—Neuritic neuralgia of the inferior alveolar nerve, expressed as mandibular toothache.

aspiration needle is then inserted into the cavity of the antrum and its contents aspirated. A normal antrum contains only air. Fluid aspirated is positive evidence of antral disease, and the patient should be transferred to the care of an otolaryngologist. Such a test is harmless if properly done. The information obtained more than justifies its use when the cause of maxillary neuritic toothache is in doubt.

Occasionally, persistent toothache may follow facial trauma. Such pains have behavioral characteristics of atypical trigeminal neuralgia. Although neurogenous, the toothache is neither typically neuritic nor neuralgic. Rather, it is both, being persistently felt as a burning sensation but interrupted at times by severe paroxysmal pain.

Bell's Palsy (Facial Neuritis)

Bell's palsy results from inflammation of the facial nerve. The location is usually, but not necessarily, within the facial canal. Although some deeply situated neuritic pain along with a persistent burning pain of the auricular area is noticeable, the predominant effects are weakness or paralysis of facial muscles because efferent fibers to the muscles of facial expression are numerically greater. Other sensory effects, autonomic effects, and taste aberrations also may be recognized.

Compression effects due to angioneurotic edema within the facial canal can also cause facial paralysis that may be indistinguishable from true facial neuritis. Clinically it may be assumed that sudden painless and otherwise nonsymptomatic facial paralysis of a transitory type that accompanies other allergic manifestations is a result of angioneurotic edema rather than true facial neuritis.

Glossopharyngeal Neuritis

Inflammation of the glossopharyngeal nerve is characterized by neuritic pain in the throat and postmandibular and auricular areas. The pain may be aggravated by throat and mandibular movement and therefore may be mistaken for masticatory pain.

Traumatic involvement of a prominent styloid process may cause glossopharyngeal neuritis that may be confused with masticatory pain because of its relationship with mandibular functioning (Case No. 15–9). Styloid process pain usually can be identified by manual palpation through the tonsillar fossa, pressure being directed laterally toward the styloid process. Elongation of the styloid process and/or calcification of the stylohyoid ligament is commonly known as Eagle's syndrome.[25] The symptoms are those of glossopharyngeal neuritis and sometimes of carotid arteritis also.

Neurogenous Pains

Oral and Facial Pain
DR. WELDEN E. BELL
8226 DOUGLAS AVENUE
DALLAS, TEXAS

Name: Female age 44

HISTORY

QUALITY	DURATION	LOCALIZATION	AFFECTED BY	LOCAL EFFECTS
(Mild) Severe	(Bright) Dull	(Continuous) Intermittent Recurrent	(Localized) Diffuse Radiating Spreading	Face Movement (Jaw Movement) (Tongue Movement) Swallowing Head Position Body Position Activities Tension Fatigue Time of Day	Sensory: Hypesthesia (Hyperesthesia) (Paresthesia) Dysesthesia — Motor: Weakness Co(ntr)action (Spasm) — Special Sense: Visual Auditory Olfactory Gustatory — Autonomic: Ocular Signs Nasal Signs Cutaneous Signs Gastric Signs
Spontaneous Triggered Induced Paroxysmal (Steady)	Pricking Itching (Burning) (Aching) Pulsating	Momentary Minutes Hours Day long (Protracted)	Enlarging Migrating Secondary Pain		

Location
Inception
Initial pain
Duration, clinical course
Therapeutic response
Physical and emotional background
Trauma, infection, etc.
Medications in use

Mild continuous variable protracted steady bright aching, stinging and burning pain located in the left ear and throat, aggravated by chewing, talking and swallowing, and accompanied by rawness of the throat and a sensation of "wetness" in the left ear.

The complaint began about 30 days ago following a severe blow to the left face. That evening she had pain in the left ear and postmandibular area that increased with opening the mouth. Her ENT physician found no aural cause for the complaint and advised a corticosteroid injection of the left TM joint. This was vetoed by her internist pending a dental examination. Her dentist found no dental or oral cause for the pain. Open and closed TM joint radiographs by her physician revealed normal translation of the condyles. Under symptomatic treatment she improved considerably. When some of the complaint persisted, she was referred for a TM joint examination on a presumptive diagnosis of "temporomandibular joint syndrome".

EXAMINATION

B/P 130/80   Neurological Survey   Psychological Survey

Oral
TM joints
Muscle system
Diagnostic blocks
Diagnostic drugs
Trial therapy

Orally: There is no dental or oral cause for the pain. The ear, throat and postmandibular pain increases with extended mandibular movements and to a lesser degree with tongue and throat movements when the mandible is stabilized by means of a bite block. All masticatory and tongue movements are normal. The palatal and pharyngeal reflexes are normal. There is deep palpable tenderness in the direction of the left styloid process via the tonsillar fossa. Radiographic visualization of the left styloid process shows a long process with an overriding fracture in its midbody.

TM joints: Both joints are structurally and functionally normal.

Muscle system: There is no palpable tenderness in any masticatory muscle and no muscular dysfunction of any kind.

Topical anesthetic applied to the throat did not arrest the pain. Analgesic blocking of the left mandibular nerve intraorally and of the left TM joint proper extraorally did not arrest the pain.

Opinion: The only masticatory relationship is extensive mandibular movement that stretches the stylomandibular ligament. The behavioral characteristics are highly suggestive of neurogenous pain involving the left glossopharyngeal nerve. Radiographic evidence of fracture of the left styloid process should confirm a diagnosis of glossopharyngeal neuritis induced by trauma.

DIAGNOSIS

Glossopharyngeal neuritis mistaken for masticatory pain.

Case No. 15-9.—Neuritic neuralgia of the glossopharyngeal nerve, due to fractured styloid process, mistaken for masticatory pain.

Herpes Zoster

Acute herpes zoster[1, 8, 14] is a self-limiting viral infection of the ganglion, sensory root, or medullary tract of a nerve. The cause of the infection is the varicella-zoster virus of chicken pox. It is unlike the virus of herpes simplex. The heterotopic neuritic pain and herpetic eruptions are located superficially in the exact anatomical peripheral distribution of the affected nerve. Until vesicles appear, the pain may be difficult to diagnose. Laboratory examination of spinal fluid shows elevated protein levels and pleiocytosis. Most patients recover within six weeks. One attack normally renders the subject immune. Occasionally, however, it may recur. Postherpetic neuralgia may follow an acute attack of herpes zoster, especially in elderly patients.

Trigeminal herpes zoster may involve any of the divisions but most frequently the ophthalmic. The maxillary and mandibular divisions may be affected individually, in conjunction with each other or with the ophthalmic. The cutaneous and mucosal eruptions are located in the superficial peripheral sensory distribution of the particular nerve affected, and the pain is felt in exactly the same area (Fig 15–3).

Fig 15–3.—Herpes zoster involving all divisions of right trigeminal nerve. Note that cutaneous herpetic lesions are confined to peripheral distribution of the nerve on right side of face.

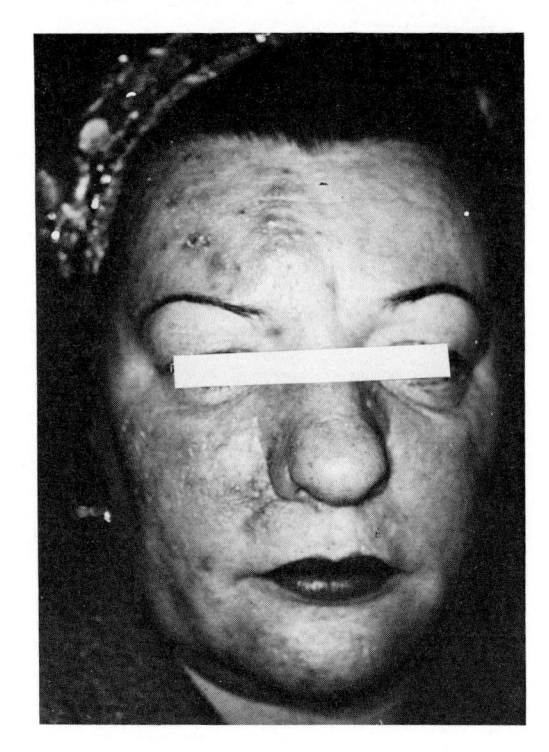

Intraoral lesions may be the only eruptions and therefore confused with aphthous stomatitis. The pain may be mistaken for mucogingival of superficial somatic type. The diagnostic clue that the condition is herpes zoster is the anatomical location of the lesions—identical to that of the peripheral superficial distribution of the sensory nerve mediating the pain. Herpes zoster pain is not arrested by application of a topical anesthetic or by regional block anesthesia. Sometimes it may occur before or after the appearance of the mucosal or cutaneous lesions and occasionally without superficial lesions (Case No. 15–10).

Ramsay Hunt syndrome is herpes zoster of the intermediate nerve of Wrisberg, the sensory component of the facial nerve. This rare syndrome causes neuritic pain and superficial herpetic lesions in the external ear, auditory canal, and mastoid area. Intraorally, the heterotopic pain and herpetic lesions affect the fauces, soft palate, and anterior tongue.[14] Herpes zoster does not display muscle symptoms.

Postherpetic Neuralgia

Occasionally, acute herpes zoster persists as an intractable, chronic, burning pain. The heterotopic pain of postherpetic neuralgia is felt superficially in the area affected by the acute attack. If it lasts as long as a year, it is likely to persist indefinitely and resist all therapy. It is thought that one reason for the extreme difficulty in managing this syndrome by trigeminal denervation is because the virus involves central pathways in the brain stem and cerebral hemispheres.[6] The pain is usually accompanied by other sensory symptoms such as dysesthesia, hypoesthesia, and hyperesthesia in the cutaneous distribution of the affected nerve. The syndrome may display episodes of exacerbated symptoms; occasionally, spontaneous subsidence occurs. Usually the pain remains moderate in intensity, but the constancy and intractability may render it intolerable.

DEAFFERENTATION PAINS OF THE MOUTH AND FACE

Crushing and lacerating injuries of the mouth and face as well as surgery and denervation procedures interrupt the flow of afferent impulses in sensory neurons. Damage to peripheral nerves causes reactions, not only in the central terminals, but also in other peripheral and central cells that are functionally related. Such deafferentation therefore may initiate a variety of symptoms, including pain. Such pains arise within the nervous system itself and are not significantly

Name Female age 66			Age	Date		Oral and Facial Pain DR. WELDEN E. BELL 8226 DOUGLAS AVENUE DALLAS, TEXAS
	QUALITY	DURATION	LOCALIZATION	AFFECTED BY	LOCAL EFFECTS	
	Mild (Severe) ——— Spontaneous Triggered Induced Paroxysmal (Steady)	(Bright) Dull ——— Pricking Itching (Burning) Aching Pulsating	(Continuous) Intermittent Recurrent Momentary Minutes Hours Day long (Protracted)	(Localized) Diffuse Radiating Spreading Enlarging Migrating Secondary Pain	Face Movement Jaw Movement Tongue Movement Swallowing Head Position Body Position Activities Tension Fatigue Time of Day	Sensory: Hypesthesia Hyperesthesia Paresthesia Dysesthesia Motor: Weakness Contraction Spasm	Special Sense: Visual Auditory Olfactory Gustatory Autonomic: Ocular Signs Nasal Signs Cutaneous Signs Gastric Signs

HISTORY

Location — Moderately severe steady bright burning pain located in the left lower jaw from the mental foramen to the ear and in the lower lip and labial gingiva from the mental foramen to the mandibular symphysis.

Inception
Initial pain — The pain began without apparent cause about 4-5 days ago and has continued

Duration, clinical course — as a protracted complaint ever since. She had a similar but milder attack about ten months ago. It lasted 5-6 weeks and finally disappeared without

Therapeutic response — therapy.

Physical and emotional background — Her dentist has checked her artificial dentures and prescribed a muscle relaxant without benefit. There appears to be no history of prior illness, infection, trauma or allergy.

Trauma, infection, etc. — Simple analgesics only are presently being used.

Medications in use

B/P 155/85   Neurological Survey   Psychological Survey

EXAMINATION

Oral — Orally: The mouth is edentulous and the artificial dentures appear to be satisfactory. There is no hyperemia or ulceration seen. The tissues around the mental foramen and the entire lower lip are hyperalgesic.

TM joints — TM joints and muscle system: Negative.

Muscle system

Diagnostic blocks — Local anesthetic mandibular block caused a mild burning sensation in the left lower lip prior to anesthesia. A few hours later, patient noticed some superficial swelling of the lower lip. This was followed by some vesiculation of the inner mucosa of the lip. About two days later, herpetic type ulceration became evident located precisely in the peripheral distribution of the left mental nerve.

Diagnostic drugs

Trial therapy — Opinion: This complaint presents the features of neuritic pain of herpetic origin. Probably recurrent.

DIAGNOSIS

Herpes zoster involving the mandibular division of the left trigeminal nerve.

Case No. 15-10.—Herpes zoster involving the mandibular nerve, expressed intraorally.

influenced by the subject's activities, nor effectively controlled by measures that reduce peripheral nociceptive stimulation. Some deafferentation symptoms may remain even when considerable regeneration takes place. Thus, sensory symptoms including anesthesia, hypoesthesia, paresthesia, dysesthesia, hyperesthesia, hyperalgesia, and spontaneous pain may be felt in the region innervated by an injured nerve. These strange sensations may actually be felt in an area larger than that subserved by the injured nerve because deafferentation causes an enlargement of the receptive field. Such symptoms may persist indefinitely. Deafferentation symptoms may follow such simple surgical procedures as tooth extraction and pulp extirpation (Case No. 15–11).

The recent discovery that an ongoing barrage of afferent signals is generated in the dorsal ganglion and propagated both orthodromically and antidromically has opened new avenues of thought concerning deafferentation syndromes. The fact that such genesis of afferent impulses is significantly increased as the result of nerve damage may do much to increase our understanding of such mechanisms.[11]

Deafferentation symptoms in the orofacial region are commonplace. Only a few such conditions, however, elicit pain. The most frequent complaint is anesthesia and paresthesia following injury of the mandibular nerve incidental to the removal of teeth. Despite considerable regeneration, some sensory abnormality may persist. Being nonpainful, such conditions are beyond the scope of this book. The painful deafferentation syndromes of the mouth and face may be classified as (1) reflex sympathetic dystrophy, (2) anesthesia dolorosa, and (3) phantom pains (Fig 15–4).

Reflex Sympathetic Dystrophy

In the past it has been difficult to decide how to classify the causalgic pains that result from nerve injury. With the continuing research on deafferentation, however, the neurogenous category is clearly indicated. The syndrome has been referred to as *autonomic reflex pain* because of its striking relationship to sympathetic autonomic activities. Whether or not the currently accepted term *reflex sympathetic dystrophy* is the most suitable one remains to be seen. It refers to the dystrophic change that accompanies protracted causalgia. Since interruption of sympathetic pathways frequently relieves the pain, causalgia has been classified as "visceral pain" on the presumption that it was mediated by sympathetic afferents of the visceral nervous system. It is now known, however, that the clinical relationship to the visceral neurons is not one of neural pathway mediation of impulses. Rather, it is due to the fact that neural sprouts at the site of injury become sensitized to norepinephrine; therefore efferent sympathetic activity induces a nociceptive response. Suppression of such activity by analgesic blocking has a definite antinociceptive effect.

Case No. 15–11

Oral and Facial Pain
DR. WELDEN E. BELL
8226 DOUGLAS AVENUE
DALLAS, TEXAS

Name: Female age 42

QUALITY	DURATION	LOCALIZATION	AFFECTED BY	LOCAL EFFECTS
(Mild) / Severe	**(Bright)** / Dull	**(Continuous)** / Intermittent / Recurrent	**(Localized)** / Diffuse / Radiating / Spreading	Face Movement / Jaw Movement / Tongue Movement / Swallowing / Head Position / Body Position / Activities / Tension / Fatigue / Time of Day	Sensory: Hypesthesia / Hyperesthesia / **(Paresthesia)** / Dysesthesia — Motor: Weakness / Contraction / Spasm — Special Sense: Visual / Auditory / Olfactory / Gustatory — Autonomic: Ocular Signs / Nasal Signs / Cutaneous Signs / Gastric Signs
Spontaneous / Triggered / Induced / Paroxysmal / **(Steady)**	Pricking / Itching / **(Burning)** / Aching / Pulsating	Momentary / Minutes / Hours / Day long / **(Protracted)**	Enlarging / Migrating / Secondary Pain		

HISTORY

Location / Inception / Initial pain / Duration, clinical course / Therapeutic response / Physical and emotional background / Trauma, infection, etc. / Medications in use

Mild continuous protracted steady bright burning pain located in the left mandibular teeth and accompanied by paresthesia described as a sensation of "high teeth" and recently as "gingival swelling."

The complaint began five years ago following the surgical removal of an impacted lower left wisdom tooth. After a few months, dental pain began in the LL6 which was extracted and replaced with a fixed bridge that felt "too high" in spite of repeated occlusal adjustment and finally remaking. A year later, the LL7 was treated endodontically because of pain and later the LL5 also. Finally, the LL5 was extracted, then the LL7, and subsequently the LL4 and LL3 as well. The replacing partial denture could not be tolerated because of pain. Then some diffuse temporal discomfort began which lead to muscle therapy by first a periodontist and then an oral surgeon unsuccessfully. Presently she has an excellent prosthesis but she cannot wear it because of pain and a sensation of gingival swelling. It feels no better when she leaves it out.

B/P 125/80   Neurological Survey   Psychological Survey

EXAMINATION

Oral / TM joints / Muscle system / Diagnostic blocks / Diagnostic drugs / Trial therapy

Orally: Missing LL3,4,5,6,7,8 replaced with an excellent partial denture which she does not wear. No dental cause is evident either clinically or radiographically. There is an acutely tender spot to finger pressure located in the mucosal scar residual to the surgery for removal of the LL8. Injection of a local anesthetic into this spot immediately gave considerable relief of pain and, therefore, it was presumed to represent a painful neuroma. Excision, however, gave only transitory relief and after a few weeks all pain was as before.

TM joints and muscles: The joints were clinically and radiographically normal. There was minor tenderness in the left temporal muscle area which was interpreted to represent muscle splinting due to missing posterior teeth. Analgesic blocking of that muscle arrested the muscle pain only.

Opinion: The behavioral characteristics of this pain problem suggest a posttraumatic pain syndrome based on degenerative neural changes located centrally in either the somatic or visceral pain conduction system. There is no evidence that the pain stems from dental, oral, or masticatory causes.

DIAGNOSIS

Multiple "toothache" in the left mandible as a manifestation of posttraumatic neuritic pain.

Case No. 15–11.—Deafferentation syndrome, expressed as sensory aberrations (postsurgical).

It should be noted that exacerbation of pain by central phenomena, such as emotional stress and visual or auditory stimuli, is characteristic of causalgic pains.[12] In the light of present knowledge of the role of neurotransmitters and opioid peptides, such behavior is better under-

OROFACIAL PAIN SYNDROMES

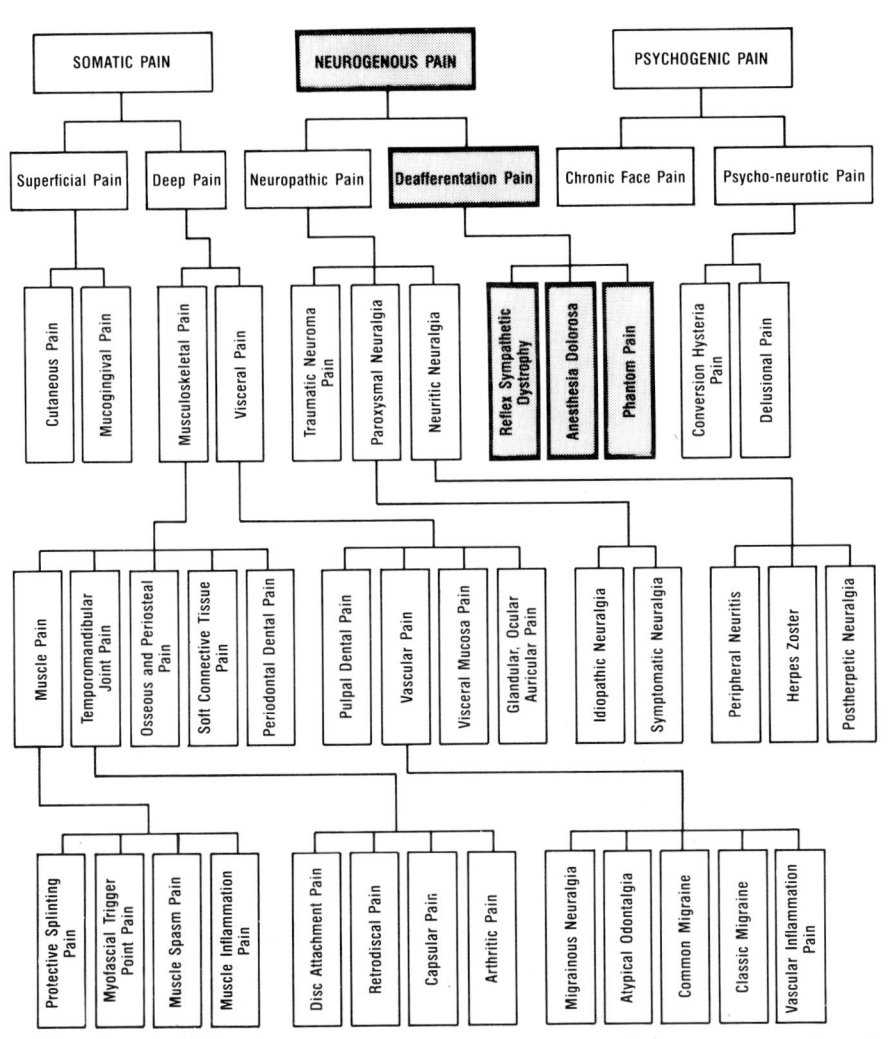

Fig 15-4.—Chart showing classification relationship of neurogenous pains of deafferentation origin to other orofacial pain syndromes.

stood. The knowledge that afferent impulses generated in the dorsal ganglion are significantly increased by nerve damage now makes more understandable the fact that painful impulses can be propagated from structures that are denervated or that no longer exist.

Classic causalgia, as initially described by Mitchell,[26, 27] had to do with extremity wounds involving injured nerves in Civil War soldiers. The word literally means "burning pain." The syndrome was dramatic, onset of pain varying from time of injury to several weeks later. It was typically a constant, diffuse, intense, burning sensation not necessarily confined to the sensory distribution of the injured nerve. The skin was sensitive, and excruciating pain could be set off by almost any stimulus such as touch, air drafts, thermal changes, vibration, noise, or emotional stress. Autonomic symptoms were seen such as changes in cutaneous temperature, color, texture, and perspiration. Trophic changes in the skin, muscles, and bones also followed in due time.

Causalgia is presently referred to as reflex sympathetic dystrophy.[28, 29] In a minor form, it may involve the mouth and face. It follows nerve injury incidental to trauma, surgery, or infection. It is described as a dull, persistent, unremitting, variable, diffuse, burning sensation. It is arrested by analgesic blocking of the stellate ganglion. Since this syndrome may follow minor oral surgery or postsurgical infection, the history of a dental relationship may be misunderstood by patient and dentist alike.

Although rare, reflex sympathetic dystrophy may cause toothache of nondental origin. Toothache from this cause has descriptive characteristics that differ from those of true pulpal pain. The pain is described as a persistent, unremitting, only slightly variable, *burning* sensation in and around the tooth—giving it a neuritic quality not characteristic of odontogenous toothache (Case No. 15–12).

Reflex sympathetic dystrophy may be confused with masticatory pain (Case No. 15–13). It may be differentiated from masticatory pain by the following criteria:

1. The similarity in these two syndromes is their tendency to induce central excitatory effects. When the syndromes are confused, the real character of the pain has probably been overlooked and only the secondarily induced muscle spasm pain observed.
2. The underlying ongoing, persistent, constant, diffusely located, burning sensation should never suggest masticatory pain, which is characterized by variability linked to functional demands and by an aching quality that can be clinically identified as to source by manual palpation and analgesic blocking.
3. This syndrome can be identified by a diagnostic stellate ganglion analgesic block.
4. As with all differential diagnosis, true masticatory pain should be identified by positive evidence, as obtained by a satisfactory and exacting examination by the dental examiner.

Oral and Facial Pain
DR. WELDEN E. BELL
8226 DOUGLAS AVENUE
DALLAS, TEXAS

Name: Female age 45

QUALITY	DURATION	LOCALIZATION	AFFECTED BY	LOCAL EFFECTS
Mild	Bright	(Continuous)	Localized	Face Movement	Sensory:	Special Sense:
Severe ✓	Dull	Intermittent	(Diffuse)	Jaw Movement	Hypesthesia	Visual
		Recurrent		Tongue Movement	Hyperesthesia	Auditory
			Radiating	Swallowing	(Paresthesia)	Olfactory
Spontaneous			Spreading	Head Position	Dysesthesia	Gustatory
Triggered	Pricking	Momentary		Body Position		Autonomic:
Induced	Itching	Minutes	Enlarging	Activities	Motor:	Ocular Signs
	Burning	Hours	Migrating	Tension	Weakness	Nasal Signs
Paroxysmal	Aching	Day long		Fatigue	Contraction	Cutaneous Signs
(Steady)	Pulsating	(Protracted)	Secondary Pain	Time of Day	Spasm	Gastric Signs

HISTORY

Location / Inception / Initial pain: Mild to severe variable but continuous protracted steady dull burning pain diffusely located in the right mandibular teeth and edentulous area described as persistent toothache in the remaining teeth as well as phantom toothache in the LR5,6,7 area which is edentulous.

Duration, clinical course / Therapeutic response / Physical and emotional background / Trauma, infection, etc. / Medications in use: The complaint began following an automobile accident in which the patient sustained injuries to the back and head. A neurological examination at the time indicated cerebral concussion and fracture of T11, plus complaints including transient leg numbness, headaches, facial paresthesias, and visual disturbance even though there were no abnormal sensory or motor nerve findings. All the cranial nerves are said to be intact.
After the accident, patient felt toothache in the LR6,7 teeth which after two weeks were extracted without benefit. Two months later, the LR5 also was extracted, but the complaint continued as before.
Percodan is used to control the pain.

EXAMINATION

B/P 135/85   Neurological Survey   Psychological Survey

Oral: Orally: Recent extraction of LR5,6,7 is evident. Healing appears to be normal. Remaining teeth and mouth are clinically and radiographically negative for cause of pain.

TM joints / Muscle system: TM joints and muscle system: Clinically normal. No dysfunction.

Diagnostic blocks: Analgesic blocking of the right mandibular and maxillary teeth did not arrest the pain even though satisfactory anesthesia was promptly obtained.

Neurological consultation for diagnostic analgesic blocking of the right stellate ganglion: Blocking appears to arrest the mandibular pains.

Diagnostic drugs / Trial therapy: Opinion: No dental, oral, or masticatory cause for the complaint. The toothache and phantom pains appear to be mediated by afferent sympathetic fibers from the head. The stimulus appears to arise central to the level of intraoral analgesic blocking of the mandibular nerve. The neuritic-like pain appears to be part of a posttraumatic pain syndrome.

DIAGNOSIS

Mandibular toothache due to so-called reflex sympathetic dystrophy.

Case No. 15–12.—Deafferentation syndrome, expressed as mandibular toothache (post-traumatic).

Oral and Facial Pain
DR. WELDEN E. BELL
8226 DOUGLAS AVENUE
DALLAS, TEXAS

	Name Female age 41 Age Date				
	QUALITY	DURATION	LOCALIZATION	AFFECTED BY	LOCAL EFFECTS
HISTORY	(Mild) Bright Severe (Dull) ——— ——— Spontaneous Triggered Pricking Induced Itching (Burning) Paroxysmal Aching (Steady) Pulsating	(Continuous) Intermittent Recurrent ——— ——— Momentary Minutes Hours Day long (Protracted)	Localized (Diffuse) ——— Radiating (Spreading) ——— ——— Enlarging Migrating ——— (Secondary Pain)	Face Movement (Jaw Movement) Tongue Movement Swallowing Head Position Body Position Activities Tension Fatigue Time of Day	Sensory: Special Sense: Hypesthesia Visual (Hyperesthesia) Auditory Paresthesia Olfactory Dysesthesia Gustatory ——— Motor: Autonomic: Weakness Ocular Signs Contraction Nasal Signs Spasm Cutaneous Signs Gastric Signs

HISTORY

Location
Inception
Initial pain
Duration, clinical course
Therapeutic response
Physical and emotional background
Trauma, infection, etc.
Medications in use

Mild continuous protracted steady dull burning pain diffusely located in the left jaw and face and aggravated by peripheral stimulation of the entire painful area as well as by masticatory movements.
The complaint began about six months ago as pain following the extraction of several left mandibular posterior teeth. Initially, it was treated as an acute alveolitis but persisted after healing occurred. Soon it was felt as earache. Her ENT physician found the ear to be normal and advised that the dentist "raise the bite". Her dentist replaced the missing teeth without benefit. As the pain spread to the masseter, temporal, and orbital areas, the dentist adjusted the occlusion several times, prescribed nicotinic acid and muscle relaxants, remade the partial denture, tried an anterior bite-plane device, and injected corticosteroid into the left joint. When the complaint persisted, she was referred for a temporomandibular joint examination.
No medications are presently being taken except ordinary analgesics.

B/P 125/85 Neurological Survey Psychological Survey

EXAMINATION

Oral
TM joints
Muscle system
Diagnostic blocks
Diagnostic drugs
Trial therapy

Orally: The teeth and mouth are clinically and radiographically negative for cause of pain. The left mandibular edentulous area is hypersensitive to touch. There is subjective increase in discomfort with all mandibular movements but there is no identifiable masticatory dysfunction of any kind. The auricular, masseter, temporal, and orbital areas all seem to be hyperalgesic to touch.
TM joints: Both joints are clinically and radiographically normal.
Muscle system: There is vague subjective discomfort in the masseter and temporal muscles with manual palpation but no muscular dysfunction of any kind.
Analgesic blocking of the left masseter and temporal muscles, followed by blocking of the left TM joint proper, did not arrest the complaint.
Consultation with an anesthesiologist was requested for the purpose of making an analgesic block of the left stellate ganglion. This block arrested all left orofacial pain and subsequently two more similar blocks eliminated the complaint without relapse.

Opinion: The history, clinical course, and present behavioral characteristics suggested an autonomic reflex pain syndrome (causalgia). This presumptive diagnosis was confirmed by analgesic blocking of the stellate ganglion.

DIAGNOSIS

Minor reflex sympathetic dystrophy mistaken for a masticatory pain-dysfunction syndrome.

Case No. 15–13.—Deafferentation syndrome, expressed as reflex sympathetic dystrophy, mistaken for masticatory pain (postsurgical).

Anesthesia Dolorosa

Deafferentation normally induces anesthesia of the area innervated by the damaged nerve. This is usually accompanied by paresthesia.

If the abnormal sensation becomes unpleasant, dysesthesia complicates the symptom picture. Hyperesthesia also may occur, or hyperalgesia and spontaneous pain. When pain occurs in an anesthetic area, the condition is termed *anesthesia dolorosa*. Such pain may follow trauma or surgery involving facial structures. It is also one of the hazards of rhizotomy for the control of facial pain. Anesthesia dolorosa is a chronic intractable pain syndrome that may persist indefinitely.

Phantom Pains

Phantom sensations about the mouth and face may be described by subjects who have lost teeth due to surgery or trauma. These sensations usually comprise a feeling of "presence" of the missing part. It is a deafferentation effect and likely relates to the generation of afferent impulses in the gasserian ganglion. Occasionally, however, the phantom sensation entails pain also. Although such pains may have psychological implications, so-called phantom toothache is no doubt a deafferentation syndrome. It may be intractable and persist indefinitely.

REFERENCES

1. Dalessio D.J.: *Wolff's Headache and Other Head Pain*, ed. 3. New York, Oxford University Press, 1972.
2. Bishop G.H.: Fiber size and myelinization in afferent systems, in Knighton R.S., Dumke P.R. (eds.): *Pain*. Boston, Little, Brown & Co., 1966, pp. 83–89.
3. Kerr F.W.L.: Peripheral versus central factors in trigeminal neuralgia, in Hassler R., Walker A.E. (eds.): *Trigeminal Neuralgia*. Stuttgart, Georg Thieme Verlag, 1970, pp. 180–190.
4. Kerr F.W.L., Miller R.H.: The pathology of trigeminal neuralgia: Electron microscopic studies. *Arch. Neurol.* 15:308, 1966.
5. Kerr F.W.L.: Fine structure and functional characteristics of the primary trigeminal neuron, in Hassler, R., Walker A.E., (eds.): *Trigeminal Neuralgia*. Stuttgart, Georg Thieme Verlag, 1970, pp. 11–21.
6. Sweet W.H.: Trigeminal neuralgia, in Alling C.C., Mahan P.E. (eds.): *Facial Pain*, ed. 2. Philadelphia, Lea & Febiger, 1977, pp. 71–93.
7. Melzack R., Wall P.D.: Pain mechanisms: A new theory. *Science* 150: 971, 1965.
8. Kerr F.W.L.: Evidence for a peripheral etiology of trigeminal neuralgia. *J. Neurosurg.* 26(suppl.):168–174, 1967.
9. Salar G., Mangrino S.: Trigeminal neuralgia and endorphins. *Pain*, suppl. 1, 1981, p. S259.
10. Calvin W.H., Loeser J.D., Howe J.F.: A neurophysiological theory for the pain mechanism of tic douloureux. *Pain* 3:147–154, 1977.
11. Wall P.D., Devor M.: Sensory afferent impulses originate from dorsal root ganglia as well as from the periphery in normal and nerve injured rats. *Pain* 17:321–339, 1983.

12. Finneson B.E.: *Diagnosis and Management of Pain Syndromes*, ed. 2. Philadelphia, W.B. Saunders Co., 1969.
13. Campbell J.B.: Painful phantom limb: Relief through peripheral nerve surgery, in Knighton R.S., Dumke P.R. (eds.): *Pain*. Boston, Little, Brown & Co., 1966, pp. 255–271.
14. Stookey B., Ransohoff J.: *Trigeminal Neuralgia*. Springfield, Ill., Charles C Thomas, Publisher, 1959.
15. Walker A.E.: The differential diagnosis of trigeminal neuralgia, in Hassler R., Walker A.E. (eds.): *Trigeminal Neuralgia*. Stuttgart, Georg Thieme Verlag, 1970, pp. 30–34.
16. McArdle M.J.: Atypical facial neuralgia, in Hassler R., Walker A.E. (eds.): *Trigeminal Neuralgia*. Stuttgart, Georg Thieme Verlag, 1970, pp. 35–42.
17. Hassler R., Walker A.E. (eds.): *Trigeminal Neuralgia*. Stuttgart, Georg Thieme Verlag, 1970.
18. Gardner W.J.: Trigeminal neuralgia, in Hassler R., Walker A.E. (eds.): *Trigeminal Neuralgia*. Stuttgart, Georg Thieme Verlag, 1970, pp. 162–165.
19. Gorlin R.J., Pindborg J.J.: *Syndromes of the Head and Neck*. New York, McGraw-Hill Book Co., 1964.
20. Walker A.E.: Neuralgia of the glossopharyngeal, vagus, and intermedius nerves, in Knighton R.S., Dumke P.R. (eds.): *Pain*. Boston, Little, Brown & Co., 1966, pp. 421–429.
21. Kaemmerer E.F.: A review of the etiologic factors in trigeminal neuralgia, in Hassler R., Walker A.E. (eds.): *Trigeminal Neuralgia*. Stuttgart, Georg Thieme Verlag, 1970, pp. 175–179.
22. Gregg J.M.: Posttraumatic pain: Experimental trigeminal neuropathy. *J. Oral Surg.* 29:260–267, 1971.
23. Wolff H.G., Wolf S.: *Pain*, ed. 2. Springfield, Ill., Charles C Thomas, Publisher, 1958.
24. LaBanc J.P., Epker B.N.: Serious inferior alveolar nerve dysesthesia after endodontic procedure: Report of three cases. *J.A.D.A.* 108:605, 1984.
25. Engle W.W.: Elongated styloid process: Further observations and a new syndrome. *Arch. Otolaryngol.* 47:630, 1948.
26. Mitchell S.W.: *Injuries of Nerves and Their Consequences*. Philadelphia, J.B. Lippincott Co., 1872.
27. Livingston W.K.: Banquet address: Silas Weir Mitchell and his work on causalgia, in Knighton R.S., Dumke P.R. (eds.): *Pain*. Boston, Little, Brown & Co., 1966, pp. 561–572.
28. Bonica J.J.: *The Management of Pain*. Philadelphia, Lea & Febiger, 1953.
29. Bonica J.J.: Management of intractable pain, in Way E.L. (ed.): *New Concepts in Pain*. Philadelpha, F.A. Davis Co., 1967, pp. 155–167.

16

Chronicity and Psychogenic Pains

THE TERM CHRONIC PAIN is presently in common use. Yet its meaning has not been well defined in the literature. It is generally recognized that the behavior as well as treatment response of chronic pain syndromes is different from that of acute pain complaints. The difference, however, seems vague, and the therapeutic implications uncertain. The term *chronic* means "persisting over a long period of time." How long? Is time the only criterion for judgment? Is duration alone the treatment problem that makes special therapy necessary?

Time of course is a factor in chronic pain. But duration alone is not a dependable basis for judgment. Do you set six months, nine months, 12 months as the determinant? There are pain syndromes that persist indefinitely without becoming a treatment problem that differs significantly from the original pain. An example is classic migraine.

Orofacial pain expresses chronicity in two clinically recognizable forms: (1) organic pains that persist due to the continuance of etiologic factors (chronic structural pains), and (2) pains, whether initially organic or not, that lose their etiologic basis but persist despite lack of adequate cause (chronic functional pains). Although these two clinical forms of chronic pain may be closely related, and in some cases form a sort of continuum with one merging into the other in a transitional phase, it is important from the management standpoint that they be differentiated diagnostically. The common denominator is the matter of psychogenesis, so-called psychogenic intensification of pain (Fig 16–1).

CHRONIC STRUCTURAL PAIN

Historically, the profound influence of emotions on suffering has been recognized by all investigators. Some have assigned more importance to it than others. Although the dual concept of pain is still

right fear form the ingredients of pain intensification through reduced central inhibitory influences. These factors are of great importance in chronic pain syndromes, especially those of the deep somatic category. Perhaps an understanding of vascular and deafferentation pain should center around this aspect of the problem. It would not be proper to label such conditions psychogenic pain, but certainly psychogenic intensification is a valid concept of the behavior of such syndromes. Likewise, chronic neuropathic pains and even persistent mucogingival pains are no doubt prolonged and intensified by similarly diminished central inhibitory influence. Thus the emotional sensitivity and reactivity of pain sufferers become inseparable from the total pain experience, and due consideration of these factors is necessary as the dental examiner accepts the task of diagnosis and management of oral and masticatory pains.

Important in the behavior of pain syndromes are the attention directed to the suffering and the *expectancy* of such suffering. The longer a pain lasts, the longer it is expected to last. The more frequently pains occur, the more often they are expected to occur. The more severe pain becomes, the more severe it will be expected to become. These factors help explain the so-called cycling of pain as well as the beneficial effect of interrupting the cycle by analgesic blocking. These and similar mentation effects help explain recurrent and periodic episodes of pain as well as spontaneous remission in neurogenous pain syndromes.

Stressful life situations, emotional tension, anxiety, and neurosis may profoundly influence and magnify pain. Pain in neurotic individuals may become necessary to interpersonal relationships. Hypochondriacal concern may so focus the subject's attention on the body part involved that the level of suffering is markedly intensified. Tension and anxiety may induce spasm of smooth muscle,[4] thus causing a variety of visceral effects. They may also lead to skeletal muscle spasm.[2] Most such induced painful local conditions may be classified as psychosomatic as long as the examiner understands that all symptoms are in fact psychosomatic because of the inseparability of psyche and soma. So perhaps it becomes a matter of degree. As the mechanism of pain is better understood, with all mentation factors and the organic influence they exert taken into consideration, the psychologic factors that seem to have preeminence in some pain syndromes actually become only problems of management.

The examiner should understand the meaning of malingered pain. Dorland[5] defines malingering as "The willful, deliberate, and fraudulent feigning or exaggeration of the symptoms of illness or injury done for the purpose of a consciously desired end." This concept of malingering makes it a sort of "game"[6, 7] and no doubt is commonplace in today's socioeconomic world. So-called compensation pain may be encountered. Head and face pains are popular socially acceptable forms of illness that serve many purposes, especially those of gain, avoidance, and retreat. Whether symptoms are feigned or simply exaggerated is unimportant; the purpose served is important—that of consciously achieving some desired end. In the present-day complexity of interpersonal relationships, the incidence of feigned or exaggerated pain can only be imagined, but it must be significantly great and the reasons numerous indeed. Such factors present serious problems in pain management.

It should be evident that psychogenic intensification is a normal part of pain modulation. It is only when such intensification advances to the point where there no longer exists any significant peripheral noxious input that the condition should be considered and managed as a psychogenic pain.

Duration alone has a positive modulating effect on the pain experience—the longer the complaint lasts, the greater the suffering. This occurs without any increase in the initiating noxious input. Chronicity therefore predisposes to increased suffering. This may be true even though the noxious input decreases with resolution of the initiating cause. As the ratio of lowered input to increased suffering due to duration is maintained, psychogenic intensification may occur. *In the chronic pain syndromes an element of psychogenesis usually must be taken into account.*

Chronicity tends to change the clinical characteristics of a pain syndrome. Nonanatomical and nonphysiologic behavioral characteristics that have come to be associated with psychogenic pain make their appearance. Thus, as different pain syndromes take on characteristics of chronicity, they tend to become more alike, and effective management methods less diverse.

The persistence of pain has a deleterious effect on the sufferer in that it tends to increase his awareness of the complaint and the anxiety it fosters. This in turn modulates the painful experience and causes the suffering to increase. With chronicity, an otherwise relatively minor noxious input may produce a level of suffering that accentuates the patient's attention to his complaint. Indeed, the pain problem may become his chief concern, causing his daily life to center around it. His preoccupation and obsession with pain may become such that little else matters. He may stop at nothing and spare no expense to find relief. Such patients may be driven from doctor to doctor seeking cure; others may become overwhelmed by suffering and retreat into a shell of inactivity and isolation.

It should be understood that anxiety and frustration normally modulate pain in an ever-increasing escalation. It is also known that duration of pain affects the endogenous antinociceptive system. As pain continues, the level of endorphins in the CSF decreases. It has been determined that this effect is greater with chronic structural than with chronic functional pains.[8]

As a natural consequence, chronic structural pain takes on a measure of psychogenic intensification. Depending on circumstances and the type of subject involved much more than on duration alone, structural pain syndromes take on the nature of psychogenesis as time passes. No time limits can be set because the circumstances vary. Thus, one subject may show symptoms of psychogenesis almost immediately while another may show none at all after many months.

Chronicity of somatic and neurogenous pain syndromes normally presents a management problem that must address the psychogenic as well as the organic features of the complaint. Effective treatment often depends on striking the proper balance between local antinociceptive therapy and systemic and psychotherapy. The point is that both are needed to resolve the patient's pain problem.

CHRONIC FUNCTIONAL PAIN

As previously indicated, the longer pain persists, the more severe it becomes. This accentuation of suffering, although part of the normal pain modulation phenomenon, may continue even as the initiating cause diminishes through the natural process of resolution. Thus, pain may continue as a real complaint as the peripheral input decreases. At some point in such psychogenic intensification, suffering may continue in the absence of adequate peripheral input. It is in such circumstances that the pain syndrome takes on the characteristics of functional pain.

Because of the strange effects wrought by the duration of pain, management of the initial cause may no longer have decisive effect. The actual peripheral input may drop to an insignificant level with the result that local therapy offers no benefit. As the condition takes on symptoms of depressive illness, effective management must shift largely to systemic and psychologic methods. Although local treatment may provide some immediate benefit due to placebo effect, in the end little or nothing is accomplished. Furthermore, relapse which is almost inevitable may escalate the suffering to a still higher level. This should be considered seriously when treatment is undertaken.

It should be understood that, as psychogenesis becomes the dominant element in a pain syndrome, there is a change in pain behavior. Although the clinical characteristics of the pain may continue to reflect the original acute pain complaint, the location and therapeutic response change. Thus, the complaint may continue to display features indicative of a somatic or neurogenous pain category. The anatomical behavior, however, is such that the location of pain may no longer bear a proper relationship to the original source of input. It may become multiple or bilateral, or it may shift in location from time to time. Also, the complaint may fail to conform reasonably to what should be expected in the form of therapy. The response to therapy may be too fast, too slow, too great, too little. Or it may relapse or recur without justifiable cause. It may display changeableness without organic justification. These are the identifying clinical characteristics of psychogenic pain. The degree to which such symptoms are displayed indicate the psychogenic content in the patient's complaint.

All chronic functional pain syndromes tend to take on features that make them resemble each other. As chronicity persists, pains about the mouth and face tend to lose their original characteristic features. As such they should be reclassified as *chronic face pains*. Although one should guard against a hasty diagnosis of psychogenesis, failure to recognize such may render therapy, not only useless, but possibly harmful. It is especially important, however, to understand that psychogenic pain does not indicate "neurosis." The pain is real; the suffering is intense. These patients need to be understood, not censured. The neuroticism that so frequently accompanies chronic pain syndromes is thought to be the result of the condition, not the cause of it.[9]

SYMPTOMS OF CHRONICITY

It is important that chronicity be identified as early as possible. Even though of much greater intensity, pains that are truly intermittent or frequently recurrent are less prone to develop into this type of depressive illness. The respite between attacks seems to prevent physical and emotional deterioration. Thus, with idiopathic neuralgia and periodic migraine, chronicity seldom becomes a problem. However, persistence of neuritic pain, reflex sympathetic dystrophy, atypical facial neuralgia, or masticatory pain should lead the examiner to iden-

tify evidence of chronicity as early as possible. Guidelines based on units of time are not dependable because chronicity is extremely variable. Rather, identification of chronicity depends on such factors as the following:
1. Constancy and continuity of peripheral input.
2. Evidence of increased suffering in spite of otherwise effective peripheral therapeutic efforts.
3. Persistence or prompt relapse of symptoms in spite of different methods of therapy used by different doctors.
4. Increasing anxiety on the patient's part.
5. Patient's obsessive concern with his suffering expressed by relief-seeking efforts of all types.
6. Progressive depression and withdrawal behavior.
7. Physical and emotional deterioration.

Some chronic pain syndromes have aptly been described as forms of *depressive* illness. The depressive mood may not be too obvious to patient or doctor because of the overshadowing pain complaint. Therefore, signs of depression should be looked for. There is loss of interest in everything that constitutes normal behavior. There may be insomnia, anorexia, weight loss, decreased libido, apathy, self-neglect, pessimism, and various hypochondriacal obsessions. It is essential in diagnostic evaluation of such complaints that the depressive nature of the illness be recognized because the most common cause of suicide is depression.[4]

The most frequently encountered chronic orofacial pain syndrome concerns the masticatory system. Every dental examiner should be alert to this possibility. As a preventive measure, it is essential that masticatory pains be managed promptly and effectively. This requires accurate identification of the source(s) of pain, likely cause(s), and rational treatment. Persistence of the complaint or prompt relapse after adequate therapy should alert the doctor to recheck the accuracy of his diagnosis and the propriety of the treatment. When true chronicity of masticatory pain is identified, the diagnosis should be revised to *chronic pain syndrome of the face* and the treatment plan modified accordingly.

CHRONIC PAIN BEHAVIOR

In a study of 40,000 patients with orofacial pain,[10] 2% to 5% had no organic disease or had exaggerated response to minimal pathologic conditions. It was noted that depressive illness occurred especially

with glossodynia, glossopyrosis, recalcitrant masticatory pain, and atypical facial pain. In one clinic that treated chronic pain patients of all types,[11] 40% complained of chronic craniofacial and neck pains. In these patients, there was little or no pathosis, or it was not consistent with the degree of discomfort. The characteristics that these patients displayed included the following:
1. A high level of stress expressed as anxiety and depression.
2. A marked tendency toward tolerance, dependence, and addiction, not only to medications, but also to surgery and treatments of all kinds.
3. A marked dependency on family, friends, and doctors.
4. Evidence of loss of self-esteem, impotence, apathy, regressive attitude, and withdrawal behavior.
5. Hostility.

Moulton[12] identified two types of patients with chronic pain: (1) people who were overtly dependent on someone who was either inadequate, overdominant, or unapproachable, and thus became angry and hostile, and (2) unusually competent people who were obsessive and domineering, and therefore became hostile secretly. She warned that local treatment in patients with chronic pain may serve to focus their attention on the area treated with the result that they would continue to seek relief on a purely peripheral level thereafter.

Beck et al[13] associated depression especially with glossodynia, myofascial pain-dysfunction syndromes, and atypical face pains. They listed the symptoms of mild depression as disappointment, lack of self-confidence, and feelings of inadequacy; a desire to be alone and inactive; undue concern for physical appearance; decreased mental and physical alertness; and loss of weight and disturbed sleep. They listed the symptoms of severe and potentially suicidal depression as apathy, self-hate, despondency, immobility, poor posture, decreased muscle tone, insomnia, and fatigue.

Fordyce[14] pointed out that pain behavior, which consists of audible and visible communications that imply suffering, is subject to the influence of conditioning or "learning." Examples of such conditioning are (1) the effect of imitating the behavior of others who suffer (social modeling), (2) the reinforcement of the "reality" of pain by medications prescribed PRN (to be used as needed) as well as by the attention received from others because of suffering, and (3) the indirect reinforcement of pain by avoidance of obligations, commitments, or duties in order to "escape or minimize pain." Pain behavior that is contingent upon expectancy or secondary gain may be reinforced by cues in the environment that suffering may be imminent when actually no noxious stimulation is ever sensed. It may be necessary only to *anticipate* that pain may occur for overt pain behavior to be displayed.

Sternbach[15] has observed that subjective improvement in a patient's pain condition follows behavioral improvement—that pain responses change if the state of mind changes. Thus, since much of the pain behavior (pain reaction) in chronic pain patients is acquired or learned, it can also be eliminated or unlearned. Chronic pain reaction is modifiable through coping strategies.

Roberts[16] focused his efforts to control chronic pain directly on the patient's behavior—not on the source of nociception nor on an attempt to change an alleged emotional state. His objective was to rehabilitate the patient rather than to alleviate the pain. He believed that it is better to teach the patient to live a normal life even though pain may still be present. In chronic pain syndromes, treatment measures that are aimed only to alleviate pain tend to reinforce the "pain concept" that the patient holds.

It should be noted that in patients with chronic pain, the endorphin system does not offer protection of any importance.[17] Although the action of tricyclic antidepressants in normal subjects has no greater effect on pain threshold than placebo,[18] in depressed individuals the analgesic effect parallels the antidepressant action.[19]

In the management of chronic pain syndromes of the face, it is important to identify the presence and extent of the psychogenic element that is embodied in the complaint. When psychogenesis is mild or moderate, the complaint should be classified as a chronic structural pain. Effective management should include therapy directed toward elimination of the peripheral nociceptive input as well as systemic and/or psychotherapy as indicated, the balance between local and systemic treatment depending on the extent of psychogenesis as displayed by the patient's pain behavior. When psychogenesis is clinically predominant, the complaint should be classified as a chronic functional pain. The clinical diagnosis should be revised to *chronic face pain*, and management should differ little from that of other chronic pain syndromes of the neck and back. It should be understood, however, that there is no hard and fast line of demarcation between the two categories of chronic pain. It is a matter of degree—and judgment. The best basis for such judgment is careful consideration of the patient's pain behavior pattern.

CONVERSION HYSTERIA PAINS

Although psychologic trauma can be converted into hallucinatory pain involving any structure of the mouth and face, usually the conversion has symbolic meaning as it relates to function on a regional basis.[4] The functioning of the mouth and jaws for speech and mastication dominates the maxillofacial region. This area has special emotional significance. The mouth is chronologically the first sex organ and never loses its emotional significance in this regard. It relates importantly to body image; to attractiveness to others, especially of the opposite sex; to satisfying interpersonal communications; and to ego-sustenance. It symbolizes pleasure and gratification of all types. It may symbolize life itself. Psychologic traumas that threaten and disturb the subject's deep emotional feelings relative to these facets of his life may become expressed physically as aberrations of the oral and masticatory system. Psychogenic regional pain syndromes involving the maxillofacial region are now recognizable by alert examiners.[20]

This interesting pain problem denotes regional functional pains evoked by psychologic factors and for which there is no evident physical lesion or peripheral cause. The regional distribution of such pains forms the basis for the syndrome. The distinctive physical signs are pain, tenderness, sensory deficits, motor weakness, and reflex and vegetative changes observed throughout a region of emotional significance that overrides purely segmental neurologic innervation. Since masticatory function is regional in character, some afflictions of this functional unit may well come within the scope of this psychogenic pain syndrome. In a review of 430 patients with psychogenic regional pain, the head and heart regions were the most frequent sites of pain.[20]

To classify a pain complaint in this particular category cannot be done by exclusion, but by positive psychiatric evaluation by someone competent in medicine, neurology, and psychiatry with broad sophistication in pain problems. With pains that occur in the maxillofacial area, still greater expertise is required because of the complicated neural arrangements and important psychologic significance peculiar to this region.

In diagnosis, one should exclude other pain mechanisms, establish the features of this syndrome, and elucidate the psychiatric setting (Case No. 16–1).

DELUSIONAL PAINS

Delusional pains of the mouth and face as a manifestation of schizophrenic hallucination are rare in open practice. No doubt they consitute a much greater problem in institutionalized patients. Ordinarily there is no problem with diagnosis owing to the presence of other psychologic symptoms that usually are already under medical or psy-

Oral and Facial Pain
DR. WELDEN E. BELL
8226 DOUGLAS AVENUE
DALLAS, TEXAS

Name: Female age 28

HISTORY

QUALITY	DURATION	LOCALIZATION	AFFECTED BY	LOCAL EFFECTS
(Mild) Severe	Bright (Dull)	(Continuous) Intermittent Recurrent	Localized (Diffuse)	Face Movement Jaw Movement Tongue Movement Swallowing Head Position	Sensory: Hyesthesia Hyperesthesia Paresthesia Dysesthesia	Special Sense: Visual Auditory Olfactory Gustatory
Spontaneous Triggered Induced Paroxysmal (Steady)	Pricking Itching Burning (Aching) Pulsating	Momentary Minutes Hours Day long (Protracted)	Radiating Spreading (Enlarging) Migrating Secondary Pain	Body Position Activities Tension Fatigue (Time of Day)	Motor: Weakness Contraction Spasm	Autonomic: Ocular Signs Nasal Signs Cutaneous Signs Gastric Signs

Location
Inception
Initial pain
Duration, clinical course
Therapeutic response
Physical and emotional background
Trauma, infection, etc.
Medications in use

Protracted continuous mild steady dull aching pain diffusely located in and about the temporomandibular joints and teeth bilaterally. It is described as an itchy uncomfortable sensation punctuated occasionally by lancinating pains through the face. These pains do not seem to relate to masticatory function. Discomfort is worse in early mornings and is accompanied by a "bad taste" in the mouth.
  It began some 9-10 months ago following her third marriage and at first seemed to involve only the teeth. She wanted them removed but her dentist found no valid reason. Then it spread to involve the entire masticatory system including the teeth, joints, muscles, lips, tongue, and floor of mouth bilaterally. She has been diagnosed by her regular dentist as a pain-dysfunction syndrome and referred for confirmation and therapy.
  Due to the vagueness of the complaint, a psychologic survey was done, revealing an emotional overlay that needed further exploration.

B/P 120/90   Neurological Survey   Psychological Survey

EXAMINATION

Oral
TM joints
Muscle system
Diagnostic blocks
Diagnostic drugs
Trial therapy

Clinical and radiographic examination of the teeth, mouth, and temporomandibular joints was entirely negative for cause of pain. No masticatory dysfunction.

Further psychological investigation revealed a traumatic childhood and a sexually traumatic first marriage which ended in divorce. A second marriage was short-lived. She then isolated herself from male companions for some time. A third marriage eleven months ago seems to have reactivated her old frigidity due she thinks to an aggressive husband. She seeks ways to avoid sexual relations with him. The face pain problem is thought to be delusional and represents a psychogenic regional pain syndrome.

DIAGNOSIS

Psychogenic regional pain syndrome mistaken for a masticatory pain-dysfunction syndrome.

Case No. 16–1.—Psychogenic pain, expressed as conversion hysteria, mistaken for structural masticatory pain.

chiatric management. Psychiatric confirmation is required for this diagnosis.

Pains due to psychologic trauma and those that are symptomatic of psychiatric illness require confirmation on a psychiatric level. Management of all such pain syndromes should be under competent psychiatric supervision. Local treatment, if any, should be directed by the chief therapist, with maximum avoidance of extensive forms of local therapy.

REFERENCES

1. Finneson B.E.: *Diagnosis and Management of Pain Syndromes*, ed. 2. Philadelphia, W.B. Saunders Co., 1969.
2. Moulton R.E.: Emotional factors in nonorganic temporomandibular joint pain, in Schwartz L., Chayes C.M. (eds.): *Facial Pain and Mandibular Dysfunction*. Philadelphia, W.B. Saunders Co., 1968, pp. 318–334.
3. Melzack R., Wall P.D.: Pain mechanisms: A new theory. *Science* 150:971, 1965.
4. Pilling L.F.: Psychosomatic aspects of facial pain, in Alling C.C., Mahan P.E. (eds.): *Facial Pain*, ed. 2. Philadelphia, Lea & Febiger, 1977, pp. 213–226.
5. *Dorland's Illustrated Medical Dictionary*, ed. 26. Philadelphia, W.B. Saunders Co., 1981.
6. Berne E.: *Games People Play*. New York, Grove Press, 1964.
7. Sternbach R.A.: Varieties of pain games, in Bonica J.J. (ed.): *Advances in Neurology*. New York, Raven Press, 1974, vol. 4, pp. 423–430.
8. Almay B.G.L., Johansson F., Von Knorring L., et al.: Endorphins in chronic pain: I. Difference in CSF endorphin levels between organic and psychogenic pain syndromes. *Pain* 5:153–162, 1978.
9. Sternbach R.A., Timmermans G.: Personality changes associated with reduction of pain. *Pain* 1:177–181, 1975.
10. Gerschman J., Burrows G., Reade P.: Chronic orofacial pain, in Bonica J.J., Liebeskind J.C., Albe-Fessard D.G. (eds.): *Advances in Pain Research and Therapy*. New York, Raven Press, 1979, vol. 3, pp. 317–323.
11. Donaldson D., Kroening R.: Recognition and treatment of patients with chronic orofacial pain. *J.A.D.A.* 99:961–966, 1979.
12. Moulton R.E.: Psychiatric considerations in maxillofacial pain. *J.A.D.A.* 51:408, 1955.
13. Beck F.M., Kaul T.J., Weaver J.M. II: Recognition and management of the depressed dental patient. *J.A.D.A.* 99:967–971, 1979.
14. Fordyce W.E.: Behavior conditioning concepts in chronic pain, in Bonica J.J., Lindblom U., Iggo A. (eds.): *Advances in Pain Research and Therapy*. New York, Raven Press, 1983, vol. 5, pp. 781–788.
15. Sternbach R.A.: Fundamentals of psychological methods in chronic pain, in Bonica J.J., Lindblom U., Iggo A. (eds.): *Advances in Pain Research and Therapy*. New York, Raven Press, 1983, vol. 5, pp. 777–780.
16. Roberts A.H.: Contingency management methods in the treatment of chronic pain, in Bonica J.J., Lindblom U., Iggo A. (eds.): *Advances in Pain Research and Therapy*. New York, Raven Press, 1983, vol. 5, pp. 789–794.
17. Lindblom U., Tegner R.: Are the endorphins active in chronic pain states? Narcotic antagonism in chronic pain patients. *Pain* 7:65–68, 1979.
18. Chapman C.R., Butler S.H.: Effects of doxepin on perception of laboratory-induced pain in man. *Pain* 5:253–262, 1978.

19. Ward N.G., Bloom V.L., Friedel R.O.: The effectiveness of tricyclic antidepressants in the treatment of coexisting pain and depression. *Pain* 7:331–341, 1979.
20. Walters A.: The psychogenic regional pain syndrome and its diagnosis, in Knighton R.S., Dumke P.R. (eds.): *Pain*. Boston, Little, Brown & Co., 1966, pp. 439–456.

17

Examination and Diagnosis

THE OVERALL OBJECTIVE OF DIAGNOSIS is to identify accurately the patient's complaint as to what is wrong, where, and why. Pain diagnosis presents difficult problems: Our understanding of pain mechanisms is rudimentary at best; pain is a dynamic, changing experience that embraces sensation, emotion, and reaction; nociception is predominantly subjective in nature; objective pain behavior reflects consequences as much as cause; complex pain modulation phenomena individualize every painful experience. The diagnosis and management of an obscure pain problem can be a sobering—and sometimes a humbling—experience for the doctor, erudite as he may be.

One difficulty is that most of us are "cause oriented." The "why" in diagnosis, important as it is, may become a stumbling block when dealing with obscure pain, for there may be no *cause* at all. If the condition seems related to an actual stimulus of some kind, then identification of the cause is essential to proper management. But pain without cause should not be considered unusual. In fact, the majority of human pains lack any identifiable cause.

Another difficulty that we should be alert to is the temptation to assume that the symptoms of which the patient complains represent the real problem that needs to be investigated and managed. Pain behavior consists of audible and visible signals exhibited by the patient that indicate his suffering. These signals have filtered down through a chain of modulating influences, not the least of which are the consequences that attend the whole experience. Thus, the complaint as manifested by suffering may bear little relevance to the real underlying problem. Yet it is the suffering itself that the patient presents for treatment. A Solomon is often needed to direct the management of such conditions.

Diagnosing a pain complaint consists essentially of three major steps:
1. An accurate identification of the location of the structure from which the pain emanates. The location of pain source (in contrast to pain site) is the chief objective of the clinical examination.

2. Determination of the correct pain category that is represented in the condition under investigation. This is a matter of recognizing the clinical characteristics that are displayed. Establishing the proper pain category is dependent upon a good understanding of the genesis and mechanisms of pain.
3. Choosing the particular pain syndrome that correctly accounts for the incidence and behavior of the patient's pain problem. This requires familiarity with the clinical symptoms displayed by pain syndromes that occur in the orofacial region.

PRELIMINARY INTERVIEW

The initial contact with the patient and his problem is important. Unless satisfactory professional rapport can be immediately established, it may be wise to refer the patient before becoming further involved. It is essential that patient and doctor communicate on an "adult-adult" level in order to avoid the "playing of games" by either party.

The rapport on which such communication must rest requires sincere effort by both patient and doctor. The patient must be willing to honestly and accurately divulge the information the doctor needs. He must do so cooperatively and with sincere desire to obtain relief from his complaint. If his intentions and objectives are anything less than this, not only will valuable time and effort be wasted, but the chances are that more harm than good will result.

The doctor must feel confident of his own competence in pain problem identification and management. Any lack of confidence will quickly be sensed by the patient and can destroy the chances of a satisfactory patient-doctor relationship. Moreover, it would be professionally dishonest for a doctor to pursue any course of action for which he felt unprepared. Competence, honesty, patience, and an earnest desire by the therapist to serve his patient are the minimal prerequisites for establishing satisfactory professional rapport.

At the preliminary interview, sufficient data should be collected to help determine the future course of the examining procedure. Some overall idea of the location, inception, duration, and clinical behavior of the complaint should be obtained and plans laid for continuing the examination, for referral to another doctor, or for planning consultation, as the case may require. Very simple pain problems such as mucogingival pain of local origin, localized pain due to obvious dental cause, and some cases of typical tic douloureux may be solved without further examination. More obscure pain complaints justify a carefully planned diagnostic procedure.

CHARTING THE EXAMINATION

An efficient examination chart helps the doctor obtain essential data with the least expenditure of time and effort. Making sure that such data are complete is an important step in the identification of pain.

An examination chart should be simple and flexible so as to be readily adaptable to the many different pain problems that may present themselves. A questionnaire type of form has not proved as useful as one that serves only to remind the examiner what data should be obtained.[1,2] The form illustrated (Fig 17–1) is of this type.

The first section gives the examiner a means of selecting applicable terms relative to the descriptive behavior of the pain complaint. When used in this way, the pain category into which the complaint falls becomes more obvious to the examiner. Inconsistencies become evident at the earliest possible moment, and the examiner is alerted to the need for extremely careful interviewing in order to obtain dependable information from the patient. There exists for each of the different categories of pain a rather consistent general relationship of the qualities of painful sensation, its temporal behavior, localization, effects created by functional influences, and symptomatic evidence of concomitant local effects, as indicated by other sensory, motor, special sense, and autonomic signs. For example, a typical narrative description of tic douloureux involving the right mandibular division of the trigeminal nerve would be as follows:

> Severe pains in right mandibular dental and alveolar process area occurring both spontaneously and triggered by light touch and movement of lower lip. The complaint is described as recurrent episodes of bright burning pain that occur intermittently in repeated paroxysms lasting a few seconds each time and felt in the same precise anatomical location with little or no variation from time to time. No secondary pains are noticed. The paroxysms are excited by all functional activities that cause minor stimulation of the lower lip. The pains are accompanied by contraction of facial muscles, but no other concomitant neurologic effects are seen.

Utilizing the chart, this description would appear as seen in Fig 17–2.

The remainder of the history section of the chart serves to remind the examiner to record the present location of the pain complaint, the

	QUALITY		DURATION		LOCALIZATION	AFFECTED BY	LOCAL EFFECTS	
	Mild	Bright	Continuous		Localized		Sensory:	Special Sense:
	Severe	Dull	Intermittent		Diffuse	Face Movement	Hypesthesia	Visual
			Recurrent			Jaw Movement	Hyperesthesia	Auditory
					Radiating	Tongue Movement	Paresthesia	Olfactory
	Spontaneous				Spreading	Swallowing	Dysesthesia	Gustatory
	Triggered	Pricking	Momentary			Head Position		
	Induced	Itching	Minutes		Enlarging	Body Position		Autonomic:
		Burning	Hours		Migrating	Activities	Motor:	Ocular Signs
	Paroxysmal	Aching	Day long			Tension	Weakness	Nasal Signs
	Steady	Pulsating	Protracted		Secondary Pain	Fatigue	Contraction	Cutaneous Signs
						Time of Day	Spasm	Gastric Signs

HISTORY

Location

Inception
Initial pain

Duration, clinical course

Therapeutic response

Physical and emotional
  background

Trauma, infection, etc.

Medications in use

B/P   Neurological Survey   Psychological Survey

EXAMINATION

Oral

TM joints

Muscle
  system

Diagnostic
  blocks

Diagnostic
  drugs

Trial
  therapy

DIAGNOSIS

Oral and Facial Pain
DR. WELDEN E. BELL
8226 DOUGLAS AVENUE
DALLAS, TEXAS

Fig 17–1.—Illustration of simple but versatile examination form used by the author for charting examinations for orofacial pains.

time it began, and a detailed description of the pain as initially felt. An evaluation of the early characteristics of the complaint may give valuable clues to its identification prior to modification. Information concerning the duration and clinical course of the complaint with special reference to efforts at treatment is valuable. The general phys-

QUALITY		DURATION	LOCALIZATION	AFFECTED BY	LOCAL EFFECTS	
Mild	(Bright)	Continuous	(Localized)	(Face Movement)	Sensory:	Special Sense:
(Severe)	Dull	(Intermittent)	Diffuse	(Jaw Movement)	Hypesthesia	Visual
		(Recurrent)		Tongue Movement	Hyperesthesia	Auditory
			Radiating	Swallowing	Paresthesia	Olfactory
(Spontaneous)			Spreading	Head Position	(Dysesthesia)	(Gustatory)
(Triggered)	Pricking	(Momentary)		Body Position		Autonomic:
Induced	Itching	Minutes	Enlarging	Activities	Motor:	Ocular Signs
	(Burning)	Hours	Migrating	Tension	Weakness	Nasal Signs
(Paroxysmal)	Aching	Day long		Fatigue	(Contraction)	Cutaneous Signs
(Steady)	Pulsating	Protracted	Secondary Pain	Time of Day	Spasm	Gastric Signs

Fig 17–2.—Illustration of a typical case of idiopathic trigeminal neuralgia (tic douloureux) as it would appear on the examination chart.

ical and emotional background for the complaint should be noted as well as the historical implications of such conditions as trauma, infections, and systemic illness. Certainly all medications currently in use should be listed.

The examination section of the chart provides a place to summarize essential and applicable data gathered by clinical, radiographic, and laboratory procedures relative to the oral cavity, masticatory system, and regional musculature. Special information derived from diagnostic analgesic blocking, the effect of diagnostic drugs, and trial therapy should be recorded.

HISTORY

There is no examination in which accurate history-taking is more important than that for identifying obscure pain. The innate subjectivity of pain makes this so. Without an accurate understanding of the inception and early clinical characteristics of the pain and its clinical course, which reflects modulation, reference, and spreading as well as its temporal and spatial behavior throughout its entire duration, the objective data obtained from clinical examination may largely be meaningless. It is by history-taking that the subjective elements of a pain syndrome can be identified. Much thought should be given to this undertaking, and skillful interviewing is prerequisite to success.

Description of Patient's Complaint

A good starting point in history-taking is to obtain an accurate description of the complaint. This should first be taken in the patient's own words and then restated in technical language as indicated. To obtain a good account of the pain problem, the interview should be guided by the doctor since few patients could know what descriptive information he really needs.

A description of the pain complaint should take into account details concerning the following:

1. Anatomical description of where pain is felt
2. Intensity of pain
3. Mode of onset
4. Manner of flow of pain
5. Quality of pain
6. Temporal behavior
7. Duration of individual pains
8. Localization behavior
9. Effect of functional activities
10. Concomitant neurologic symptoms

The *intensity of pain* should be established by differentiating between mild and severe pain. This can be based on how the patient appears to react to his suffering—*mild* pain being what the patient describes but to which he displays no visible physical reactions, and *severe* pain being what causes muscular and autonomic effects that are objectively evident to the examiner.

The *mode of onset* of individual pains is important. The onset may be wholly *spontaneous*. It may be *induced* by certain activities such as yawning, chewing, drinking hot or cold liquids, or bending over. It may be *triggered* by minor superficial stimulation such as touch or movement of the skin, lips, face, tongue, or throat. When triggered by such activities, it is well to distinguish between stimulation of overlying tissues that are only incidentally stimulated and the result of functioning of the joints and muscles themselves. The former is true triggering; the latter is pain induction. This distinction usually can be made by stabilizing the joints and muscles with a bite-block to prevent their movement while the other structures are stimulated or moved. If uncertainty exists, the distinction can be made more positively by utilizing local anesthesia. Topical anesthesia of the throat effectively arrests triggering in the glossopharyngeal nerve distribution. Mandibular block anesthesia stops triggering from the lower lip and tongue. Infraorbital anesthesia arrests triggering from the upper lip and maxillary skin. None of these procedures prevents the induction of true masticatory pain.

The *manner of flow* yields important information by determining whether the individual pains are *steady* or *paroxysmal*. A flowing type of pain, even though variable in intensity or distinctly intermittent, is described as steady. Such pain is to be distinguished from paroxysmal pain, which characteristically consists of sudden volleys of jabs. The volleys may vary considerably in both intensity and duration. When they occur frequently, the pain may become nearly continuous.

The *quality of pain* should be classified according to how it makes the patient feel. This classification is usually termed bright or dull. When pain has a stimulating or exciting effect on the patient, it is classified as *bright*. When the pain has a depressing effect, causing the patient to withdraw to some extent, it is classified as *dull*. It is important that such judgment be wholly independent of pain intensity and variability, its temporal characteristics, or any accompanying lancinating exacerbations that may punctuate the basic underlying painful sensation.

Further evaluation of the quality of pain that constitutes the patient's complaint should be made to classify it as pricking, itching, stinging, burning, aching, or pulsating. Many pains of course require more than a single designation. Bright, tingling pain is classified as a *pricking* sensation, especially when mild and stimulating. Superficial discomfort that does not reach pain threshold intensity may be described as *itching*. As intensity increases, it may take on a pricking, stinging, aching, or burning quality. Deep discomfort that does not reach pain threshold intensity may be described as a vague, diffuse sensation of pressure, warmth, or tenderness. As intensity increases, it may take on a sore, aching, throbbing, or burning quality. When the discomfort has an irritating, hot, raw, caustic quality, it is usually described as *burning*. Most pains have an *aching* quality. Some noticeably increase with each heart beat and are described as *pulsating* or throbbing.

The *temporal behavior* of the pain complaint should be evaluated. If the suffering distinctly comes and goes, leaving pain-free intervals of noticeable duration, it is classified as *intermittent*. If such pain-free intervals do not occur, it is classified as *continuous*. Intermittency should not be confused with variability, in which there may be alternate periods of high and low level discomfort. Intermittent pain implies the occurrence of true intermissions or pain-free periods during which comfort is complete. This temporal behavior should not be confused with the effect of medications that induce periods of comfort by analgesic action.

When episodes of pain, whether continuous or intermittent, are separated by an extended period of freedom from discomfort, only to be followed by another similar episode of pain, the syndrome is said to be *recurrent*. The duration of individual pains in an episode is an important descriptive feature that aids in pain identification. A pain is said to be *momentary* if its duration can be expressed in seconds.

Longer-lasting pains are classified in minutes, hours, or a day. A pain that continues from one day to the next is said to be *protracted*.

The *localization behavior* of the pain should be included in its description. If the patient is able to define the pain to an exact anatomical location, it is classified as *localized* pain. If such description is less well defined and somewhat vague and variable anatomically, it is termed *diffuse* pain. Rapidly changing pain is classified as *radiating*. A momentary cutting exacerbation is usually described as *lancinating*. More gradually changing pain is described as *spreading*, and, if it progressively involves adjacent anatomical areas, the pain is called *enlarging*. If it changes from one location to another, the complaint is described as *migrating*. Referred pain and secondary hyperalgesia are clinical expressions of *secondary pain*.

The *effect of functional activities* should be observed and described. Common biomechanical functions include such activities as movement of the face, jaw, or tongue and the effect of swallowing, head position, and body position. The effect of such activities as talking, chewing, yawning, brushing the teeth, shaving, washing the face, turning the head, stooping over, or lying down should be noted. The effect of tension, fatigue, and time of day also should be recorded.

All *concomitant neurologic symptoms* such as sensory, motor, or autonomic effects that accompany the pain should be included. Sensations such as hyperesthesia, hypoesthesia, anesthesia, paresthesia, or dysesthesia should be mentioned. Any concomitant change in the *special senses* affecting vision, hearing, smell, or taste should be noted. *Motor* changes expressed as muscular weakness, muscular contractions, or actual spasm should be recognized. Various localized *autonomic* symptoms should be observed and described. Ocular symptoms may include lacrimation, injection of the conjunctiva, pupillary changes, and edema of the lids. Nasal symptoms include nasal secretion and congestion. Cutaneous symptoms have to do with skin temperature, color, sweating, and piloerection. Gastric symptoms include nausea and indigestion.

Chronological History

After the descriptive behavior of the patient's current pain complaint is completed, a more general review of the past behavior of the entire pain problem should be obtained. Special attention should be given to the initial pain as to time of inception, location, and early behavioral characteristics, since these data more accurately reflect the true nature of the pain before appreciable modulation or central excitatory effects have altered it.

A chronological account of the complaint should then be obtained to accurately reflect its complete clinical course from the beginning to the present. Examinations and therapeutic attempts by other practitioners should be noted, with a recording, if possible, of the diagnosis and effectiveness of therapy. Any related physical illness, emotional situations, injuries, surgical operations, or infections should be recorded. All medications currently in use should be identified and their effectiveness noted.

McGILL PAIN QUESTIONNAIRE

To evaluate the patient's pain in terms of what it means to him, it is necessary to obtain specific and meaningful descriptors from the patient that accurately describe his complaint. Many patients may not have at their disposal an adequate means of communicating such exact information. In his McGill Pain Questionnaire, Melzack[3] has arranged descriptive adjectives in several groups. Each series of words is arranged in an order of increasing intensity. The patient is instructed to select *one word* in each series, the word that best describes the complaint. If none in a series is truly applicable, none should be selected.

The first group is composed of *sensory* descriptors that help describe what the discomfort feels like to the patient:
1. *Temporal:* flicking, quivering, pulsing, throbbing, beating, pounding.
2. *Spatial:* jumping, flashing, shooting.
3. *Punctate pressure:* pricking, boring, drilling, stabbing, lancinating.
4. *Incisive pressure:* sharp, cutting, lacerating.
5. *Constrictive pressure:* pinching, pressing, gnawing, cramping, crushing.
6. *Traction pressure:* tugging, pulling, wrenching.
7. *Thermal:* hot, burning, scalding, searing.
8. *Brightness:* tingling, itchy, smarting, stinging.
9. *Dullness:* dull, sore, hurting, aching, heavy.
10. *Miscellaneous:* tender, taut, rasping, splitting.

The second group consists of *affective* descriptors that yield information about how the patient is reacting to the pain:
1. *Tension:* tiring, exhausting.
2. *Autonomic:* sickening, suffocating.
3. *Fear:* fearful, frightful, terrifying.
4. *Punishment:* punishing, gruelling, cruel, viscious, killing.
5. *Miscellaneous:* wretched, blinding.

The third group is a series of *evaluative* descriptors that tend to classify the intensity of pain:
　1. Annoying, troublesome, miserable, intense, unbearable.

A fourth group of general descriptors has been added to the questionnaire:
　1. Spreading, radiating, penetrating, piercing.
　2. Tight, numb, drawing, squeezing, tearing.
　3. Cool, cold, freezing.
　4. Nagging, nauseating, agonizing, dreadful, torturing.

Patients who cannot verbalize the description of their complaint may find use for these descriptors. The questionnaire is designed to be scored and used for statistical and research purposes. So used, it serves to estimate intensity levels more precisely and gives a better means of judging effectiveness of therapy.

TENTATIVE CLINICAL DIAGNOSIS

When a complete history has been taken, an examiner knowledgeable in the mechanisms of pain should be able to classify the complaint in its proper general category and to arrive at a reasonably accurate tentative diagnosis on which to base the next step in his procedure—whether to immediately refer the patient to another doctor or pursue the clinical examination himself. At the very least, the examiner at this point should be able to narrow the various diagnostic possibilities to two or three that require differentiation.

If confusing neurologic signs are present, a cursory neurologic survey would be indicated at this point to determine if immediate reference to a neurologist is in order. If definite lack of anatomical and physiologic consistency is evident, a psychologic survey might be indicated to determine if immediate reference for further psychologic evaluation is needed.

NEUROLOGIC SURVEY

When some neurologic abnormality in the maxillofacial region is recognized, it is the examining dentist's right and duty to make a cursory survey of cranial and upper cervical spinal nerve function. The purpose of this survey is to determine with certainty if referral to a neurologist is essential and justified. When one or more of the following conditions are observed, immediate neurologic consultation is indicated:

1. Areas of facial hypoesthesia
2. Loss of normal corneal reflex
3. Persistent muscular weakness or paralysis
4. Simultaneous involvement of otherwise unrelated nerve trunks

CHECKING SENSORY FUNCTION.—Sensory elements of the trigeminal (fifth cranial), glossopharyngeal (ninth cranial), and upper cervical spinal nerves can readily be tested by pin prick, light touch, and palpation of the cutaneous and mucosal structures innervated by peripheral sensory branches of these respective nerve trunks. Dental sensory response can be checked by an electric pulp tester. It is obvious that accuracy depends on the examiner's knowledge of the neuroanatomy of the maxillofacial region (Fig 17–3).

CHECKING SPECIAL SENSES.—The olfactory (first cranial) nerve is tested by the patient's ability to perceive different odors. Oil of orange can be used for this purpose. The optic (second cranial) nerve is tested by checking the acuity and range of vision. The stato-acoustic (eighth cranial) nerve is tested for sense of hearing by means of watch tick and for equilibrium by standing with the eyes closed. The gustatory function of the facial (seventh cranial) and the glossopharyngeal (ninth cranial) nerves is tested by checking the patient's ability to discern well-known taste sensations such as sweet, salty, or acrid flavors. Honey, saline, or bitters can be used for this purpose.

CHECKING MOTOR FUNCTION.—Motor function of the oculomotor (third cranial), trochlear (fourth cranial), and abducent (sixth cranial) nerves is tested by checking the voluntary ocular movements—upward, downward, to the right, to the left—as well as binocularity. The motor elements of the trigeminal (fifth cranial) nerve are tested by checking the movements of the mandible—opening, closing, protrusion, right lateral excursion, left lateral excursion. The facial (seventh cranial) nerve motor function is tested by face movements—wrinkling the forehead, lifting the eyebrows, winking, puckering the lips, smiling. The throat motor functioning of the glossopharyngeal (ninth cranial), vagus (tenth cranial), and accessory (11th cranial) nerves is tested by swallowing and speech. The neck motor elements of the accessory (11th cranial) and upper cervical spinal nerves are tested by checking the voluntary head movements. The functioning of the hypoglossal (12th cranial) nerve is tested by observing tongue movements—protruding the tongue, lifting the tip, depressing the tip, turning it to the right, and turning it to the left.

Neurological Survey
Mouth and Face

DR. WELDEN E. BELL
MEDICAL ARTS BUILDING
DALLAS, TEXAS

Name Age Date

SENSORY:		Right	Left	Nerve
Hyperalgesia (A+), Hypalgesia (A-), Hyperesthesia (E+), Hypoesthesia (E-)	Corneal Reflex Forehead Upper Lid Nose			5th N. Ophthalmic Div.
	Lateral Orbit Lower Lid Zygomatic Maxilla Upper Lip			5th N. Maxillary Div.
	Temple Tragus Cheek Lower Lip Chin			5th N. Mandibular Div.
Paresthesia (P), Dysesthesia (D), Reflex Absent (R)	Occipital Post-auricular Parotid Mand. Angle Neck			2nd and 3rd Cervical Nerves
	Lip Mucosa Cheek Mucosa Gingiva Hard Palate			5th N.
	Fauces Pharyngeal Reflex Palatal Reflex			9th N.
	Deep Sensation of Face			7th N.

MOTOR:	Right	Left	Nerve
Pupils Centered Ocular Movements			3rd, 4th, 6th N.
Wrinkle Forehead Wink Smile Pucker			7th N.
Mandibular Movements			5th N.
Tongue Movements			12th N.
Swallowing Speech			9th, 10th, 11th N.

SPECIAL SENSE:	Right	Left	Nerve
Odor Perception			1st N.
Visual Range			2nd N.
Taste (Ant. 2/3)			7th N.
Taste (Post. 1/3)			9th N.
Hearing Distance			8th N.

AUTONOMICS:	Right	Left	Nerve
Pupillary Accommodation			3rd N.
Lacrimation Saliva (sub-max.-sub-ling)			7th N.
Saliva (Parotid)			9th N.
Carotid Sinus Reflex			10th N.
Horner's Syndrome			Cerv. Sympath.

TEETH (Pulpal Sensation):

UR 1	2	3	4	5	6	7	8
UL 1	2	3	4	5	6	7	8
LR 1	2	3	4	5	6	7	8
LL 1	2	3	4	5	6	7	8

EVALUATION:

Fig 17–3.—Illustration of a neurologic survey form used by the author for checking nerve function in the maxillofacial area.

CHECKING AUTONOMIC FUNCTION.—The parasympathetic functioning of the oculomotor (third cranial) nerve is checked by testing pupillary accommodation to light. That of the facial (seventh cranial) and glossopharyngeal (ninth cranial) nerves is by checking lacrimation and salivation. The parasympathetic functioning of the vagus (tenth cranial) nerve is checked by testing the carotid sinus reflex by which the heart rate is reduced in response to pressure on the internal carotid artery at the level of the cricoid cartilage. A deficit in cranial sympathetic functioning is recognized by the presence of Horner's syndrome, which presents narrowing of the palpebral fissure with ptosis of the upper lid and elevation of the lower lid, constriction of the pupil, and facial anhidrosis.

CHECKING SUPERFICIAL REFLEXES.—The corneal reflex consists of closure of the eyelids in response to irritation of the cornea by touching with a sterile cotton applicator. It involves afferent impulses transmitted by the trigeminal (fifth cranial) nerve and efferent motor impulses via the facial (seventh cranial) nerve. The palatal reflex is involuntary swallowing in response to stimulation of the soft palate. It involves afferent impulses transmitted by the trigeminal (fifth cranial) and glossopharyngeal (ninth cranial) nerves and efferent motor impulses via the glossopharyngeal (ninth cranial) and vagus (tenth cranial) nerves. The pharyngeal or gag reflex is contraction of the constrictor muscle of the pharynx elicited by touching the posterior wall of the pharynx. It involves afferent impulses transmitted by the glossopharyngeal (ninth cranial) nerve and efferent motor impulses via the glossopharyngeal (ninth cranial) and vagus (tenth cranial) nerves.

Only a few minutes are required to make such a neurologic survey, and frequently the information gained is essential to proper management of the patient who presents a pain complaint.

PSYCHOLOGIC SURVEY

When the symptom complex is inconsistent anatomically and physiologically, the question of psychogenic pain may arise and the advisability of referral of the patient for psychologic evaluation should be considered. To help arrive at the proper decision, simple psychologic testing may be done by the dentist.

One such test is to evaluate how the patient responds to an attempt to induce pain purely by suggestion. This may be done by pressing firmly on the painful site and strongly suggesting to the patient that he will feel the pain simultaneously in the corresponding site on the opposite normal side. If he does in fact complain of similar pain on the opposite side, the emotional overlay is probably great. Or the reverse may be tried. This consists of attempting to relieve the pain purely by suggestion. The examiner presses firmly at the corresponding site on the opposite normal side and strongly suggests that by doing so the patient will sense relief of pain at the site in question. If the pain is thus substantially relieved by this maneuver, the psychogenic component presumably is high.

Another testing device is trial placebo therapy, even though this method has not been looked upon with favor by some investigators.[4] It is to be remembered that normal placebo effect may account for up to 40% of the effectiveness of any form of treatment, especially in tense individuals.[5] Therefore, to evaluate placebo therapy, the results up to this percentage must be discounted. Testing this therapy can be done by prescribing a definite plan of treatment utilizing only placebo medications and suggesting to the patient that definite benefit will occur at a specified time. If such benefit occurs according to the specified time schedule and the benefit is substantially greater than 40%, it may be presumed that the purely psychologic element is important.

Patients who appear to need further evaluation on a psychologic level should first be cleared medically or neurologically. *Verbalizing a tentative diagnosis of psychogenic pain to the patient should be avoided by the dentist since he usually is not competent to make this judgment.* It is not an easy one to make even for a pain-knowledgeable psychiatrist.

PAIN EXAMINATION

The clinical examination should be preceded by a general evaluation of the patient's physical condition to determine if a medical consultation is needed. This may be facilitated by using a screening medical history questionnaire routinely filled out by the patient when he registers for examination. Since such a form is intended only to help the examiner decide if medical data can be useful in arriving at a correct diagnosis and is not intended as a medical examination in itself, it may be short and simple. The form illustrated in Fig 17–4 has proved quite satisfactory for this purpose.

The patient's blood pressure should be recorded routinely. Temperature, pulse rate and respiratory rate should be checked if illness is suspected.

The indications for a medical consultation are as follows:
1. Obvious illness, as indicated by the patient's appearance and behavior and by the medical history questionnaire.
2. The presence of obscure illness, as indicated by the medical history questionnaire.
3. Evidence obtained during the history-taking interview that the pain complaint may relate to physical or emotional illness.
4. Evidence obtained during the clinical examination that systemic factors may be present and need investigating.
5. Determination that the pain syndrome does not stem from dental, oral, or masticatory causes.
6. Indication that the pain syndrome coexists with or is aggravated by some systemic condition that should be approached on a medical level.

Examination of the Teeth and Mouth

No doubt pains about the mouth and face stem frequently from local dental causes, and thorough examination of the teeth is an indispens-

MEDICAL HISTORY QUESTIONNAIRE:	Name_____ Date_____
Are you under the care of a doctor?_____	Do you have: High blood pressure?_____
If so, his name:_____	Prolonged bleeding?_____
For what is he treating you?_____	Arm, chest, or neck pain with exercise?_____
What medicines do you take?_____	Heart trouble?_____
Do you take a "blood thinner"?_____	Diabetes?_____
Are you allergic to any drug?_____	Rheumatic fever?_____
Have you ever taken cortisone?_____	Arthritis?_____
	Kidney trouble?_____
	Anemia?_____

Fig 17-4.—Simple form used for medical screening.

able first step. Odontogenous pains have the propensity to simulate many other pain syndromes, and very careful examination is needed to arrive at a correct differential diagnosis.

The teeth, especially on the side in question, should be examined individually to yield the following data:

1. Sensitivity or tenderness without provocation.
2. Sensitivity or tenderness due to occlusal function.
3. Sensitivity to touch, percussion, or probing with a dental explorer.
4. Tenderness from pressure directed down the long axis of the tooth.
5. Tenderness from pressure exerted laterally on the tooth.
6. Response to thermal shock. Warmth may be applied via a heated instrument. Chilling may be done by applying ethyl chloride on a cotton applicator. The tooth should be isolated with celluloid strips, especially when adjacent metallic fillings are present or when covered with an artificial dental crown.
7. Response to electric pulp tester. Each tooth should be isolated with celluloid strips, especially when adjacent metallic fillings are present. Care should be taken to differentiate between pulpal and gingival responses.[6]
8. Radiographic evidence of pathologic change.
9. Evidence of occlusal disharmony.
10. Evidence to justify direct exploration of the tooth.

The gingiva and entire oral mucosa should be tested by touch, pin prick, and manual palpation to identify areas of abnormal sensibility. Manual palpation of the face, lips, cheeks, tongue, palate, throat, sublingual areas, and submandibular areas, as well as the auricular, preauricular, infra-auricular, postauricular, and cervical areas, should be done to identify pain triggers, painful areas, local tenderness, swelling, induration, fluctuation, or other abnormality. Visual inspection of the superficial skin as well as the mucogingival tissues of the mouth and throat is done to identify any hyperemia, inflammation, abrasion, ulceration, neoplasm, or other abnormality.

Radiographic visualization should include lateral oblique and transfacial projections of the maxillary bones as well as an occlusal film through the floor of the mouth (Fig 17–5). A panoramic projection of the maxillofacial structures is useful.

Examination of the Masticatory System

Examination of the masticatory system is required to determine if pain emanates from the temporomandibular joints or the masticatory musculature. Clinically, the masticatory system should function painlessly within the ranges of movement needed for chewing and talking. These ranges are tested by opening and closing the mouth, clenching the teeth in firm occlusal position, biting on a tongue blade separator ipsilaterally and contralaterally, and moving the mandible protrusively and laterally. The temporomandibular joints and the masticatory muscles should be carefully palpated or manipulated for evidence of discomfort arising from them. Pain sources may be confirmed by careful analgesic blocking.

The following criteria have been found useful and dependable for accurate identification and localization of masticatory pain sources[7]:
1. The pain should relate directly and logically to the movements and functioning of the mandible incidental to mastication.
2. Tenderness in the masticatory muscles or over the temporomandibular joints should be discernible by manual palpation or functional manipulation.
3. Analgesic blocking of a tender muscle or joint should confirm the presence and precise location of such pain.

If masticatory pain is identified clinically, it is important that the true source of pain be located accurately. Masticatory myalgia should be differentiated from arthralgia. The type of muscle pain should be established as to whether the condition represents protective muscle splinting, myofascial trigger point pain, muscle spasm pain, or muscle inflammation pain. The particular muscle(s) involved should be identified by manual palpation or functional manipulation, and, if necessary, by analgesic blocking. If arthralgia is present, the pain source should be determined as to whether it emanates from the discal attachments, the retrodiscal tissue, or joint capsule, or occurs as the result of arthritis.

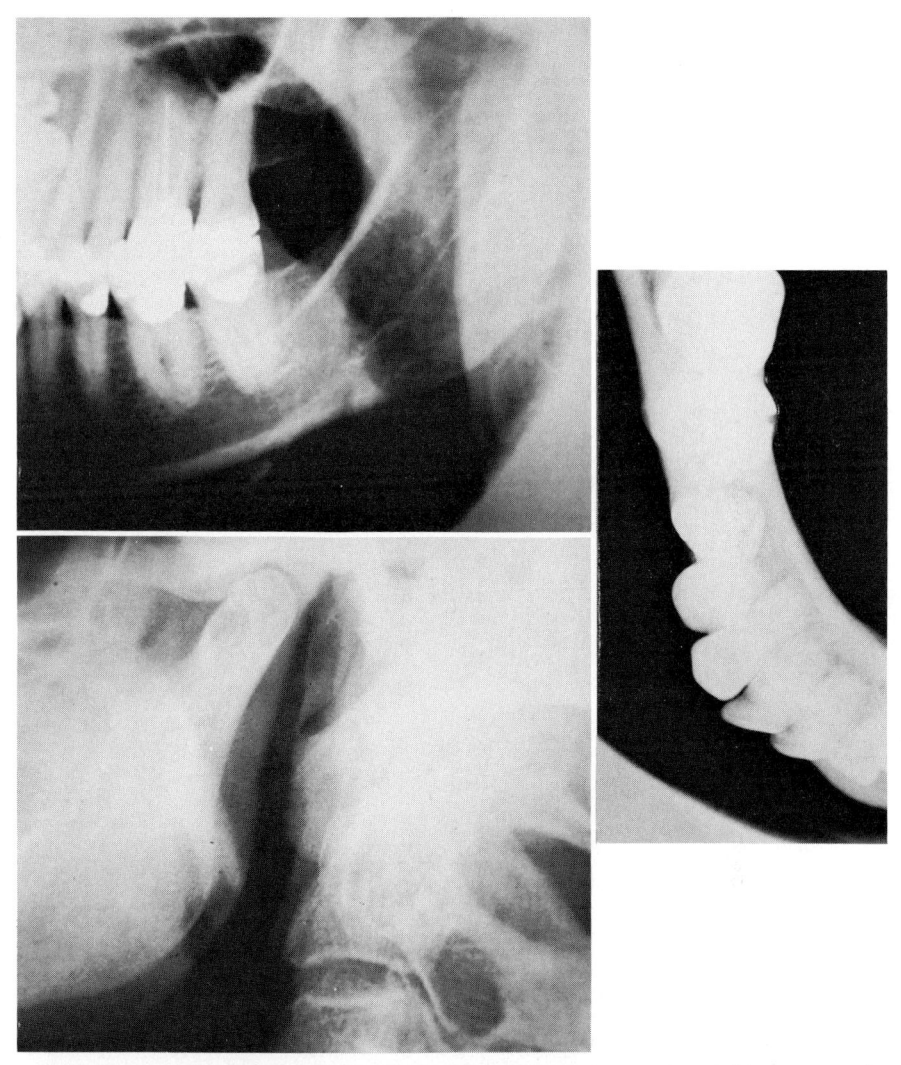

Fig 17-5.—Radiographic projections of facial structures (in addition to usual radiographic survey of the teeth) that are useful in pain examinations. *Top,* lateral oblique film of maxillary bones. *Bottom,* transfacial film of mandibular ramus and condyle. *Right,* lower occlusal film to visualize sublingual structures.

Although pain alone may at times involve the masticatory muscles, joints, or both, frequently some biomechanical dysfunction is also present. Thus, more than a pain examination is usually needed.[8] A good history of the complaint is essential. It should begin with the inception of the complaint. Each symptom should be traced chronologically from its beginning, special notice being taken of any relationship between the various symptoms. It should be determined if, prior to the beginning of each symptom, there has been any related injury, abusive use, dental treatment, illness, or emotional crisis, or if such conditions have been aggravating factors during the clinical course. The temporal behavior of each symptom should be noted in order to determine continuity, episodic or periodic timing, intermittency, and recurrence. Whether or not the symptoms have progressed and the rate of change should be recorded. All conditions that have had bearing on the complaint should be explored. The effectiveness of therapy by other doctors should not be overlooked. When the history of the complaint has been investigated and its clinical course defined, a fairly detailed description of the current behavioral characteristics of each symptom and that of the total complaint should be summarized. Finally, several background conditions that might have bearing on the problem should be explored, including the following:

1. The *medical history*, to determine if there is any related disease, especially arthritis or muscular complaints.
2. The *emotional state* of the individual and noticeable changes in emotional stress that might relate to the clinical course of the complaint.
3. *Habits of use*, especially clenching the teeth, that might be abusive.
4. *Traumatic incidents*, even from childhood, that might have caused injury to the masticatory system.
5. The *condition of the dentition* should be examined especially for evidence of occlusal disharmony.

When a radiographic examination of the temporomandibular joints is needed to confirm the clinical diagnosis, the following criteria should be met if the radiographic method is to yield maximal results:

1. It should clearly visualize both condylar and fossa-eminence surfaces of the joint with the least distortion and superimposition of other osseous structures.
2. It should permit the subject to be examined in a comfortable erect sitting position that does not inhibit mandibular movements.
3. It should permit films to be made by the examining dentist or under his direct supervision, utilizing standard dental x-ray equipment.
4. It should permit making series of films in different mandibular positions with sufficient precision that they can be exactly su-

perimposed for reading. This requires a film-holder of some type so that the entire series of one joint can be accomplished with no movement or change of position of tube, patient, or film between exposures.

In order to visualize functional movements as well as joint structure, a series of four films is needed (Fig 17–6):
1. With the teeth fully occluded but unclenched.
2. With the teeth fully occluded and firmly clenched.
3. With the jaw moved to the opposite side in maximum but unstrained lateral excursion, teeth not separated.
4. With the mouth wide open, maximum but unstrained.

Interpretation of the condylar positions thus recorded should be done by superimposing the upper articular surfaces while directly observing or tracing the condyle outlines. Although direct observation may be slightly more accurate due to the width of a tracing line, the tracing method has the advantage of making a graphic record. It facilitates visualizing condylar movements and making measurements of each (Fig 17–7).

Unfortunately, neither the articular disc nor the actual articular surfaces are seen radiographically. Only the subarticular bone and the intervening "space" are seen on the film. Also, usually the central articulating relationship of these subarticular osseous structures is not recorded (except by the tomographic method). Rather, what is seen on the film is the lateral contour of the joint. This interarticular space may not accurately represent the true thickness of the articular disc. If actual osseous disease is observed on the flat plate, tomographic visualization is the best technique for accurate evaluation. The usual open and closed views of the joint give some information about joint structure and the extent of condylar movement as restricted by all factors, intracapsular, and extracapsular, but more usable information comes from a series of films, as previously indicated.

A confirmed working diagnosis should precede all definitive therapy of masticatory pain. When the clinical symptoms, history of the inception and chronologic course of those symptoms, clinical evaluation of the masticatory system, and radiographic evidence fall reasonably and logically into place, leaving little room for diagnostic error, a good working diagnosis has been reached. Final confirmation of that diagnosis is judged by clinical response to trial therapy. Once this has been accomplished, a prognosis of the effectiveness of definitive therapy becomes possible and planning for such therapy is in order.

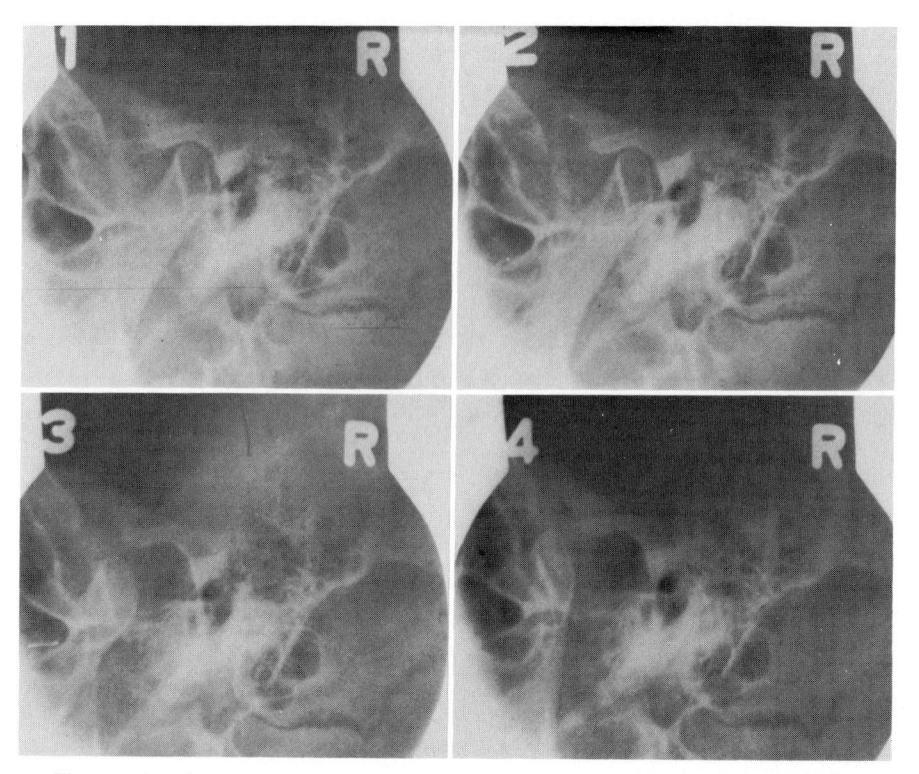

Fig 17–6.—Series of films needed to satisfactorily visualize the temporomandibular joint structurally and functionally. *Top left*, transparietal projection in primary occlusal contact position (POC). This records joint with teeth in so-called centric position. *Top right*, transparietal projection in fully occluded position (OP). This records the joint in so-called centric occlusion. *Bottom left*, transparietal projection in contralateral excursion (LP). This records condylar movement when mandible is moved laterally to opposite side. *Bottom right*, transparietal projection in full open position (MTO). This records condylar movement when mouth is opened widely. (From Bell W.E.: Management of temporomandibular joint problems, in Goldman H.M., Gilmore H.W., Royer R.Q., et al. (eds.): *Current Therapy in Dentistry.* St. Louis, C.V. Mosby Co., 1970, vol. 4. Reproduced with permission.)

Regional Musculature

All the muscles in the maxillofacial region should be palpated manually to identify sites of muscle pain. Besides the masticatory muscles already mentioned, this examination should include facial muscles, sublingual and suprahyoid muscles, occipital muscles, and cervical muscles, especially the sternomastoid and trapezius. Confirmation of

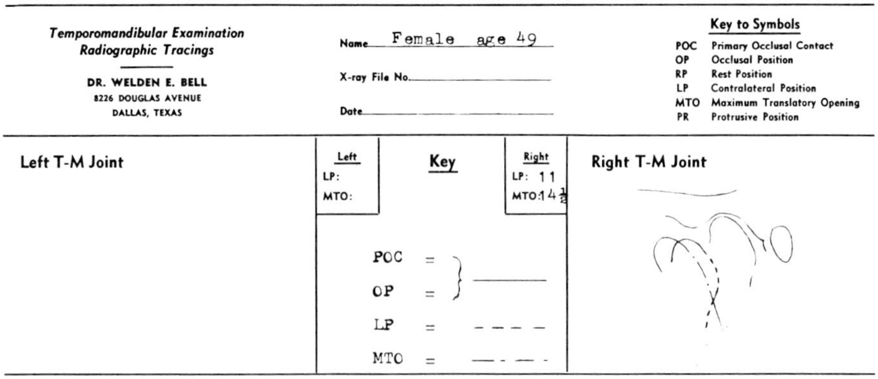

Fig 17-7.—Radiographic tracings made from four transparietal films of the temporomandibular joint (see Fig 17–6). The joint surfaces are well defined and smoothly contoured. The interarticular space is minimal in width but does not decrease in width under biting stress (from POC to OP). There is good superimposition in POC and OP, indicative of no gross displacement of condyle when teeth are fully occluded. Translatory movement of condyle in LP is adequate (10 mm or more). Translatory movement in MTO exceeds that of LP. By established standards of normal, this joint is radiographically within normal limits both structurally and functionally.

myalgia by analgesic blocking can be done if required for proper identification and localization.

IDENTIFYING THE PROPER PAIN CATEGORY

To identify properly the type of pain that constitutes the patient's complaint is an essential step toward diagnosis. Several questions help to make this determination:
1. Is the pain structural (organic) or functional (psychogenic)?
2. If structural, is it somatic or neurogenous?
3. If somatic, is it primary or secondary?
4. If primary, is it superficial or deep?
5. If deep, is it musculoskeletal or visceral?

The degree of accuracy reflected in the answers will set the guidelines toward correct identification of the pain complaint (Fig 17–8).

Structural or Functional? (clinical criteria)

STRUCTURAL
1. Pain behavior relates reasonably to adequate peripheral input.

OROFACIAL PAIN SYNDROMES

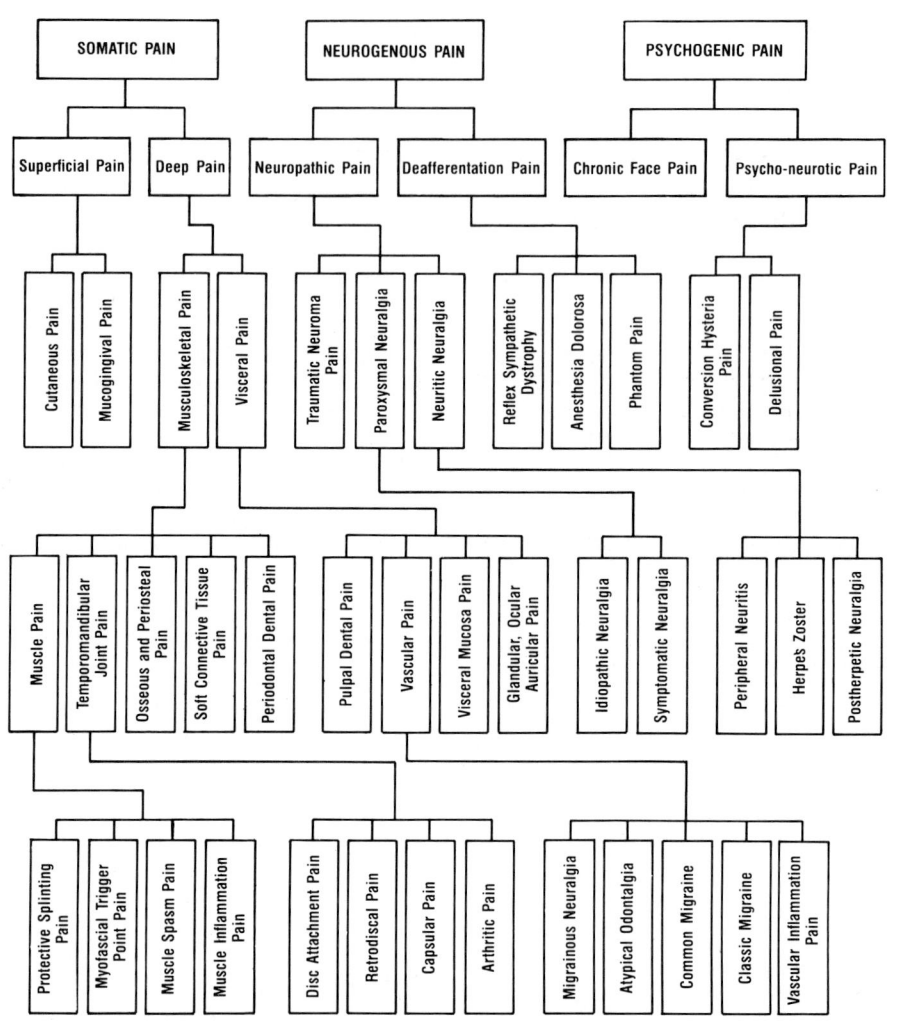

Fig 17-8.—Classification of orofacial pain syndromes.

  2. Site of pain makes anatomical sense relative to the source of input.
  3. Response to therapy is physiologic.

FUNCTIONAL
  1. Lacks adequate peripheral input.
  2. Site of pain does not make anatomical sense relative to the presumed source of input.

3. Response to therapy is not reasonable or physiologic.

Somatic or Neurogenous? (clinical criteria)

SOMATIC
1. Incidence of pain relates reasonably to the stimulation of peripheral structures.
2. Response to provocation at the site of pain is in keeping with the applied stimulus.
3. Pain is not accompanied by symptoms of neural deficits (anesthesia, paresthesia, paralysis, etc.)

NEUROGENOUS
1. Incidence of pain is not dependent on stimulation of peripheral structures. The pain may be ongoing, spontaneous, or triggered.
2. Response to provocation at the site of pain is disproportionate to the applied stimulus.
3. May be accompanied by other sensory or motor symptoms.

Primary or Secondary? (clinical criteria)

PRIMARY
1. Site of pain is located at the source of pain input.
2. Provocation at the site of pain accentuates it.
3. Analgesic blocking at the site of pain arrests it.

SECONDARY
1. Site of pain is not located at the source of input.
2. Provocation at the site of pain does not accentuate referred pain, but it does initiate secondary hyperalgesia.
3. Analgesic blocking at the site of pain does not completely arrest the pain.

Superficial or Deep? (clinical criteria)

SUPERFICIAL
1. Pain is bright, stimulating, and precisely localizable.
2. Pain is "clean-cut," with no accompanying effects.
3. Pain is arrested by application of topical anesthetic at the site of pain.

DEEP
1. Pain is dull, depressing, and variably localizable.
2. Pain may be accompanied by central excitatory effects.
3. Pain is arrested by analgesic blocking at the site of pain.

Musculoskeletal or Visceral? (clinical criteria)

MUSCULOSKELETAL
1. The pain relates reasonably to biomechanical function.
2. Responds proportionately to intensity of a stimulus applied at the site of pain.

VISCERAL
1. The pain is independent of biomechanical function.
2. Responds at threshold level to a stimulus applied at the site of pain.

CONFIRMATION OF CLINICAL DIAGNOSIS

At this stage, the true source of pain input should be identified and the general category of the pain established. A reasonably accurate clinical diagnosis should be forthcoming by comparing the information obtained in the history and clinical examination with the clinical characteristics and overall behavior of the various pain syndromes described in previous chapters. Caution should be exercised that true primary sources of pain constitute the condition under consideration. Heterotopic pains can be deceiving. Chronicity should be recognized; neurogenous pains should be identified; the difference between visceral and musculoskeletal pains should be established; vascular pain syndromes should be recognized; odontogenous toothache should be distinguished from nondental tooth pain; masticatory pains should be differentiated from those of nonmasticatory origin. If all such questions are settled with assurance, the clinical diagnosis should require little confirmation.

Before undertaking *definitive* therapy, however, confirmation of the clinical diagnosis is advisable. There are four methods that can help confirm the diagnosis:
1. Diagnostic analgesic blocking
2. Utilization of diagnostic drugs
3. Consultations
4. Trial therapy

DIAGNOSTIC ANALGESIC BLOCKING.—The value of local anesthetic injections and application of topical anesthetics to identify and localize pain cannot be overemphasized. It is essential when differentiating primary and secondary pains. It is equally useful to identify the pathways that mediate peripheral pain and to localize pain sources. The examiner should therefore become skilled in the use of this valuable diagnostic tool, using not only the routine injections common to dental practice but also infraorbital, pterygopalatine canal, second division, third division, and cervical plexus blocks.[9] Skillful analgesic blocking of muscles of the masticatory system (Figs 17–9 to 17–12) and maxillofacial region, as well as anesthetizing the temporomandibular joint proper, is especially useful in diagnosing masticatory pains and nonmasticatory myofascial pain syndromes. Although the area is outside the scope of dental practice, the examiner should be familiar with the indications for analgesic blocking of the stellate ganglion for the diagnosis of face and head pains that are mediated by the afferent sympathetic pathways.[10] *An anesthesiologist or neurologist should be called upon to make this injection.*

The usual fundamental rules for local anesthesia should be observed:
1. Knowledge of the neuroanatomy of all structures injected.
2. Knowledge of the pharmacology of all solutions used.
3. Avoidance of injection into inflamed or diseased tissues.
4. Maintenance of strict asepsis at all times.
5. Unfailing aspiration before injection to be sure the needle is not in a blood vessel.

Since prolongation of the anesthetic effect is unimportant diagnostically, use of short-acting drugs is desirable. Usually one without a vasoconstricting agent is best. Good anesthesia for skeletal muscle requires a nonvasoconstricting solution due to the vasodilating effect of epinephrine-like substances on such tissue. This reverse effect on muscle tissue is sometimes forgotten and may account for the transient anesthesia of poor quality sometimes obtained when muscles are injected for diagnostic purposes.

It has been demonstrated that local anesthetics have a measure of myotoxicity. Procaine appears to be the least myotoxic of the local anesthetics in common use.[11] Mild inflammatory reactions follow the injection of 1% and 2% procaine hydrochloride as well as isotonic sodium chloride.[12] Single injections of either procaine or isotonic saline cause no muscle necrosis.[13] The longer-acting and stronger anesthetics induce more severe inflammation and occasional coagulation necrosis of muscle tissue.[11] Regeneration takes place in about seven days. Solutions containing epinephrine cause greater muscle damage.[14] To minimize the danger of muscle damage in analgesic blocking for both diagnostic and therapeutic purposes, low concentrations of procaine are advisable, and such injections should be spaced at least seven days apart. The diagnostic use of local anesthetics on muscles should be curtailed to actual need.

It should be noted that, despite some myotoxicity, the diagnostic and therapeutic use of local anesthesia in the management of my-

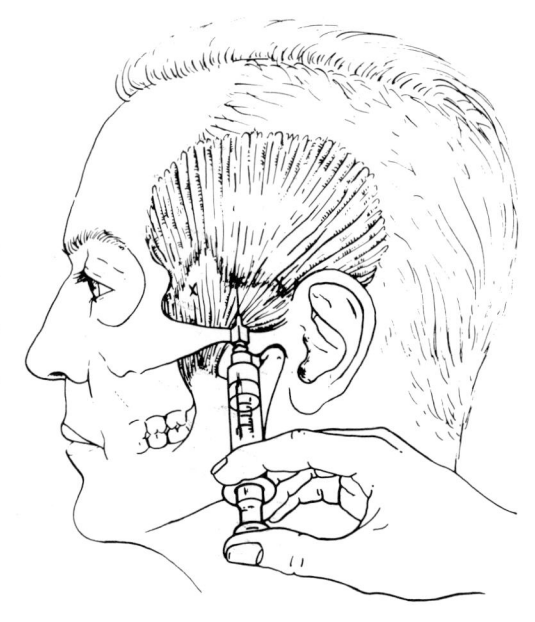

Fig 17-9.—Drawing to illustrate technique for extraoral injection of masseter muscle. The needle enters the muscle at the anterior border about midbody and is passed through the muscle at several angles and depths so as to reach the deep and superficial layers. With each pass of the needle, after aspirating it, the solution is slowly deposited as the needle is withdrawn. (From Bell W.E.: Management of masticatory pain, in Alling C.C., Mahan P.E. (eds.): *Facial Pain*, ed. 2. Philadelphia, Lea & Febiger, 1977. Reproduced with permission.)

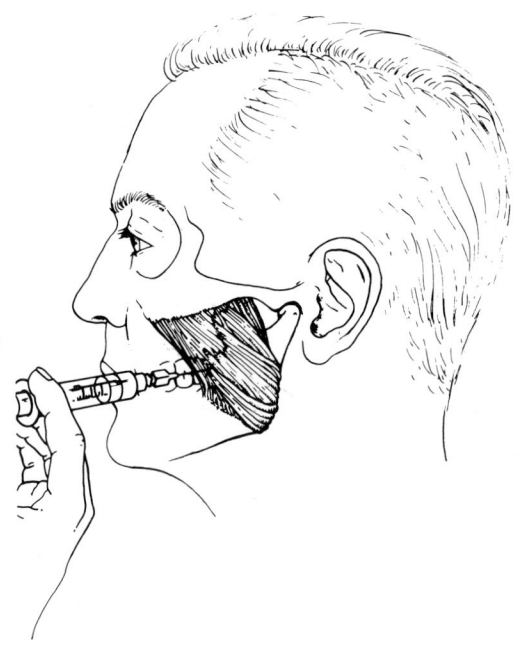

Fig 17-10.—Drawing to illustrate technique for injecting temporalis muscle. The needle penetrates the muscle at several points (X's) just above the zygomatic arch so as to reach most of the fibers. With each penetration, after aspiration of the needle, the solution is slowly deposited. (From Bell W.E.: Management of masticatory pain, in Alling C.C., Mahan P.E. (eds.): *Facial Pain*, ed. 2. Philadelphia, Lea & Febiger, 1977. Reproduced with permission.)

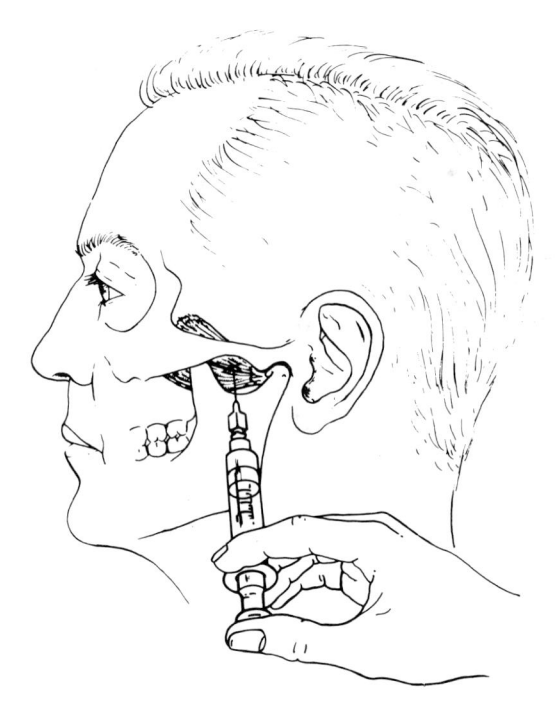

Fig 17–11.—Drawing to illustrate technique for extraoral injection of lateral pterygoid muscle. After the needle is carefully passed through the mandibular sigmoid notch, it is directed slightly upward and inward to a total depth of 35 to 40 mm. After aspiration of the needle, the solution is slowly deposited. Motor fibers of the facial nerve also may be anesthetized. (From Bell W.E.: Management of masticatory pain, in Alling C.C., Mahan P.E. (eds.): *Facial Pain*, ed. 2. Philadelphia, Lea & Febiger, 1977. Reproduced with permission.)

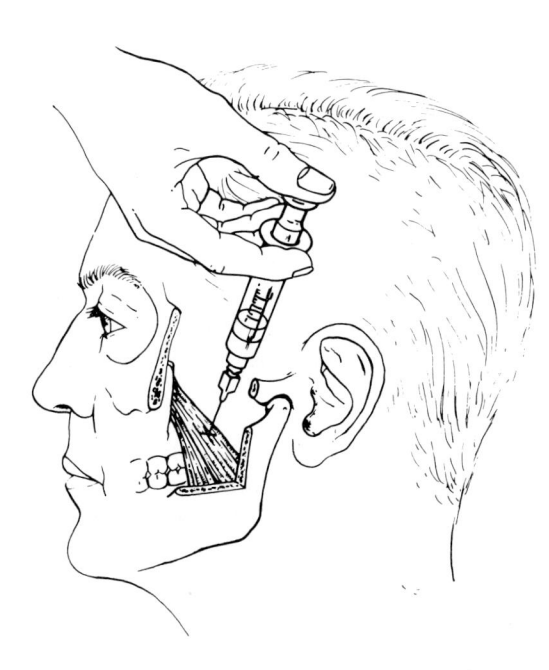

Fig 17–12.—Drawing to illustrate technique for extraoral injection of medial pterygoid muscle. After the needle is carefully passed through the mandibular sigmoid notch, it is directed boldly downward and inward to a total depth of about 40 mm. After aspiration of the needle, the solution is slowly deposited. Motor fibers of the facial nerve may also be anesthetized. (From Bell W.E.: Management of masticatory pain, in Alling C.C., Mahan P.E. (eds.): *Facial Pain*, ed. 2. Philadelphia, Lea & Febiger, 1977. Reproduced with permission.)

ogenous pain syndromes is clinically justified. Many diagnostic procedures and therapeutic modalities are attended by some risk. Note the destructive effects of radiation in radiography. All anesthetics and most medications are toxic to some degree. The inherent risks therefore must be weighed against the benefits derived. Reasonable judgment should be exercised in the application of all procedures that entail a measure of risk to the patient.

DIAGNOSTIC DRUGS.—Since at least part of the discomfort of vascular pain syndromes derives from the dilatation and amplitude of pulsation of the blood vessels involved, the diagnostic use of drugs that temporarily constrict blood vessels may help confirm the diagnosis. For this purpose ergotamine tartrate is used, administered as 0.5 to 1 mg of drug injected intramuscularly or 2 mg via a sublingual tablet. The drug constricts the cranial blood vessels and decreases the amplitude of pulsation. Relief of pain relates only to that portion that comes from distended vessels and does not affect concomitant pain due to edema of the vessels or to pain of muscle origin. The effect therefore is only partial and relates especially to pain that has a throbbing quality. The temporary benefit occurs within 30 to 45 minutes and may last for an hour or longer. A single intramuscular injection usually suffices for testing purposes. If the sublingual route is used, a second tablet should be placed beneath the tongue if no response is noticed within 30 minutes. Neither mode of administration should be repeated within a 24-hour period. *The drug is contraindicated with peripheral vascular disease, coronary heart disease, hypertension, impaired hepatic or renal function, sepsis, and pregnancy.* Side effects may include paresthesia of the fingers and toes, muscle pain and weakness in the extremities, precordial distress, transient tachycardia or bradycardia, nausea, and vomiting. Ordinarily such side effects are not seen from a single testing dose unless the patient is hypersensitive to the drug or a specific contraindication is violated. Intravenous infusion of histamine is known to precipitate headache only in "migraine patients."[15] This substance may become a useful test for vascular pain syndromes.

Confirmation of pain due to myocardial ischemia is usually accomplished by using a testing dose of nitroglycerin beneath the tongue. The drug relaxes smooth muscle principally in the smaller blood vessels and therefore dilates the arterioles, especially in the coronary circulation. *The drug is contraindicated in early myocardial infarction, severe anemia, glaucoma, increased intracranial pressure, and idiosyncrasy.* Occasionally it causes a transient headache. Overdose may cause flushing, headaches, tachycardia, and vertigo.

Confirmation of acute muscle spasm can sometimes be accomplished by testing with methocarbamol. One 10-cc ampule is used intravenously at an injection rate that does not exceed 3 cc per minute. *It is specifically contraindicated in renal disease, pregnancy, children under 12 years of age, epilepsy, and hypersensitive patients.* Adverse reactions include vertigo, hypotension, syncope, drowsiness, gastrointestinal upset, metallic taste, thrombophlebitis, sloughing at injection site, anaphylaxis, allergy, various autonomic effects, muscular incoordination, and fever. Speed of injection and alcoholism increase the incidence of these symptoms. Convulsive seizures have been reported. It goes without saying that this type of medication should be used with caution, and the examiner must be prepared to properly manage any adverse reaction. *The more potent intravenous muscle relaxant succinylcholine chloride should be used only when apparatus for assisted or controlled respiration with oxygen is available and only by persons skilled in the use of such apparatus.*

CONSULTATIONS.—There are occasions when pain problems require medical, otolaryngologic, orthopedic, neurologic, or psychologic consultation for proper identification of the pain syndrome. It requires judgment, therefore, on the part of the examiner to guide the patient through the examining procedure to arrive at a firm diagnosis in the most direct, time-saving, and economical manner. Elaborate diagnostic and consultative procedures should not be routine. Yet if the problem justifies it, every avenue of exploration should be used to arrive at a confirmed working diagnosis.

TRIAL THERAPY.—A short period of trial therapy is a good means of confirming a diagnosis provided the examiner is familiar with the effectiveness of placebo therapy, particularly with patients who are under considerable stress. This must be taken into account when evaluating the results. One form of trial therapy is the use of phenytoin (Dilantin) to help confirm a doubtful diagnosis of paroxysmal neuralgia. This medication has no analgesic action and therefore does not relieve pain per se. If relief well beyond the 40% maximum placebo effect is obtained with this medication within a few days, it is presumptive evidence that the syndrome in question is in fact paroxysmal neuralgia. *One should guard against assuming that absence of effect from this drug excludes neuralgia.* This would be a serious error since not all such neuralgias respond to this medication. Its exact mode of action is not known.

Trial therapy with a medication that constricts the cranial arteries can do much to confirm a diagnosis of vascular pain. One of the many ergotamine tartrate preparations available may be utilized for this purpose. If the drug used does in fact diminish the pain, especially the throbbing component, even though some muscle pain and tender edematous vessels still cause discomfort, it is highly suggestive that a vascular pain syndrome exists.

Trial therapy for muscular pains is useful to help confirm the diagnosis. This includes the use of vapocoolants, analgesic blocking of painful muscles, controlled physiotherapy, and use of muscle relaxants. If definite benefit accrues from such therapy, a firm diagnosis of muscle pain becomes justified.

Temporomandibular arthralgia suspected to be due to hyperuricemia can be subjected to a period of trial therapy consisting of colchicine, if the condition is an acute attack, or colchicine combined with a uricosuric agent such as probenecid in subacute and chronic conditions. Such medications should be given under medical supervision. If the arthralgia responds favorably to such therapy, the diagnosis should stand confirmed, and further medical care would be in order.

CONFIRMED WORKING DIAGNOSIS

A confirmed working diagnosis upon which effective therapy can be planned is the objective of any pain examination. On a dental level, it is essential to establish whether the pain problem stems from dental, oral, or masticatory causes. This is a primary responsibility. If the cause is amenable to dental therapy only, proper treatment should be planned and the patient so advised. If the cause has medical implications or complications, a multidisciplinary approach should be suggested. If the cause lies clearly outside the scope of dental practice, proper referral of the patient is indicated. If a confirmed diagnosis cannot be made by the examining dentist, referral would be in order prior to any attempt at definitive therapy.

Until a confirmed working diagnosis has been reached, definitive therapy should be withheld. Temporary palliative treatment, including the use of analgesic agents, preferably non-narcotic, may be prescribed pending confirmation of the diagnosis or transfer of the patient to other professional care. The patient should understand that such treatment is not meant to be definitive and curative. *All serious definitive therapy should await a confirmed working diagnosis, otherwise the effect may cause more harm than good.* Chance therapy, process-of-elimination therapy, and desperation measures cannot be condoned; at the very least, they are unnecessary.

REFERENCES

1. Bell W.E.: *Synopsis: Oral and Facial Pain and the Temporomandibular Joint.* Dallas, Welden E. Bell, Publisher, 1967.
2. Bell W.E.: Management of masticatory pain, in Alling C.C., Mahan P.E. (eds.): *Facial Pain*, ed. 2. Philadelphia, Lea & Febiger, 1977, pp. 181–199.
3. Melzack R.: The McGill Pain Questionnaire: Major properties and scoring methods. *Pain* 1:277–299, 1975.
4. Keats A.S.: Use of analgesics at bedside, in Way E.L. (ed.): *New Concepts in Pain.* Philadelphia, F.A. Davis Co., 1967, pp. 143–154.
5. Beecher H.K.: The use of chemical agents in the control of pain, in Knighton R.S., Dumke P.R. (eds.): *Pain.* Boston, Little, Brown & Co., 1966, pp. 221–239.
6. Mumford J.M.: *Toothache and Related Pain.* Edinburgh, Churchill Livingstone, 1973.
7. Bell W.E.: Management of temporomandibular joint problems, in Goldman H.M., Gilmore H.W., Royer R.Q., et al. (eds.): *Current Therapy in Dentistry.* St. Louis, C.V. Mosby Co., 1970, vol. 4, 398–415.
8. Bell W.E.: *Clinical Management of Temporomandibular Disorders.* Chicago, Year Book Medical Publishers, 1982.
9. Kramer H.S. Jr., Schmidt W.H.: Regional anesthesia of the maxillofacial region, in Alling C.C., Mahan P.E. (eds.): *Facial Pain*, ed. 2. Philadelphia, Lea & Febiger, 1977, pp. 237–256.
10. Moore D.C.: *Stellate Ganglion Block.* Springfield, Ill., Charles C Thomas, Publisher, 1954.
11. Travell J.G., Simons D.G.: *Myofascial Pain and Dysfunction.* Baltimore, Williams & Wilkins Co., 1983.
12. Pizzolato P., Mannheimer W.: *Histopathologic Effects of Local Anesthetic Drugs and Related Substances.* Springfield, Ill., Charles C Thomas, Publisher, 1961.
13. Burke G.W. Jr., Fedison J.R., Jones C.R.: Muscle degeneration produced by local anesthesia. *Va. Dent. J.* 49:33, 1972.
14. Yagiela J.A., Benoit P.W., Buoncristiani R.D., et al.: Comparison of myotoxic effects of lidocaine with epinephrine in rats and humans. *Anesth. Analg.* 60:471–480, 1981.
15. Krabbe A.A., Olesen J.: Headache provocation by continuous intravenous infusion of histamine: Clinical results and receptor mechanisms. *Pain* 8:253–259, 1980.

18

Management of Patients in Pain

PAIN SERIOUSLY IMPAIRS THE LIVES of millions of people around the world. Bonica[1] has reported that nearly a third of the population of industrialized nations suffers to some extent from chronic pain. This, he estimated, costs the American people more than $65 billion annually for health care services, loss of work, decreased productivity, and disability compensation, a sum that is 15 times the total national expenditure for all biomedical research.

The conditions that generate pain are susceptible to modification. The treatment of people who suffer pain entails (1) the manipulation of those factors that initiate and accentuate pain, and/or (2) the institution of means and methods by which patients can better cope with their complaint. The conditions that we as pain therapists set out to manipulate, therefore, comprise on the one hand such factors as the elimination of etiologic noxious stimuli, the interruption of nociceptive circuits, and the enhancement of our natural mechanisms of pain inhibition. On the other hand, we may elect to direct the main attention toward the patient rather than his problem in an effort to help him contend more successfully with his "disease." Sternbach[2] has shown that, whereas "pain" in *acute pain* is a symptom of disease, "pain" in *chronic pain* is the disease itself. Instantly, it should be obvious that pain management is a complex undertaking. Unfortunately, we are just beginning to learn the rules of the game.

The first step in the treatment of any condition is accurate and complete diagnostic evaluation of what the problem is, what structures are involved, and what conditions account for it. The diagnosis of pain is not a "naming process." It is an understanding of pain genesis, of modulating conditions, of inhibitory and excitatory mechanisms, of secondary effects, of accompanying symptoms, of physical and emotional reactions that occur in human beings as distinct individuals. Every patient who presents a pain complaint has a problem that is peculiar to him. Yet we as dentists are trained as therapists more than as diagnosticians. We are conditioned to *treat*— and our patients are conditioned to expect decisive and effective treatment from us. We are more mouth-oriented than patient-oriented. We do well as long as everything is obvious; when we face obscure problems our conditioning may fail us. Therefore, when we meet an obscure pain complaint, we need to call forth all our best diagnostic capabilities.

It is essential at the very outset to decide if we are dealing with an acute pain or a chronic pain. We must decide if the behavioral characteristics suggest somatic or neurogenous pain; if the pain emanates from superficial or deep structures; if the pain is primary or secondary. To skip these ABCs is to invite failure. Very early we need to decide if the complaint appears to be stimulus-evoked. Will our therapy be directed toward the elimination of a source of noxious stimulation? Will it use techniques that manipulate modulating influences? Will it entail the management of neurogenous pain sources? Will it employ the use of systemic medications? Will psychotherapy likely be utilized? A decision is needed: Is this a problem that I can handle alone, or do I need help? What kind of help? Who? Ultimate success or failure may well rest upon such early decisions. They should form the overall guidelines for managing the problem at hand. Each case should be individualized. We are not dealing so much with different kinds of problems as with different kinds of people. Genuine caring on the part of the doctor is the one indispensable attribute necessary for good pain management.[3]

TREATMENT MODALITIES

Management of a patient suffering with orofacial pain may require one or several kinds of treatment. For purposes of discussion, therapeutic modalities may be grouped as follows:
1. *Cause-related therapy.*—This consists of the identification and elimination of etiologic factors.
2. *Sensory stimulation.*—This is utilizing the pain-inhibitory effects of stimulating certain afferent neurons. This may be classified as cutaneous, transcutaneous, or percutaneous nerve stimulation.
3. *Analgesic blocking.*—This is the use of local anesthesia to (a) arrest pain input, (b) interrupt cycling, (c) resolve myofascial trigger point activity, or (d) induce sympathetic blockade.
4. *Physiotherapy.*—This includes cutaneous and deep massage, exercises, deep heat therapy, trigger point therapy, and physical activity to increase "up-time."

5. *Relaxation training.*—This includes autosedation, biofeedback training, and occlusal disengagement.
6. *Placebo therapy.*
7. *Psychotherapy.*—This includes counseling, hypnotherapy, and contingency management and formal psychotherapy.
8. *Neurosurgery.*—Such procedures include (a) peripheral therapy, (b) gangliolysis, rhizotomy, and decompression, and (c) trigeminal tractotomy.
9. *Medicinal therapy.*—This includes (a) analgesics, (b) anti-inflammatory agents, (c) analgesic balms, (d) antibiotics, (e) antiherpes agents, (f) local anesthetics, (g) anticonvulsants, (h) neuroactive drugs, (i) tranquilizers and muscle relaxants, (j) antidepressant drugs, and (k) vasoactive agents.
10. *Dietary supplement therapy.*

CAUSE-RELATED THERAPY

Many patients who experience orofacial pain have organic structural cause that is responsible for the suffering. The main thrust of therapy for such complaints is to identify the cause and eliminate it. The extent to which one achieves this will determine his success in the management of the pain problem. The cause of pain emanating from somatic structures (superficial and deep somatic pain) is thought to be chiefly, if not exclusively, due to the action of algogenic substances such as prostaglandins, bradykinin, histamine, serotonin, potassium, and phosphates.[4] The etiology of neurogenous pains is less well understood.

Somatic-Generated Pain

Much somatic pain results from trauma, intrinsic injury, infections, and disease that induce inflammatory reactions. The variety of traumatic conditions as to the type of agent as well as the extent and location of injury is nearly endless. Inflammatory conditions reactive to abusive use, intrinsic strains, microtraumas, bacterial, fungal, and viral infections, pathologic lesions, and biomechanical dysfunctions are almost without number. At a dental level, inflammatory conditions of the teeth, the supporting structures, and the mucogingival tissues, as well as dysfunctional and inflammatory conditions of the temporomandibular joints and masticatory musculature, are commonplace. It is known that ischemia liberates bradykinin,[5] that hemolyzed red blood cells in muscle tissue liberate potassium ions, and that phosphates, histamine, and serotonin are liberated from blood platelets.[4] Some of the visceral somatic structures elicit pain without such evident cause. Vascular pain involves more than simple vasodilatation; it is likely that algogenic substances are involved.

There are occasions when the somatic condition that generates pain is refractory to therapy, and the complaint persists as chronic *structural* pain. Cancer presents this problem. Some masticatory pains such as inflammatory arthritis may also fall into this category. Somatic pains, especially poorly managed myogenous pains, may gradually develop into a chronic *functional* pain syndrome. Chronic face pain that evolves from temporomandibular dysfunction may follow this course. Such chronic face pains have a dominant component of psychogenic pain and therefore require some systemic or psychological therapy or both. Chronic functional pains do not respond to cause-related therapy.

Neurogenous Pain

The matter of eliminating the cause of neurogenous pain presents problems. A traumatic neuroma in accessible scar tissue can be excised. Some benefit may come from anti-inflammatory therapy for inflammatory neuritis pain, and symptomatic neuralgia may respond to neurosurgical elimination of the neuropathy. But, on the whole, pains due to idiopathic neuralgia and deafferentation cannot be managed by cause-related therapy.

SENSORY STIMULATION

Cutaneous Stimulation

Although the stimulation of skin has been used to obtain relief from pain since ancient times, it has only been during the last two decades that some understanding of the mechanism involved has come to light, and with it a revival of many old remedies. By the gate control theory, the effect occurs through stimulation of thick myelinated cutaneous afferents, A-beta neurons chiefly. Whether other inhibitory mechanisms are involved remains to be determined.

There are many forms of cutaneous stimulation that effectively attenuate pain. Perhaps the oldest and most natural is pressing or rubbing the skin over the site of injury. Superficial massage is an important means of reducing pain. It is enhanced by adding a stimulating substance such as alcohol or menthol ointment.

Counterirritation is an age-old pain remedy.[6] Mustard plasters can still be remembered by many. It is well known that mild stimulation of nociceptors also increases pain inhibitory mechanisms. A mixture of aconite and iodine has been used for this purpose by dentists. Presently, vapocoolant therapy is an important element in myofascial trigger point pain therapy. Initially thought to be effective through its local anesthetic action, it is now recognized that the vapocoolant mildly stimulates the cutaneous nociceptors as well as the thicker A-beta fibers. Thus, the body's own pain inhibitory system is activated. As long ago as 1902, ethyl chloride was sprayed on the eardrum to alleviate the pain of otitis media.[7] Kraus[8] introduced the use of ethyl chloride spray for the treatment of painful motion in 1941. Travell advocated its use for the treatment of somatic trigger areas in 1949[9] and for treating skeletal myospasms in 1952.[10] Schwartz[11] applied it for the treatment of painful mandibular movement in 1954.

Intermittency is an essential element in vapocoolant therapy and probably is the reason why it is more effective than other forms of thermal therapy. Thick afferents adapt quickly to stimulation and therefore are more reactive to gradient changes. The application of heat and cold to obtund pain is very old. It has long been known to be more effective when the heat and cold are applied alternately for brief periods. Infrared heat is another form of cutaneous stimulation.

An old pain remedy has recently reentered the experimental laboratory—the use of mechanical vibration to relieve pain. It has been reported that at least one third of patients obtain complete relief from dental pain by this method, and the period of relief outlasts the stimulation by several hours.[12,13] Mechanical vibration also enhances the effect of transcutaneous electrical stimulation in about half the subjects.[14]

Hydrotherapy is another form of cutaneous stimulation, especially for neck and back pains of muscle origin. Agitated circulating bath water has therapeutic effect, and a brisk stream of shower water directed against the neck and back gives considerable relief. On the whole, cutaneous stimulation as a therapeutic tool for the management of pain has not been fully utilized.

Transcutaneous Stimulation

In ancient times, electric fish are said to have been used to relieve pain.[15] During the last century there have been several attempts to utilize electrical stimulation for this purpose. The method was resurrected by Wall and Sweet[16] in 1967 as the result of the gate control theory, verbalized by Melzack and Wall[17] two years before. Soon, transcutaneous electrical nerve stimulation became a popular form of pain control. The units employed a low-intensity faradic current at high frequency (50 to 100 Hz) applied to the skin through electrodes attached by conduction paste. No discomfort was felt. It was remarkably effective in relieving pains of various types. It was innocuous except for an occasional rash from the conduction paste. Being portable, the mechanism could be worn and used by subjects at will.

In 1972 the American public became aware of traditional Chinese acupuncture methods through media coverage. This initiated a wave of nociceptive research to explain this "miracle from the orient." It was really not until the discovery of the endogenous antinociceptive system in 1975 that some plausible explanation for the action of acupuncture became available. Research into electroacupuncture on a worldwide scale established a relationship between it and the newly discovered endorphins. Although some confusion still exists and conflicting reports appear, the following summarizes the present understanding of transcutaneous stimulation methods[18]:

1. *Transcutaneous electrical nerve stimulation* (TENS) utilizes high-frequency (50 to 100 Hz) but very low-intensity electric current. It is used to stimulate the nonnociceptive A-beta cutaneous afferents that activate the descending pain inhibitory mechanism without involving the opioid peptides. It may be felt as a tingling or vibratory sensation with no phasic muscle contraction even though some minor tonic contraction may occur in nearby muscles. Its action is immediate, is generally restricted to the segment that is stimulated, and induces little or no after effects. Therapeutic benefit is negligible. It does not depend on skin location where impedance is low, but, if applied at such sites (acupoints), an electroacupuncture (EA) effect may result. The analgesic effect ranges from 50% to 70%. [19, 20]

2. *Electroacupuncture* utilizes low-frequency (2 Hz) but high-intensity electric current. It is applied at specific cutaneous sites where impedance is low, so-called acupoints. It is used to stimulate the muscle nociceptors (group III and group IV afferents), which in turn activate the endogenous antinociceptive system. Phasic muscle contraction and pulsing muscle pain are required. The antinociceptive effect is not immediate but requires an induction period of 15 to 20 minutes. Some therapeutic effect may result. The analgesia may be either segmental or general. The segmental relief of pain is thought to involve the CSF enkephalin level, while the general effects appear to involve

the hormonal action of endorphins secreted by the pituitary gland into the blood stream.

Antinociception of the teeth and mouth occurs segmentally by applying EA at the infraorbital acupoint; more general effects come from the HoKu acupoint located between the thumb and index finger. Best results are obtained by simultaneously using both acupoints bilaterally.

Muscle pulsing with the Myo-monitor (Myo-Tronics Research, Inc.) has been reported to yield favorable results with the myofascial pain-dysfunction syndrome.[21]

A comparison of the two methods of transcutaneous sensory stimulation on a clinical level indicates that both are effective if properly applied, yielding satisfactory relief from pain in 50% to 70% of the subjects. The antinociceptive mechanism that is involved in either case is of more academic than clinical value. The two techniques have much in common and often overlap. It seems to matter little whether they are used separately or conjointly.[22-26] Cold laser (helium-neon) stimulation at acupoints is as effective as electroacupuncture and has the advantage of being practically painless.[27,28]

Although Sweet[29] did not find transcutaneous sensory stimulation useful in the management of tic douloureux, Melzack[30] reported significant relief from peripheral nerve injury pain, phantom limb pain, shoulder-arm pain, and low-back pain. Sodipo[31] reported acupuncture to be beneficial in 60% of patients with chronic pain. It has been reported useful in the management of tension headache.[32] It can also effect mood changes that resemble those of opioids.[33]

Electric current is also said to have favorable influence on growth and healing. Alteration in the volume of callus and in the direction of trabecular orientation occurs when electrodes are applied externally at a fracture site.[34-37] Also, reports of the use of pulsating electric currents to induce sleep, coming from Russia especially, indicate a still broader possible application of electrotherapy.[38]

Percutaneous Stimulation

Percutaneous stimulation is done by electrodes that penetrate the skin. Such methods have been used by neurosurgeons for many years. Subcutaneous nerve stimulation (SCNS) by an electric current produces prolonged analgesia that is not reversible by naloxone, indicating that it does not recruit the opioid peptides. Tolerance is not developed, and it can be administered with other analgesic medications, including narcotics.[39]

Lawrence[40] has introduced a new, but as yet experimental, form of percutaneous stimulation. It is electric stimulation of the periosteum by insulated needles. He used 9 to 12 volts at 100 to 300 Hz for 45 minutes. He kept the stimulation intensity at a level just perceived by the subject. He reported results subjectively superior to EA and TENS for the relief of chronic pain.

ANALGESIC BLOCKING

The use of local anesthesia to control surgical pain, and diagnostically to identify nociceptive pathways and primary sources of pain, is commonplace. The therapeutic use of analgesic blocking is less well known. Four facets of this modality of pain control are useful at a clinical level, namely, (1) to arrest primary pain input, (2) to interrupt pain cycling, (3) to resolve myofascial trigger point activity, and (4) to induce a sympathetic blockade.

Arresting Primary Pain Input

Primary deep pain input is an important factor, not only initiating heterotopic pains and secondary myospastic activity, but also in perpetuating them. For example, the pain of muscle spasm by its own central excitation tends to perpetuate the spasm as a cycling muscular complaint. To arrest the pain of myospasm by analgesic blocking has marked therapeutic value; it shuts off this perpetuating influence. This can be done by anesthetizing the muscle itself. Since myotoxicity of local anesthetics may restrict the choice of agent to short-acting anesthetics of low potency, it is preferable to block the nociceptive pathway rather than the muscle proper. Long-acting potent anesthetics can then be used with relative impunity, and thus the benefits of arresting the deep pain input can be extended.

Interruption of Pain Cycling

On the basis of clinical evidence, a cycling mechanism appears to complicate several pain syndromes that occur in the orofacial region. When such cycling is effectively interrupted by local anesthetic blockage of nociceptive impulses at the primary source or somewhere along its mediating pathway, remission of pain may significantly outlast the period of anesthesia. Such remission indicates that a therapeutic effect has been achieved. When such an effect can be obtained with a short-acting anesthetic, a still greater therapeutic effect usually results from the use of a longer-acting drug.

Repeated analgesic blocking of the pathway that subserves the peripheral receptors that trigger trigeminal neuralgia may induce an extended period of remission. Analgesic blocking of the primary source of pain input may effectively arrest some myofascial trigger point pains in the facial region. Remission of migrainous neuralgia can sometimes be achieved by local anesthesia at the site of pain. Myospasm of masticatory muscles can be influenced favorably, if not completely resolved, by one or more analgesic blocks of the nociceptive pathway that subserves the muscle.

Trigger Point Therapy

It is well known that the injection of a short-acting, aqueous local anesthetic of low myotoxicity at a myofascial trigger point located in muscle tissue effectively resolves the referred pain phenomena that characterizes myofascial pain syndromes.[41] Kraus[42] believed that such therapy is *required* when the trigger point is located in a muscle tendon.

Sympathetic Blockade

The diagnostic analgesic blocking of afferent sympathetic pathways to identify pain mediated by such neurons is well known. The stellate ganglion block is the one usually used for afferent sympathetic routes from the head.[43] Analgesic blocking at the same site also arrests the efferent sympathetic impulses and constitutes a sympathetic blockade as far as the orofacial region is concerned. It is reported that daily stellate ganglion analgesic blocking is as effective as guanethidine for the treatment of reflex sympathetic dystrophy.[44] Thompson[45] reported that half of his 120 cases of causalgia were relieved by repeated sympathetic analgesic blocks. Procacci et al[46] reported that, in 11 of their 30 subjects with reflex sympathetic dystrophy of the limbs, a significant increase in cutaneous pain threshold developed after analgesic blocking of the sympathetic ganglia on the affected side. Wetchler and Wyman[47] reported that all 23 of their patients with acute herpes zoster of the ophthalmic nerve had excellent pain relief and freedom from cutaneous scarring by treatment with daily analgesic blocks of the stellate ganglion. Three of this group, however, complained of postherpetic neuralgia at the six-month follow-up.

PHYSIOTHERAPY

MASSAGE.—Although physiotherapy is used primarily to improve biomechanical function, there are indications for its use in conjunction with pain management. The merit of cutaneous stimulation has already been discussed. This includes the use of surface massage with and without added medicaments, mechanical vibration, surface thermal applications, and hydrotherapy. Deep massage especially of muscles is another important therapeutic measure in pain management.

EXERCISES.—Forceful contraction of antagonist muscles causes reflex relaxation of an agonist muscle. This principle of reciprocal inhibition is useful in the treatment of masticatory myospasms.[48] For example, a spastic elevator muscle is relaxed by exercises that open the mouth *against resistance*. Retruding the protruded mandible *against resistance* tends to relax a spastic inferior lateral pterygoid muscle.

It has been reported that stimulation of muscle proprioceptors tends to normalize excessive EMG activity in painful spastic skeletal muscles.[49] Using this principle, resumption and maintenance of *normal muscular activity* in masticatory muscles is beneficial as long as pain is not generated by the activity.

For a muscle to maintain its normal resting length, occasional stimulation of the inverse stretch reflex is necessary. This is accomplished by occasionally stretching the muscle. An immobilized muscle not only loses its strength by disuse atrophy, it also shortens due to myostatic contracture.[50] Exercises that stimulate both the muscle spindles (contraction) and the Golgi tendon organs (stretching) are therefore needed to maintain normality of muscles. So-called functional manipulation is useful physiotherapy.

DEEP HEAT THERAPY.—Physiotherapy in the form of penetrating heat has value in treating patients with pain. Diathermy and ultrasound are used for this purpose. The judicious use of deep heat is beneficial in treating inflammatory pain. Although it has been employed to help relieve myospasm activity, its effects are equivocal. It is reported to be a useful adjunct in the treatment of myofascial trigger point pain.[41]

TRIGGER POINT THERAPY.—The primary physiotherapeutic technique for the treatment of myofascial trigger points is so-called stretch and spray.[41] A mixture of fluorocarbons is used as the vapocoolant (Fluori-Methane, Gebauer Chemical Co.). A spring-capped bottle with a calibrated nozzle that delivers a fine stream is needed. While the muscle is moderately stretched just short of pain, the vapocoolant is applied using parallel sweeps in one direction, traveling toward the reference area. The nozzle is held 15 to 18 inches away from the skin, and the stream is directed at an acute angle of about 30°. The sweeps are made at the rate of about 4 in. per second. After two or three sweeps, the muscle should be rewarmed. At the end of the treatment, moist heat should be applied and range-of-motion exercises instituted. The best results are obtained by first spraying, then stretching, using care not to stretch to the point of pain, and then spraying again. It is thought that the vapocoolant modulates the pain so that more manipulation is possible without discomfort. It should be noted that painfully stretching a muscle with myofascial triggers may induce muscle spasm. Other forms of physiotherapy applicable to the treatment of myofascial trigger points include ischemic compression, deep massage and kneading, and ultrasound. Ischemic compression is done by applying 20 to 30 lb of pressure at the trigger site for one minute while the muscle is stretched just short of pain.[41]

PHYSICAL ACTIVITY.—In patients with chronic pain, the maintenance of physical activity is an important part of therapy. Patients tend to withdraw and take to their beds. Fordyce et al[51] have found that, during periods when the pain is increased, extending exercises to the limit of patient tolerance is significantly beneficial: the more exercises performed, the fewer the pain behaviors displayed. The maintenance of physical activity keeps the body in better condition and reduces bed time.

RELAXATION

To the extent that tension and stress are etiologic factors in pain problems, the ability to relax may be beneficial. If tension and anxiety, however, are the result rather than the cause of the condition, relaxation may accomplish very little. Relaxation techniques have been used extensively in the treatment of headache complaints.

Autosedation

Biofeedback techniques have demonstrated that some functions heretofore thought to be wholly automatic and beyond volitional influence can in fact be manipulated by conscious mental processes. This applies to heart rate, body temperature, and EMG activity in skeletal muscles. There are a number of relaxation techniques that involve mental discipline and self-training. Illustrations are yoga techniques and systems of meditation. There should be little doubt that the modulating effects of conscious mental autosuggestion are very real and should be actively utilized in pain management. The effectiveness of Christian Science techniques, for example, testifies to the worth of autosedation.

Biofeedback Training

Although mental techniques such as meditating on a pleasant relaxing memory induce muscular relaxation and reduce anxiety,[52] biofeedback training appears to be the method that is most popular at this time. Appenzeller,[53] however, considered biofeedback to be no more than placebo effect. Jessup et al[54] believed that although biofeedback worked better for muscle contraction headache than placebo, it seemed to be no more effective than other relaxation training. To them, its application to migraine and other pain syndromes remained of unproven value. To this position Sternbach[55] took issue. He said that biofeedback could not be expected to help unless the clinical condition presented symptoms of peripheral vasomotor origin. He considered that too "scientific" an evaluation of biofeedback without due consideration for patient selection and individualization of treatment technique could be misinterpreted and misleading. Turner and Chapman[56] reported that, although biofeedback may be helpful with some headaches and some temporomandibular joint pain, it was not helpful in chronic pain. Sherman et al[57] reported substantial benefit from muscle relaxation training in the treatment of phantom limb. Half of their patients obtained virtually complete relief from pain.

Of some significance in the management of chronic muscle pain are two recent studies: (1) Large and Lamb[58] reported that a significant correlation existed between subjective pain levels and surface EMG activity; that EMG feedback was superior to other methods of relaxation, but not in reducing the subjective pain level; and (2) Nouwen[59] reduced significantly the EMG activity in paraspinal muscles by EMG feedback training, but it did not reduce the pain. Brooke and Stenn[60] reported on 174 patients with myofascial pain-dysfunction syndrome who were randomly treated by physiotherapy, occlusal splinting, biofeedback, and relaxation training without biofeedback. The biofeedback-assisted relaxation was reported to be as effective as either physiotherapy or occlusal splinting, but it was no more effective than relaxation training without the feedback assistance.

Relaxation training with or without the aid of biofeedback training appears to have merit in the overall management of masticatory problems in that it does reduce EMG activity. Its actual value in reduction of pain, however, is equivocal. Relaxation of muscles seems to be accomplished more readily by using biofeedback techniques.

Training devices generally monitor either body temperature or surface EMG activity. A home training device in the form of a ring has been devised to monitor finger temperature (BIO-Q, Futurehealth, Inc.) It is said to be accurate within one-half degree Fahrenheit and reads like a clock.

Occlusal Disengagement

For many years it has been clinically obvious that occlusal disengagement induces a substantial beneficial effect on the discomfort of temporomandibular disorders. This constituted the treatment used by Costen when he inserted thin cork wedges between the teeth. Disengagement sets the occlusion "at rest" and does for the masticatory system what restricted function does for other musculoskeletal systems. It constitutes a form of relaxation.

Occlusal disengagement can be accomplished in several ways: (1) by voluntarily leaving the teeth apart or ajar, (2) by a variety of simple habit-training devices such as a thin pat of chewing gum between the molar teeth, (3) by the use of muscle-relaxing medications, and (4) by interocclusal devices.

Christensen et al[61] showed that voluntary isometric contraction of elevator masticatory muscles induced pain and muscle fatigue. The pain seemed not to be due to cumulative EMG activity alone, because delay in pain was achieved by *elongating* the elevator muscles with a splinting device. Solberg and co-workers[62] showed that interocclusal devices significantly decreased the nocturnal EMG activity of bruxism. Kemper and Okeson[63] showed that "TMJ patients" complained of frequent headaches more than twice as often as a control group, and the frequency of such headaches was cut in half by occlusal splinting. Referring again to the work of Brooke and Stenn[60] it may well be assumed that much of the benefit of occlusal splinting derives from muscular relaxation.

Occlusal splints may be classified according to their intended function as (1) disengaging splints, (2) occlusion correcting splints, and (3) mandibular repositioning splints. Disengaging splints are particularly useful in the management of masticatory pain. Both disengaging and occlusion correcting splints tend to normalize sensory and proprioceptive impulses generated by occlusal dysfunction and thus shut off afferent input that initiates muscle splinting and aggravates myospastic activity. Repositioning splints are used to correct masticatory dysfunction primarily—not to relieve pain per se. It should be noted that all such interocclusal devices, regardless of how well they may be planned and made, have the propensity to generate altered sensory and proprioceptive signals that can accentuate the condition for which they are intended to benefit. Thus, careful monitoring is essential in the early phase of such therapy so as to be certain that the benefit derived is not offset by detrimental effects.

PLACEBO THERAPY

The effect of placebo on pain reaction has been known for many years. Beecher[64] pointed out that up to 40% of the benefit from any type of therapy may be attributed to placebo effect. Levine et al[65] determined that the effectiveness of placebo on postoperative pain equaled the effect of 4 to 6 mg of morphine, and patients with more intense initial pain showed greater probability of responding to placebo. Lewith et al[66] reported that acupuncture and placebo were equally effective for the relief of pain in postherpetic neuralgia.

It has been demonstrated that placebo is a useful antinociceptive modality. In years past, it was assumed that placebo effect was a psychological phenomenon; no doubt it is. But from the volume of evidence accumulating in the area of neurochemistry, it is becoming obvious that emotional behaviors are organic—that psyche and soma are inseparable facets of being human. So it is also with placebo. It is known that placebo responders are primed to release endorphins, and the entire effect of placebo is naloxone reversible.[67] With the knowledge that placebo analgesia is endorphin mediated, placebo therapy may be confidently incorporated into regimens for the management of pain.

PSYCHOTHERAPY

Psychological management has powerful influence on pain. It works both ways. Pain is intensified by fear and anxiety; it is accentuated by inept patient management, while adept therapy does much to lower the level of suffering.

Counseling

Most patients with acute pain respond favorably to informal counseling by a caring, pain-knowledgeable doctor. Fear can be allayed and anxiety diminished by words of assurance, particularly if the doctor possesses sure knowledge of pain management. An explanation that gives the patient insight into the pain behavior of the particular case at hand in language that he understands has powerful modulating influence.

The patient's attention should be directed away from his complaint as much as possible. He should be made to understand that there is little relationship between the level of suffering and the true seriousness of its cause. Reasonable physical activities commensurate with the patient's condition should be encouraged. Learning to cope with pain—living with it in peace—helps to offset psychogenic intensification, and thus to forestall chronicity. Suggestion has powerful modulating influence on pain.

Hypnotherapy

Hypnotherapy can be a useful antinociceptive method provided the pain does not stem from a purely psychogenic cause. Some suffering is too "valuable" to the patient to be given up; personality disintegration may follow the sudden withdrawal of pain.[68] Some form of psychiatric screening therefore should precede the use of hypnosis in the management of a pain problem.

The effectiveness of hypnosis depends largely on the susceptibility of the subject to suggestion. Direct induction technique may be quite satisfactory in highly susceptible subjects. Indirect induction, however, is equally effective and is superior in less susceptible individuals.[69] Hypnosis is clinically effective for a large number of patients presenting symptoms of severe pain of organic origin.[70] Almost all patients derive some benefit through placebo effect and relaxation. Some well-hypnotized individuals can block high-intensity pain of organic origin. Chronic pain usually requires behavioral modification also.[71] Hypnotherapy is especially useful in the management of pain associated with burns.[72]

Although the issue is still unsettled, there is some evidence that long-term reduction of pain by hypnotherapy involves the endorphins.[73]

Contingency Management and Formal Psychotherapy

Some formal psychotherapy is needed in many chronic pain syndromes, particularly those classified as chronic functional pains. All conversion hysteria and delusional pains require psychiatric consultation. A small percentage of temporomandibular disorders that are refractory to nonsurgical therapy may need psychotherapy rather than more aggressive surgical treatment.[74] In chronic face pain syndromes, local peripheral therapy, including surgery, should be restricted to a secondary role in management. The chief therapeutic effort should be systemic, psychologic, or both.

Fordyce[75] considered that some pains were behavioral and for the most part *learned*. To a considerable degree, pain is controlled by consequences in the environment. The modification of such consequences may be needed for pain management to be effective. Pain behavior may be unlearned by manipulation of consequences such as withdrawing positive reinforcers and by rewarding better behavior. Such contingency management usually requires full knowledge and cooperation, not only of the patient, but also of all those in close personal contact with him. This includes family members, doctors, nurses, therapists, and aids.[76]

Melzack[77] pointed out the importance of coping strategies in chronic pain, because some pains may last a lifetime. The objective in such cases is not to abolish the pain, but to make it bearable. Melzack trained his subjects to reach a meditational state, thus gaining the benefits of distraction, response to suggestion, relaxation, and the development of voluntary control over the pain. Strong suggestion is essential to psychological approaches for pain management.

Sternbach[78] assumed that pain behavior was acquired and therefore modifiable. Subjective improvement followed behavioral improvement. He utilized social modeling, conditioning, and cognitive forms of therapy.

Roberts[79] focused therapy, not on nociceptive sources or the alteration of an emotional state, but directly on patient behavior. His objective was to rehabilitate the patient rather than to alleviate the pain. He avoided all strategies that focus on pain per se, e.g., analgesics, electrical stimulation, analgesic blocking, and biofeedback training.

NEUROSURGERY

In managing pain problems about the mouth and face, a neurological consultation should be obtained when symptoms indicate the pres-

ence of a lesion that lies central to the orofacial structures. When one or more of the following symptoms are present, such a consultation is usually needed:
1. Depressed corneal reflex
2. Areas of hypoesthesia about the face
3. Persistent muscular weakness or paralysis
4. Simultaneous involvement of two or more cranial nerves

Peripheral Therapy

Peripheral neurosurgical procedures such as peripheral neurectomy and neurolytic block are now less enthusiastically undertaken because of better understanding of the problems that attend deafferentation of peripheral nerves. The benefit of such procedures must be weighed against the possibility of dysesthesia and anesthesia dolorosa. Although such procedures do give long-term relief from pain, the benefit is not lasting. They usually serve only to postpone a more definitive neurosurgical approach to the problem.

As another temporary alternative to invasive neurosurgery for trigeminal neuralgia, radiofrequency thermolysis of the peripheral nerve is available. Although pain threshold and tolerance are significantly raised, it is said that sensory threshold to tactile-discriminative stimuli is not permanently altered. This suggests that the method is somewhat selective for small myelinated and unmyelinated fibers.[80]

Microsurgical repair of injured peripheral sensory nerves of the face is being accomplished successfully. Trauma-induced paresthesia of several months' duration and recently lacerated nerves offer opportunities for oral surgery of this type. Regeneration of afferent fibers may be sufficient to restore useful sensation.[81] Surgical decompression and other microneurosurgical techniques may be helpful in the treatment of mandibular nerve paresthesia and neuritis due to surgical trauma to the inferior alveolar nerve or to accidental involvement of the nerve canal during endodontic procedures.[82, 83]

Suzuki et al[84] reported the use of cryocautery of sensitized skin areas in refractory postherpetic neuralgia. Their success rate was reported to be good.

Gangliolysis, Rhizotomy, Decompression

Although trigeminal rhizotomy is still practiced for the management of trigeminal neuralgia, it appears that the destruction of gasserian ganglion cells may also be required to completely arrest nociceptive impulses mediated by the trigeminal nerve. This is thought to be due to the mediation of some sensory afferents from the ganglion through the ventral root.[85] Sweet and Wepsic[86] used controlled thermocoagulation of the gasserian ganglion for trigeminal neuralgia. An alternative to denervation is decompression of the ganglion and dorsal root. This was described in 1952 by Taarnhoj[87] in Denmark and by Love[88] in this country. Janetta[89] has refined and popularized the operation.

Trigeminal Tractotomy

Spinal trigeminal nucleotomy is used to control the pain of postherpetic neuralgia, painful dysesthesia, and deafferentation anesthesia dolorosa with variable levels of success.[90,91]

MEDICINAL THERAPY

Medications of different kinds play an important role in the management of patients with pain. Their proper use is a major concern. It is the doctor's responsibility to be adequately familiar with the drug being administered and with the patient who is receiving it so that safety and effectiveness are assured. Individualization is necessary.

Many things need to be known about a medication: indications and contraindications for its use, drug incompatibilities, modes of administration, safe and toxic dosage, side effects, and possible complications. The doctor should be prepared to recognize and effectively deal with such things as sensitivity to the drug, undesirable side effects, toxicity, idiosyncrasy, anaphylaxis, or other untoward reactions to its use. He should know about the possibility of potentiation of other medications being used, synergisms, dependence, and the probability of addiction. Adequate medical supervision and emergency care should always be available if needed. All these responsibilities rest firmly upon the prescribing doctor, and they cannot be abrogated. If one is not prepared to accept these responsibilties, he should place the medicinal management of his patient in the hands of someone who is.

Analgesics

Medications that reduce pain are only one class of drugs that are useful in pain control. As a general rule, the objective of analgesics should not be to eliminate pain altogether. Pain has some value in estimating progress in the patient's condition. It helps inform the patient when his actions are excessive or abusive. The objective of analgesics should be to make the pain tolerable.

Analgesics are divided into two main groups: (1) the nonsteroid anti-inflammatory analgesics, typified by aspirin, and (2) the opioid analgesics, typified by morphine. Aspirinlike drugs strongly inhibit the action of cyclo-oxygenase, thus interferring with the biosynthesis of prostaglandins from arachidonic acid that occurs as part of an inflammatory process. The resulting decreased concentration of prostaglandins in inflamed tissue coincides with the alleviation of pain.[92,93] This helps explain the anti-inflammatory effect of the drug and no doubt has some bearing on its analgesia action. It does not, however, fully explain the analgesic action of aspirin. Age-related changes modify the response to aspirin. A higher incidence of drug reaction occurs in the aged. Some caution is indicated, therefore, in the use of aspirin in geriatric patients.[94]

Morphinelike drugs act through CNS receptors to induce a peripheral analgesic effect.[95] They depress nociceptive neurons while stimulating nonnociceptive cells.[96] Both aspirin and morphine inhibit the release of bradykinin, but aspirin inhibits its release regardless of the type of noxious stimulus, while morphine inhibits its release when mediated by neural mechanisms.[97] There is evidence that part of morphine-induced analgesia is contributed indirectly by the release of endogenous opioid peptides.[98] There is also some evidence that opiates exert an inhibitory influence on substance P release.[99]

Anti-Inflammatory Agents

In addition to the anti-inflammatory analgesics, there are several similar nonsteroid medications that are used solely for their anti-inflammatory effect. They are mildly analgesic and antipyretic. The specific action of all such medications is not known. The therapeutic effect appears to relate to the inhibition of prostaglandins biosynthesis. All such drugs should be used with caution, especially when protracted therapy is needed. Good medical supervision is appropriate. These agents do not alter the course of disease; they only suppress the symptoms of inflammation, hence their usefulness in the management of inflammatory pain.

Corticosteroids exert potent anti-inflammatory effect, presumably by acting to inhibit prostaglandins biosynthesis. However, in addition they cause profound and varied metabolic effects and modify the body's immune responses to diverse stimuli. They are eminently useful medications but require considerable care in administration. Extended use should be under close medical supervision. Their suppressive effect on inflammation may mask infection. They are contraindicated for systemic fungal and herpes simplex infections. Corticosteroid ointments are available in different strengths and with different bases. They are useful for topical application of the drug.

Antihyperuricemic agents are needed in the treatment of hyperuricemia involving the temporomandibular joints. Although its specific action is unknown, colchicine suppresses acute attacks of gout and relieves the pain that such attacks generate. For the treatment of chronic gouty arthritis, probenecid is useful. It is a uricosuric and renal tubule blocking agent that inhibits the reabsorption of urates in the tubules of the kidney. By thus increasing the excretion of uric acid, the serum urate level is lowered. It may induce exacerbations of acute gout, however, and should not be used until the acute symptoms are controlled with colchicine. A combination of the two medications is useful in treating chronic gouty arthritis that is complicated by occasional recurrent attacks of acute gout.

Analgesic Balms

Analgesic balms are agents that give soothing, palliative relief of inflammatory pain of both superficial and deep somatic categories when applied topically to exposed or ulcerated tissue. Aloe vera juice is an ancient remedy for superficially generated inflammatory pain. It is an ingredient of compound benzoin tincture. Balsam of Peru, eugenol, and guaiacol are other well-known balms. Applied in various forms as liquid, ointment, cementlike, or adhesive dressings, analgesic balms are extremely useful in the palliative control of pain emanating from exposed or ulcerated cutaneous and mucogingival tissues, exposed dentine, and acute alveolitis.

Antibiotics

A variety of antibiotic drugs for both topical and systematic administration is available. The choice depends on the type of organism represented in the infection. Culturing and susceptibility testing to identify the best-suited drug are good practice. The antinociceptive benefit of such agents relates to the resolution of infection that causes pain.

Antiherpes Agents

A topical antiviral agent, *acyclovir*, appears to be significantly beneficial in the treatment of primary infections due to herpes simplex. It is not effective, however, in the treatment of recurrent herpetic lesions.[100]

Local Anesthetics

Local anesthetics have an essential role in pain management both diagnostically and therapeutically. Topical anesthetics may be used as solutions, sprays, ointments, or lozenges. Water-soluable ointments containing a topical anesthetic and a germicide are useful for managing dental alveolitis.

A variety of injectable local anesthetics are available in different concentrations, with and without a vasoconstricting agent. Long-acting local anesthetics such as bupivacaine hydrochloride (Marcaine) are useful even though they entail a higher risk of toxicity. Proper dosage, correct technique, adequate precautions, and readiness for emergencies are essential to the safety and effectiveness of all local anesthetics. Resuscitative equipment, oxygen, and other resuscitative drugs should be instantly available, and adequate training in their proper use is necessary. Extreme caution is required when vasopressor agents are used in patients receiving monoamine oxidase inhibitors or antidepressants of the triptyline or imipramine types, because severe prolonged hypertension may result. Since most untoward reactions with local anesthetics follow accidental intravascular injection, aspiration prior to injecting any medication is a standard *must*.

The local injection of 0.02% morphine sulphate around peripheral nerves has been reported to yield a level of local anesthesia that is equal to that of bupivacaine in onset, profundity, and duration.[101] This small dose of 1 mg or less did not produce systemic opiate effects.

Anticonvulsants

Phenytoin (Dilantin) is an anticonvulsant and cardiac depressant that also has the capability of suppressing the pain of paroxysmal neuralgia in about 20% of the cases.[102] There is wide interpatient variability, and dosage must be individualized. The extended use of this medication should be under medical supervision.

A considerably more effective drug, but also more toxic, is carbamazepine (Tegretol). Pretreatment blood studies are necessary, and careful monitoring at regular intervals during treatment is essential for patient safety. Active medical supervision is prerequisite to its use. It is an anticonvulsant that appears to be specific for suppression of paroxysmal neuralgia. There are a number of contraindications and drug incompatibilities with which one must be familar before prescribing. When tolerated, however, this medication gives surprising benefit in about 70% of trigeminal and glossopharyngeal neuralgias.[102]

Neuroactive Drugs

The most common neurolytic drug used to destroy peripheral nerves is 95% ethyl alcohol. Sometimes phenol is added. Although an effective neurolytic, its denervating effect does not preclude regeneration of the peripheral axons and therefore gives only long-term temporary relief. The hazards of neuritis, extensive local fibrosis, and deafferentation effects restrict its use in modern practice.

The successful use of glycerol (0.30 ml) injected into the retrogasserian space for the treatment of trigeminal neuralgia has been reported.[103] About 90% of the patients remained pain-free after one or two injections. About 60% noticed slight numbness, but otherwise there was no significant sensory effects. No dysesthesia or anesthesia dolorosa was observed. It is thought that glycerol acts upon demyelinated axons assumed to be involved in the triggering mechanism of neuralgia.

In lieu of analgesic blocking of the stellate ganglion for the control of causalgic pains about the orofacial region, the adrenergic blocking agent guanethidine has been used. It appears to block the uptake of epinephrine by sensitized deafferented axons. The clinical benefit outlasts the pharmacologic action.[104] Bonelli et al [44] reported that intravenous guanethidine every four days for four times was equal in effectiveness to daily stellate ganglion analgesic blocks for eight days.

Tranquilizers and Muscle Relaxants

Numerous sedative and tranquilizing medications are available, some of which have muscle relaxant action as well. The major tranquilizers such as the phenothiazines are very useful in pain control by reducing the modulating effects of anxiety and apprehension. They are not addictive. They may display some objectionable side effects, however, and therefore require careful monitoring. Extrapyramidal effects are not uncommon. Protracted use has caused tardive dyskinesia.

The minor tranquilizers such as meprobamate and diazepam have the advantage of fewer side effects. Their muscle relaxant action is also useful. But they present a serious potentiality for drug tolerance and for dependence, if not outright addiction. Abuse of such drugs is commonplace. When utilized in pain control, they should be prescribed for limited periods only. When protracted use is needed, different drugs should be used periodically so that neither dependence nor tolerance is permitted to occur. Tranquilizers appear to exert some potentiating effect on narcotic analgesics.[105]

Medications that tend to relax skeletal muscle have some value in the management of myogenous pains especially. They are helpful in obtaining occlusal disengagement. If prescribed in sufficient dosage to induce real muscle relaxation, however, the patient cannot remain ambulatory or safely continue his usual activities. The potent relaxants such as succinylcholine chloride should be restricted to hospitalized patients and administered under expert supervision. The intravenous use of methocarbamol also requires special care. Some muscle relaxants are anticholinergic and therefore display physical symptoms incidental to that action. There are also some incompatibilities with which the prescribing doctor should be familiar. Although the use of muscle relaxants with fully ambulatory patients has some value, if no more than placebo effect, the actual amount of relaxation achieved is equivocal.

Antidepressant Drugs

Some patients with vascular pain and patients with chronic pain who verbalize reactive depression may respond to the judicious use of antidepressant medications. The tricyclic antidepressants increase the availability of serotonin and norepinephrine in CNS. The dimethylated tricyclics make serotonin proportionately more available and induce some sedative effect. They are useful in treating agitated depression. The monomethylated tricyclics make norepinephrine proportionately more available and induce some CNS stimulation. They are used more for retardant depression.[106] Although tricyclic antidepressants increase the available serotonin in the CNS, they do not have inherent analgesic properties. In normal subjects, they have no greater effect on pain than placebo.[107] Ward et al[108] reported that all moderately to severely depressed individuals complained also of pain, headache being the most frequent complaint. Patients who obtained minimal antidepressant effect from tricyclics also obtained minimal analgesic effect.

The monoamine oxydase inhibitors increase the available serotonin, norepinephrine, and dopamine in the CNS by inhibiting their breakdown. They potentiate the action of sympathomimetic substances and may induce a hypertensive crisis. The use of all antidepressant agents should be under adequate medical supervision.

Vasoactive Agents

Vascular pain syndromes may be favorably influenced by the alpha-adrenergic blocking action of ergotamine tartrate, which causes a stimulating effect on the smooth muscle of peripheral and cranial blood vessels. It is available in several different preparations, with and without the addition of caffeine. The caffeine enhances the vasoconstricting effect without increasing the dosage. Its effect appears to be greatest on the pulsatile component of vascular pain. The drug has several contraindications, including peripheral vascular and coronary heart disease, hypertension, and pregnancy.

Coronary vasodilators may be useful in some coronary complaints, but have little application in orofacial pain syndromes.

Antihistamines counteract the vasodilator action of histamine by blocking certain histamine receptors. Many antihistamine preparations are available. They may be useful in allergic responses and some vascular pain syndromes.

Beta-adrenergic blocking agents that decrease vasodilator responses to beta-adrenergic receptor stimulants may have value in vascular pain syndromes even though the mechanism for the antimigraine effect has not been established. The successful use of beta-blockers in the treatment of phantom limb pain has also been reported.[109]

Somatostatin has been reported to inhibit the effect of the release of substance P from peripheral sensory nerve terminals. Since substance P induces effects that resemble some of the symptoms of vascular pain syndromes such as cluster headache, the use of somatostatin has been investigated as a possible treatment modality. It is reported to be as effective as ergotamine tartrate in the treatment of cluster headache.[110]

DIETARY SUPPLEMENT THERAPY

The possibility of dietary manipulation to influence a number of physical complaints including pain has come under serious investigation in recent years. The chief relationship between diet and pain appears to be with L-tryptophan, which converts into serotonin. Brain and spinal cord serotoninergic neurons are actively involved in nociceptive responses as well as in the analgesic effects of opiates. Based on pharmacologic, surgical, electrophysiologic, and dietary manipulative data, it is evident that increased activity of serotonin interneurons is associated with analgesia and enhanced drug potency.[111] Hosobuchi et al[112] reported that, when patients with chronic pain, who were unable to obtain pain relief from 30 mg of IV morphine in divided doses due to drug tolerance, were placed on diets supplemented with 4 g of L-tryptophan a day for several weeks, they were able to achieve significant pain relief from opiates. They were also able to lead more active lives even while reducing their daily opiate intake. Seltzer et al.[113,114] have reported significant elevation of pain tolerance by the dietary supplementation of L-tryptophan. Cheng and Pomeranz[115] reported that naloxone-reversible analgesia induced by electroacupuncture was significantly increased when dietary D-phenylalanine and D-leucine were added.

The dietary considerations in pain therapy, especially for vascular and chronic pain syndromes, open new vistas. As more is learned about the role of neurotransmitters and protein fractions, such as glutamic acid, substance P, glycine, gamma aminobutyric acid (GABA), cholecystokinin, and somatostatin, a variety of dietary manipulations and additional medicinal forms of therapy likely will become available.[116] The dietary approach would not be expected to influence the management of acute pain complaints, however, because of the time factor. Like other nutritional approaches to disease, it usually requires several weeks for the effects of dietary therapy to become apparent clinically.

THERAPEUTIC GUIDELINES

The great majority of orofacial pain complaints that occur in dental practice are of such a type that the diagnosis is obvious, and treatment is nearly mandatory. It is the unusual or obscure pain condition, the refractory, the recurrent, the tormentingly mocking-type pain condition, that requires diagnostic effort and careful treatment planning.

Since a primary principle in pain management is individualization of therapy, there is no way that specific guidelines can be offered for the various pain syndromes that occur in the orofacial region. If, however, one has at hand the usual options from which therapeutic choices can be made, he has a better chance of selecting what is best for the

case under consideration at the moment. The guidelines that are suggested therefore represent little more than lists of treatment options from which choices can be made. As previously discussed, treatment options can be broadly classed as follows:
1. Cause-related therapy
2. Sensory stimulation
3. Analgesic blocking
4. Physiotherapy
5. Relaxation training
6. Placebo therapy
7. Psychotherapy
8. Neurosurgery
9. Medicinal therapy
10. Dietary supplement therapy

It should be understood that pain management as far as somatic pain is concerned applies only to primary sources. Heterotopic pain whether expressed as spontaneous referred pain or as evoked secondary hyperalgesia, cannot be treated directly. Only through identification of the primary source and treatment of that source can such heterotopic manifestations be managed. It is mandatory, therefore, that all heterotopic pains be recognized and the primary source of input determined.

It should be understood that pain management seldom is isolated from other treatment. Since cause-related therapy is an appropriate treatment option for most pain syndromes, it becomes the therapist's responsibility to properly integrate the pain therapy into the total treatment regimen needed to resolve the patient's complaint.

PAINS OF CUTANEOUS AND MUCOGINGIVAL ORIGIN

DIFFERENTIAL DIAGNOSIS
    Referred pain (spontaneous)
    Secondary hyperalgesia (evoked)
    Neurogenous pains
THERAPEUTIC OPTIONS
    Cause-related therapy
    Analgesics, anti-inflammatory agents, analgesic balms, antibiotics, antiherpes agents, topical anesthetics, tranquilizers, synthetic saliva
    Elimination of all surface irritants
    Therapy for salivary deficiency

PAINS OF DENTAL ORIGIN

DIFFERENTIAL DIAGNOSIS
  Referred pain and/or secondary hyperalgesia from other deep pain sources
  Vascular pains (atypical odontalgia, migrainous neuralgia)
  Neurogenous pains
THERAPEUTIC OPTIONS
  Cause-related therapy
  Sensory stimulation (cutaneous, transcutaneous)
  Physiotherapy (deep heat)
  Relaxation (occlusal disengagement)
  Analgesics, analgesic balms, antibiotics, tranquilizers

PAINS OF MUSCLE ORIGIN (Including masticatory muscle pain)

DIFFERENTIAL DIAGNOSIS
  Secondary hyperalgesia from myofascial trigger point pain (especially tension headache) or from other deep pain input
  Temporomandibular arthralgia
  Vascular pains
  Neurogenous pains
  Chronic face pain
  Conversion hysteria
THERAPEUTIC OPTIONS
  Cause-related therapy
  Sensory stimulation (cutaneous, transcutaneous)
  Analgesic blocking (trigger point therapy, interrupt cycling)
  Physiotherapy (massage, exercises, deep heat, trigger point therapy)
  Relaxation (autosedation, biofeedback, occlusal disengagement)
  Psychotherapy (counseling)
  Analgesics, anti-inflammatory agents, antibiotics, local anesthetics, tranquilizers and muscle relaxants

TEMPOROMANDIBULAR JOINT PAINS

DIFFERENTIAL DIAGNOSIS
  Masticatory myalgia
  Referred pain from other deep pain sources
  Pseudoankylosis

Adjacent pathosis
Vascular pains
Neurogenous pains
Chronic face pain
THERAPEUTIC OPTIONS
Cause-related therapy
Sensory stimulation (cutaneous, transcutaneous)
Physiotherapy (deep heat)
Relaxation (autosedation, habit training, occlusal disengagement)
Psychotherapy (counseling)
Analgesics, anti-inflammatory agents, antibiotics, tranquilizers

OTHER MUSCULOSKELETAL PAINS (osseous, periosteal, soft ct.)

DIFFERENTIAL DIAGNOSIS
Myalgia
Arthralgia
Tumors, cysts
Visceral and vascular pains
Neurogenous pains
THERAPEUTIC OPTIONS
Cause-related therapy
Sensory stimulation (transcutaneous)
Physiotherapy (deep heat)
Analgesics, anti-inflammatory agents, analgesic balms, antibiotics, tranquilizers

VASCULAR PAINS

DIFFERENTIAL DIAGNOSIS
Pains of dental origin
Masticatory pains
Neurogenous pain (paroxysmal neuralgia)
Chronic face pain
Conversion hysteria
THERAPEUTIC OPTIONS
Cause-related therapy (if pain is inflammatory)
Sensory stimulation (cutaneous and transcutaneous)
Analgesic blocking (arrest cycling)
Relaxation (autosedation, biofeedback training)
Placebo therapy

Psychotherapy (hypnotherapy, formal psychotherapy)
Analgesics, anti-inflammatory agents, local anesthetics, tranquilizers, antidepressants, vasoactive agents
Dietary supplement therapy

OTHER VISCERAL PAINS (mucosal, glandular, eye, ear)

DIFFERENTIAL DIAGNOSIS
Heterotopic manifestations may simulate "toothache," "sinusitis," "TMJ pain"
Musculoskeletal pains
Neurogenous pains (neuritic and paroxysmal neuralgia)
THERAPEUTIC OPTIONS
Cause-related therapy
Analgesic blocking (topical)
Physiotherapy (deep heat)
Psychotherapy (counseling)
Analgesics, anti-inflammatory agents, analgesic balms, antibiotics, topical anesthetics, tranquilizers, vasoactive agents (antihistamines)

NEUROGENOUS PAINS (neuropathy pains, deafferentation pains)

DIFFERENTIAL DIAGNOSIS
Somatic heterotopic pains
Pains of dental origin
Masticatory pains
Vascular pains
Chronic face pain
Conversion hysteria
THERAPEUTIC OPTIONS
Cause-related therapy
Sensory stimulation (cutaneous, transcutaneous, percutaneous)
Analgesic blocking (arrest cycling, sympathetic blockade)
Placebo therapy
Neurosurgery
Analgesics, anti-inflammatory agents, antiherpes agents, anesthetics, anticonvulsants, neuroactive drugs, tranquilizers, antidepressants

CHRONIC AND PSYCHOGENIC PAINS

DIFFERENTIAL DIAGNOSIS
  Structural pains, both somatic and neurogenous
THERAPEUTIC OPTIONS
  Sensory stimulation (cutaneous, transcutaneous, percutaneous)
  Physiotherapy (physical activity)
  Relaxation (autosedation, biofeedback training)
  Psychotherapy (contingency management and formal therapy)
  Analgesics, tranquilizers, antidepressants
  Dietary supplement therapy

MASTICATORY MYALGIA

The effective treatment of masticatory muscle pain depends on the accuracy of diagnostic identification of the particular type of myalgia present—protective muscle splinting pain, myofascial trigger point pain, myospasm pain, or muscle inflammation pain.

In addition to cause-related therapy, the following guidelines should be helpful in managing different types of masticatory muscle pain:
PROTECTIVE MUSCLE SPLINTING PAIN
  Set the muscle at rest
  No therapy other than a muscle relaxant (for placebo effect)
MYOFASCIAL TRIGGER POINT PAIN
  Stretch and spray
  Inject and stretch
  Ischemic compression
  Massage and knead
  Ultrasound
MUSCLE SPASM PAIN
  Restrict use within painless limits
  Maximum *normal* use, but restrained well within painless limits
  Occlusal disengagement
  Analgesic blocking and functional manipulation
  Exercises to reflexly relax spastic muscle
  Biofeedback training
MUSCLE INFLAMMATION PAIN
  Until acute symptoms subside
    Restrict use within painless limits
    No exercises, massage, or injections
    Anti-inflammatory therapy

Deep heat judiciously applied with increasing use as acute symptoms subside

When the acute symptoms have subsided
Stop anti-inflammatory therapy
Institute active exercise therapy, increasing vigorously as resolution occurs

Near the end of resolution period
Add therapy to counteract muscle atrophy (isometric exercises) and myostatic contracture (momentary stretching exercises)

DO'S AND DON'TS OF MUSCLE EXERCISE THERAPY

1. Don't exercise fatigued or painful muscles
2. Do a "warm-up" before vigorous exercise
3. Don't induce muscle pain
4. Don't fatigue the muscles (rest between exercises; rest time should equal exercise time)
5. Do a "cool-down" after vigorous exercise

REFERENCES

1. Bonica J.J.: Pain research and therapy: Recent advances and future needs, in Kruger L., Liebeskind J.C. (eds.): *Advances in Pain Research and Therapy.* New York, Raven Press, 1984, vol. 6, pp. 1–22.
2. Sternbach R.A.: Chronic pain as a disease entity. *Triangle* 20:27–32, 1981.
3. Degenaar J.J.: Some philosophical considerations in pain. *Pain* 7:281–304, 1979.
4. Keele K.D.: A physician looks at pain, in Weisenberg M. (ed.): *Pain, Clinical and Experimental Perspectives.* St. Louis, C.V. Mosby Co., 1975, pp. 45–52.
5. Foreman R.D., Blair R.W., Weber R.N.: Effects on T3 to T5 primate spinothalamic tract cells of injecting bradykinin into the heart. *Pain*, suppl 1, 1981, p. S212.
6. Gammon G.D., Starr I. Jr.: Studies on the relief of pain by counterirritation. *J. Clin. Invest.* 20:13, 1941.
7. Politzer A.: *A Textbook of Diseases of the Ear*, ed. 4. Philadelphia, Lea Bros. & Co., 1902.
8. Kraus H.: The use of surface anesthesia in the treatment of painful motion. *J.A.M.A.* 116:2582, 1941.
9. Travell J.: Basis for the multiple uses of local block of somatic trigger areas. *Miss. Valley Med. J.* 71:13, 1949.
10. Travell J.: Ethyl chloride spray for painful muscle spasm. *Arch. Phys. Med.*, May 1952, p. 291.
11. Schwartz L.L.: Ethyl chloride treatment of limited painful mandibular movement. *J.A.D.A.* 48:497, 1954.

12. Ottoson D., Ekblom A., Hansson P.: Vibratory stimulation for the relief of pain of dental origin. *Pain* 10:37–45, 1981.
13. Lundeberg T., Ottoson D., Hakansson S., et al.: Vibratory stimulation for the control of intractable chronic orofacial pain, in Bonica J.J., Lindblom U., Iggo A. (eds.): *Advances in Pain Research and Therapy.* New York, Raven Press, 1983, vol. 5, pp. 555–561.
14. Hansson P., Ekblom A.: Transcutaneous electrical nerve stimulation (TENS) as compared to placebo TENS for the relief of acute orofacial pain. *Pain* 15:157–165, 1983.
15. Kane K., Taub A.: A history of local electrical analgesia. *Pain* 1:125–138, 1975.
16. Wall P.D., Sweet W.H.: Temporary abolition of pain in man. *Science* 155: 108–109, 1967.
17. Melzack, R., Wall P.D.: Pain mechanisms: A new theory. *Science* 150:971–979, 1965.
18. Anderson S.A.: Pain control by sensory stimulation, in Bonica J.J., Liebeskind J.C., Albe-Fessard D.G. (eds.): *Advances in Pain Research and Therapy.* New York, Raven Press, 1979, vol. 3, pp. 569–585.
19. Augustinsson L., Bohlin P., Bundsen P., et al.: Pain relief during delivery by transcutaneous electrical nerve stimulation. *Pain* 4:59–65, 1977.
20. Mannheimer C., Carlsson C.: The analgesic effect of transcutaneous electrical nerve stimulation (TNS) in patients with rheumatoid arthritis: A comparative study of different pulse patterns. *Pain* 6:329–334, 1979.
21. Wessberg G.A., Carroll W.L., Dinham R., et al.: Transcutaneous electrical stimulation as an adjunct in the management of myofascial pain-dysfunction syndrome. *J. Prosthet. Dent.* 45:307–314, 1981.
22. Fox E.J., Melzack R.: Transcutaneous electrical stimulation and acupuncture: Comparison of treatment for low-back pain. *Pain* 2:141–148, 1976.
23. Eriksson M.B.E., Sjolund B.H., Nielzen S.: Long-term results of peripheral conditioning stimulation as an analgesic measure in chronic pain. *Pain* 6:335–347, 1979.
24. Willer J.C., Boureau F., Luu M.: Differential effects of electroacupuncture (EA) and transcutaneous nerve stimulation (TNS) on nociceptive component (R2) of the blink reflex in man. *Pain,* suppl. 1, 1981, p. S280.
25. Sodipo O.A.: Transcutaneous electrical nerve stimulation (TENS) and acupuncture: Comparison of therapy for low-back pain. *Pain,* suppl. 1, 1981, p. S277.
26. Chapman C.R., Colpitts Y.M., Benedetti C., et al.: Evoked potential assessment of acupunctural analgesia: Attempted reversal with naloxone. *Pain* 9:183–197, 1980.
27. Bischko J.J.: Use of laser beam in acupuncture. *Int. J. Acupuncture and Electro-Therapeut. Res.* 5:29, 1980.
28. Barnes J.F.: Electronic acupuncture and cold laser therapy as adjunct to pain treatment. *J. Craniomand. Pract.* 2:148, 1984.
29. Sweet W.H.: Some current problems in pain research and therapy. *Pain* 10:297–309. 1981.
30. Melzack R.: Prolonged relief of pain by brief, intense transcutaneous somatic stimulation. *Pain* 1:357–373, 1975.
31. Sodipo J.O.A.: Therapeutic acupuncture for chronic pain. *Pain* 7:359–365, 1979.

32. Ahonen E., Hakumaki M., Mahlanaki S., et al.: Acupuncture and physiotherapy in the treatment of myogenic headache patients: Pain relief and EMG activity, in Bonica J.J., Lindblom U., Iggo A. (eds.): *Advances in Pain Research and Therapy.* New York, Raven Press, 1983, vol. 5, pp. 571–576.
33. Toyama P.M., Heyder C.: Acupuncture-induced mood changes reversed by narcotic antagonist naloxone. *Pain* suppl. 1, 1981, p. S279.
34. Piekarski K., Demetriades D., Mackenzie A.: Orthogenic stimulation by externally applied DC current. *Acta Orthop. Scand.* 49:113–120, 1978.
35. Klapper L., Stallard R.E.: Mechanism of electrical stimulation of bone formation. *Ann. N.Y. Acad. Sci.* 238:530–542, 1974.
36. Rowley B.A., McKenna J.M., Chase G.R., et al.: The influence of electrical current on an infecting microorganism in wounds. *Ann. N.Y. Acad. Sci.* 238:543–551, 1974.
37. Becker R.O.: The basic biological data transmission and control system influenced by electrical forces. *Ann. N.Y. Acad. Sci.* 238:236–241, 1974.
38. Weinberg A.: Clinical observations in the use of electrosleep. *J. Am. Soc. Psychosom. Dent. Med.* 16:35, 1969.
39. Walker J.B., Katz R.L.: Nonopioid pathways suppress pain in humans. *Pain* 11:347–354, 1981.
40. Lawrence R.M.: Stimulation of the periosteum of the bone for chronic pain reduction. *Pain*, suppl. 1, 1981, p. S112.
41. Travell J.G., Simons D.G.: *Myofascial Pain and Dysfunction.* Baltimore, Williams & Wilkins Co., 1983.
42. Kraus H.: *Clinical Treatment of Back and Neck Pain.* New York, McGraw-Hill Book Co., 1970.
43. Moore D.C.: *Stellate Ganglion Block.* Springfield, Ill., Charles C Thomas, Publisher, 1954.
44. Bonelli S., Conoscente F., Movilia P.G., et al.: Regional intravenous guanethidine vs. stellate ganglion block in reflex sympathetic dystrophies: A randomized trial. *Pain* 16:297–307, 1983.
45. Thompson J.E.: The diagnosis and management of post-traumatic pain syndromes (causalgia). *Aust. N.Z. J. Surg.* 49:299–304, 1979.
46. Procacci P., Francini F., Zoppi M., et al.: Cutaneous pain threshold changes after sympathetic block in reflex dystrophies. *Pain* 1:167–175, 1975.
47. Wetchler B.V., Wyman T.M: The role of stellate ganglion block in the treatment of acute herpes zoster ophthalmicus. *Pain*, suppl.1, 1981, p. S120.
48. Schwartz L.: *Disorders of the Temporomandibular Joint.* Philadelphia, W.B. Saunders Co., 1959.
49. De Steno C.V.: The pathophysiology of TMJ dysfunction and related pain, in Gelb H. (ed.): *Clinical Management of Head, Neck and TMJ Pain and Dysfunction.* Philadelphia, W.B. Saunders Co., 1977, pp. 1–31.
50. Bechtol C.O.: Muscle physiology, in American Academy of Orthopedic Surgeons: *International Course Lectures*, vol. 5. St. Louis, C.V. Mosby Co., 1948, Chap. 11.
51. Fordyce W., McMahon R., Rainwater G., et al.: Pain complaint-exercise performance relationship in chronic pain. *Pain* 10:311–321, 1981.
52. French A.P., Tupin J.P.: Therapeutic application of a simple relaxation method. *Am. J. Psychother.* 28:282–287, 1974.

53. Appenzeller O.: Headache: Clinical and pathogenetic aspects, in Bonica J.J., Liebeskind, J.C., Albe-Fessard D.G. (eds.): *Advances in Pain Research and Therapy.* New York, Raven Press, 1979, vol. 3, 345–355.
54. Jessup B.A., Neufeld R.W.J., Merskey H.: Biofeedback therapy for headache and other pain: An evaluative review. *Pain* 7:225–270, 1979.
55. Sternbach R.A.: Letter to the editor. *Pain* 9:111, 1980.
56. Turner J.A., Chapman C.R.: Psychological intervention for chronic pain: A critical review. I. Relaxation training and biofeedback. *Pain* 12:1–21, 1982.
57. Sherman R.A., Gall N., Gormly J.: Treatment of phantom limb pain with muscular relaxation training to disrupt the pain-anxiety-tension cycle. *Pain* 6:47–55, 1979.
58. Large R.G., Lamb A.M.: Electromyographic (EMG) feedback in chronic musculoskeletal pain: A controlled trial. *Pain* 17:167–177, 1983.
59. Nouwen A.: EMG biofeedback used to reduce standing levels of paraspinal muscle tension in chronic low back pain. *Pain* 17:353–360, 1983.
60. Brooke R.I., Stenn P. G.: Myofascial pain-dysfunction syndrome: How effective is biofeedback-assisted relaxation training? in Bonica J.J., Lindblom U., Iggo A. (eds.): *Advances in Pain Research and Therapy.* New York, Raven Press, 1983, vol. 5, pp. 809–812.
61. Christensen L.V., Mohamed S.E., Harrison J.D.: Delayed onset of masseter muscle pain in experimental tooth clenching. *J. Prosthet. Dent.* 48:579–584, 1982.
62. Solberg W.K., Clark G.T., Rugh J.D.: Nocturnal electromyographic evaluation of bruxing patients undergoing short-term splint therapy. *J. Oral Rehabil.* 2:215–223, 1975.
63. Kemper J.T. Jr., Okeson J.P.: Craniomandibular disorders and headaches. *J. Prosthet. Dent.* 49:702–705, 1983.
64. Beecher H.K.: The use of chemical agents in the control of pain, in Knighton R.S., Dumke P.R. (eds.): *Pain.* Boston, Little, Brown & Co., 1966, pp. 221–239.
65. Levine J.D., Gordon N.C., Smith R., et al.: Analgesic responses to morphine and placebo in individuals with postoperative pain. *Pain* 10:379–389, 1981.
66. Lewith G.T., Field J., Machin D.: Acupuncture compared with placebo in postherpetic pain. *Pain* 17:361–368, 1983.
67. Levine J.D., Gordon N.C., Fields H.L.: The role of endorphins in placebo analgesia, in Bonica J.J., Liebeskind J.C., Albe-Fessard D.G. (eds.): *Advances in Pain Research and Therapy.* New York, Raven Press, 1979, vol. 3, pp. 547–551.
68. Pilling L.F.: Psychosomatic aspects of facial pain, in Alling C.C., Mahan P.E. (eds.): *Facial Pain,* ed. 2. Philadelphia, Lea & Febiger, 1977, pp. 213–226.
69. Fricton J.R.: The effects of direct and indirect hypnotic suggestion for analgesia in high and low susceptible subjects. *Pain,* suppl. 1, 1981, p. S175.
70. Hilgard E.R.: The alleviation of pain by hypnosis. *Pain* 1:213–231, 1975.
71. Orne M.T.: Hypnotic methods for managing pain, in Bonica J.J., Lindblom U., Iggo A. (eds.): *Advances in Pain Research and Therapy.* New York, Raven Press, 1983, vol. 5, pp. 847–856.

72. Toomey T.C., Larkin D.: Trance as a pain control strategy for the nurse in the burn unit setting. *Pain*, suppl. 1, 1981, p. S113.
73. Finer, B., Terenius L.: Endorphin involvements during hypnotic analgesia in chronic pain patients. *Pain*, suppl. 1, 1981, p. S273.
74. Speculund B., Goss A.N., Hughes A., et al.: Temporomandibular joint dysfunction: Pain and illness behavior. *Pain* 17:139–150, 1983.
75. Fordyce W.E.: Pain viewed as learned behavior, in Bonica J.J. (ed.): *Advances in Neurology*. New York, Raven Press, 1974, vol. 4, pp. 415–422.
76. Fordyce W.E.: Treating chronic pain by contingency management, in Bonica J.J. (ed.): *Advances in Neurology*. New York, Raven Press, 1974, vol. 4, pp. 583–589.
77. Melzack, R.: Psychological concepts and methods for the control of pain, in Bonica J.J. (ed.): *Advances in Neurology*. New York, Raven Press, 1974, vol. 4, pp. 275–280.
78. Sternbach R.A.: Fundamentals of psychological methods in chronic pain, in Bonica J.J., Lindblom U., Iggo A. (eds.): *Advances in Pain Research and Therapy*. New York, Raven Press, 1983, vol. 5, pp. 777–780.
79. Roberts A.A.: Contingency management methods in the treatment of chronic pain, in Bonica J.J., Lindblom U., Iggo A. (eds.): *Advances in Pain Research and Therapy*. New York, Raven Press, 1983, vol. 5, pp. 789–794.
80. Gregg J.M., Banerjoe T., Ghia J.N., et al.: Radiofrequency thermoneurolysis of peripheral nerves for control of trigeminal neuralgia. *Pain* 5:231–243, 1978.
81. Mozsary P.G., Middleton R.A.: Microsurgical reconstruction of the infraorbital nerves. *J. Oral Maxillofac. Surg.* 41:697, 1983.
82. Merrill R.G.: Oral neurosurgical procedures for nerve injuries, in Walker R.V. (ed.): *Oral Surgery*. London, E. & S. Livingstone, 1970, pp. 131–140.
83. LaBanc J.P., Epker B.N.: Serious inferior alveolar dysesthesia after endodontic procedure: Report of three cases. *J.A.D.A.* 108:605, 1984.
84. Suzuki H., Ogawa S., Nakagawa H., et al.: Cryocautery of sensitized skin areas for the relief of pain due to postherpetic neuralgia. *Pain* 9:355–362, 1980.
85. Hosobuchi Y.: The majority of unmyelinated afferent axons in human ventral roots probably conduct pain. *Pain* 8:167–180, 1980.
86. Sweet W.H., Wepsic J.G.: Controlled thermocoagulation of trigeminal ganglion and rootlets for differential destruction of pain fibers: I: Trigeminal neuralgia. *J. Neurosurg.* 39:143–156, 1974.
87. Taarnhoj P.: Decompression of the trigeminal root as treatment in trigeminal neuralgia: Preliminary communication. *J. Neurosurg.* 9:288, 1952.
88. Love J.G.: Decompression of the gasserian ganglion and posterior root (A new treatment for trigeminal neuralgia: Preliminary report). *Proc. Staff Meet. Mayo Clinic*, July 2, 1952, p. 27.
89. Janetta P.J.: Treatment of trigeminal neuralgia by suboccipital and transtentorial cranial operations. *Clin. Neurosurg.* 24:538, 1977.
90. Kunc Z.: Vertical trigeminal partial nucleotomy, in Bonica J.J., Liebeskind J.C., Albe-Fessard D.G. (eds.): *Advances in Pain Research and Therapy*. New York, Raven Press, 1979, vol.3, pp. 325–330.

91. Schvarez J.R.: Stereotactic spinal trigeminal nucleotomy for dysesthetic facial pain, in Bonica J.J., Liebeskind J.C., Albe-Fessard D.G. (eds.): *Advances in Pain Research and Therapy.* New York, Raven Press, 1979, vol. 3, pp. 331–336.
92. Granstrom E.: Biochemistry of the prostaglandins, thromboxanes, and leukotrienes, in Bonica J.J., Lindblom U., Iggo A. (eds.): *Advances in Pain Research and Therapy.* New York, Raven Press, 1983, vol. 5, pp. 605–615.
93. Higgs G.A., Moncada S.: Interaction of arachidonate products with other pain mediators, in Bonica J.J., Lindblom U., Iggo A. (eds.): *Advances in Pain Research and Therapy.* New York, Raven Press, 1983, vol. 5, pp. 617–626.
94. Baskin S.I., Smith L., Hoey L.A., et al.: Age-associated changes of responses to acetyl salicylic acid. *Pain* 11:1–8, 1981.
95. Ferreira S.H.: Prostaglandins: Peripheral and central analgesia, in Bonica J.J., Lindblom U., Iggo A. (eds.): *Advances in Pain Research and Therapy.* New York, Raven Press, 1983, vol. 5, pp. 627–634.
96. Belcher G., Ryall R.W.: Differential excitatory and inhibitory effects of opiates on nociceptive and nonnociceptive neurons in the spinal cord of the cat. *Brain Res.* 145:303–314, 1978.
97. Inoki R., Hayashi T., Kudo T., et al.: Effects of opium and morphine on the release of a bradykinin-like substance into the subcutaneous perfusate of the rat paw. *Pain* 5:53–63, 1978.
98. Schlon H., Bentley G.A.: The possibility that a component of morphine-induced analgesia is contributed indirectly via the release of endogenous opioids. *Pain* 9:73–84, 1980.
99. Tamsen A., Sakurada T., Wahlstrom A., et al.: Postoperative demand for analgesics in relation to individual levels of endorphins and substance P in cerebrospinal fluid. *Pain* 13:171–183, 1982.
100. Rowe N.H., Shipman C. Jr., Drach J.C.: Herpes simplex virus disease: Implications for dental personnel. *J.A.D.A.* 108:381, 1984.
101. Mays K.S., Schnapp M., Lipman J.J., et al.: Pain relief after peripheral perineural injection of morphine. *Pain,* suppl. 1, 1981, p. S 120.
102. Loeser J.D.: The management of tic douloureux. *Pain* 3:155-162, 1977.
103. Hakanson S.: Retrogasserian glycerol injection as a treatment of tic douloureux, in Bonica J.J., Lindblom U., Iggo A. (eds.): *Advances in Pain Research and Therapy.* New York, Raven Press, 1983, vol. 5, pp. 927–933.
104. Noordenbos W.: Sensory findings in painful traumatic nerve lesions, in Bonica J.J., Liebeskind J.C., Albe-Fessard D.G. (eds.): *Advances in Pain Research and Therapy.* New York, Raven Press, 1979, vol. 3, pp. 91–101.
105. Morichi R., Pepeu G.: A study of the influence of hydroxyzine and diazepam on morphine antinociception in the rat. *Pain* 7:173–180, 1979.
106. Allen G.D.: *Dental Anesthesia and Analgesia,* ed. 2. Baltimore, Williams & Wilkins Co., 1979.
107. Chapman C.R., Butler S.H.: Effects of doxepin on perception of laboratory-induced pain in man. *Pain* 5:253–262, 1978.
108. Ward N.G., Bloom V.L., Friedel R.O.: The effectiveness of tricyclic antidepressants in the treatment of coexisting pain and depression. *Pain* 7:331–341, 1979.

109. Marsland A.R., Weekes J.W.N., Atkinson R.L., et al.: Phantom limb pain: A case for beta blockers? *Pain* 12:295–297, 1982.
110. Sicuteri F., Geppetti P., Marabini S., et al.: Pain relief by somatostatin in attacks of cluster headache. *Pain* 18:359–365, 1984.
111. Messing R.B., Lytle L.D.: Serotonin-containing neurons: Their possible role in pain and analgesia. *Pain* 4:1–21, 1977.
112. Hosobuchi Y., Lamb S., Bascom D.: Tryptophan loading may reverse tolerance to opiate analgesics in humans: A preliminary report. *Pain* 9:161–169, 1980.
113. Seltzer S., Marcus R., Stoch R.: Perspectives in the control of chronic pain by nutritional manipulation. *Pain* 11:141–148, 1981.
114. Seltzer S., Stoch R., Marcus R., et al.: Alteration of human pain thresholds by nutritional manipulation and L-tryptophan supplementation. *Pain* 13:385–393, 1982.
115. Cheng R.S.S., Pomeranz B.: A combined treatment with D-amino acids and electroacupuncture produces a greater analgesia than either treatment alone; naloxone reverses these effects. *Pain* 8:231–236, 1980.
116. Yaksh T.L., Hammond D.L.: Peripheral and central substrates involved in the rostral transmission of nociceptive information. *Pain* 13:1–85, 1982.

Index

A

Abducent nerves, 40
Abscess
 dental, 138
 of molar
  mandibular second, 126
  mandibular third, 296
 periapical, 123, 124, 131
 periodontal, 123
  lateral, 131
 subperiosteal, 233
Acetylcholine, 28
Aching pain, 7, 331
Acid phosphatase: fluoride-resistant, 82
Acupoints, 56, 150, 361
Acupuncture, 54, 361
 discussion of, 56
Acute pain vs. chronic pain, 7–8
Acyclovir, 376
Adhesions: restricting condylar movement, 213
Affective descriptors, 333
Affective-motivational property: of pain, 4, 52
Afferent fibers: cranial parasympathetic, 34
Afferent impulses: transmission of, 21–23
Afferent neuron, 17
 primary, 23–24
Afferents
 parasympathetic, 41
 sacral, 34
 sympathetic, 34, 41–42
Alarm reaction, 94

Alcohol: ethyl, 377
Algogenic substances, 358
Allergic responses: and mucogingival pain, 107–110
Allergic rhinitis, 245, 247, 252, 262
 in nasal mucosa pain, 261
Allodynia, 64
Aloe vera, 375
Alpha-endorphin, 55
Alpha fibers, 18
Alveolar nerve
 inferior, neuritic neuralgia of, 297
 neuritic neuralgia of, 295
Alveolar neuritis (see Neuritis, alveolar)
Alveolitis, 232, 376
Analgesia
 endorphin, 27
 hypnoanalgesia, 56
 placebo, 56
 stimulation-produced, 26, 56
Analgesic balms, 54–55, 375
Analgesic blocking, 97, 115, 128, 357, 363–364
 to arrest primary pain input, 363
 in causalgia, 364
 of dental pain, 120
 diagnostic, 348–352
 in elevator muscle spasm, 164
 for interruption of pain cycling, 363–364
 of masticatory system, 340
 of muscle pain, 146, 354
 in muscle spasm pain, 363
  pterygoid muscle, 169
 of musculature, regional, 345
 in nasal mucosa pain, 263

Analgesic blocking (*cont.*)
  of neuralgia, 289
    idiopathic, 280
    trigeminal, 296
  in peripheral neuritis, 292–293
  in reflex sympathetic dystrophy, 364
  in tic douloureux, 281, 282
  in tooth pain from hyperalgesia, 142
  in toothache referred from muscles, 136
Analgesics, 373–374
  antiinflammatory, nonsteroid, 374
  objective of, 373
  opioid, 374
Anemia, 110
Anesthesia, 82, 265
  dolorosa, 82, 99, 101, 303, 308–309, 372, 373
    absent after glycerol, 377
  local, rules for, 349
  topical, 94, 97, 104, 105, 107, 330
    in glossopharyngeal neuralgia, 228
    in sinus headache toothache, 140
Anesthetics
  local, 376
  topical, 376
    for dental pain, 120
    in nasal mucosa pain, 263
    in neuralgia, idiopathic, 280
    in neuralgia, ninth nerve, 286
Aneurysm
  arteriovenous, 291
  neuralgia in, symptomatic, 274
Angina: Vincent's, 260
Angioneurotic edema, 298
Ankylosis, 197
  fibrous, 214
    arthritic pain due to, 218
    of temporomandibular joint, 206
Antagonists: muscle, 147
Antibiotics, 375
Anticholinergic action, 106
Anticonvulsants, 376–377
Antidepressants, 378–379
  tricyclic, 27, 320, 378
    dimethylated, 378
    monomethylated, 378

Antidromic activity, 23
Antiherpes agents, 376
Antihistamine, 379
Antihyperuricemic agents, 375
Anti-inflammatory agents, 374–375
Anti-inflammatory analgesics: nonsteroid, 374
Antinociceptive mechanism: endogenous, 27, 83–84
Antinociceptive system, 77
  endogenous, 54, 55–56, 113, 242, 316, 361
Antiviral agent, 376
Anxiety, 57
  assurance in, 370
  tranquilizers for, 377
Apprehension: tranquilizers for, 377
Arachidonic acid, 26
Arteriovenous aneurysm, 291
Arteritis
  carotid, 227, 298
  cranial, 255
  temporal, 239, 254
Arthralgia, 163, 275
  inflammatory, 226
  intermittent, differential diagnosis, 225–226
  of nonmasticatory origin, differential diagnosis, 227
  temporomandibular (*see* Temporomandibular arthralgia)
Arthritic pain, 100, 182
Arthritic pain of temporomandibular joint, 205–224
  degenerative joint disease causing, 214
  hyperuricemia causing, 216
  inflammatory, 205, 217
  rheumatoid, 205
  symptoms of, 220–222
  traumatic, 205
Arthritis
  degenerative, 206
  infectious, 212
  inflammatory, 359
  osteoarthritis, 206
  rheumatoid (*see* Rheumatoid arthritis)
  temporomandibular joint (*see* Temporomandibular joint, arthritis)

traumatic, 209, 212
Aspirin, 374
Assurance, 57
  for fear and anxiety, 370
Atrophy
  disuse, 76, 365
  muscle, 149
Attention, 57, 370
  to pain, 4
Auricular pain, 100, 268–270
  (*See also* Earache)
  central excitatory effects, 270
  diagnosis, differential, 384
  therapeutic options, 384
Auriculotemporal
  nerve paroxysmal neuralgia, 283
  neuritis, 293
Autonomic(s)
  function checking, 336
  nerves of head, 37
  nervous system, 35
  parasympathetic, 35
  reflex pain, 303
  sympathetic, 35
  symptoms, 332
Autosedation, 366
Axolemma, 16
Axon(s), 16
  classification by size, 18–19
  degeneration, 79
  -receptor mismatch, 83
  reflex, 68
  transport system, 23
Axoplasma, 16

B

Bacterial infection: causing nasal mucosa pain, 261
Balms: analgesic, 54–55, 375
Balsam of Peru, 375
Behavior
  chronic pain, 318–320
  localization, of pain, 332
  temporal, of pain, 33
Behçet's syndrome, 108
Bell's palsy, 298
Beta-blockers, 379
Beta-endorphin, 55
Beta fibers, 18
Beta-lipotropin, 55

Bicuspid: second, maxillary, 127
Biofeedback training, 367–369
Block
  neurolytic, 372
  of stellate ganglion, 364
Blockade: sympathetic, 364
β-Blockers, 379
Blocking
  analgesic (*see* Analgesic blocking)
  of stellate ganglion, 259, 306, 349
Blood cells: hemolyzed red, 358
Body image, 12, 313
Bradykinin, 27, 74, 77, 150, 242, 358, 374
Brain
  old reptilian, 15
  primitive mammalian, 15
  tumors, 85
Bright pain, 6
Bruxism, 107, 131, 147, 148
  occlusal disengagement in, 368
Bupivacaine hydrochloride, 376
Burning
  mouth, 106–107
  pain, 7, 18, 331
  tongue, 106–107
Bursa, 177
Bursitis, 175
Bypass circuits, 23

C

Caffeine, 379
Cancer, 85, 359
  of temporomandibular joint, 217, 224
Capsaicin, 82
Capsular pain, 100
Capsulitis, 190, 206, 217
Carbamazapine, 377
Cardiac
  arrest, 286
  muscle, pain referred from, 139
  origin of toothache, 137–138
Caries
  of molar, second, maxillary, 128
  with pulpal and periodontal pain, 127
  rampant, 121
  recurrent, beneath mesial filling, 127

Carotid
  arteritis, 227, 298
  nerve, internal, 42
  pressure, 140, 247
  sinus reflex, 336
Carotidynia, 227, 255
  central excitatory effects, 255
Causalgia
  (*See also* Reflex, sympathetic dystrophy)
  classic, 306
  pain of, 303, 377
Cause-related therapy, 357, 358–359
Cell(s)
  blood, hemolyzed red, 358
  ganglion, dorsal root, 24
  nerve, 16–18
    body, 16, 23
Cellulitis, 134, 232, 234, 239
  chronic, 234
  inframylohyoid, 234
  pain of, 229
  palatal, 234
  supramylohyoid, 234
Central
  excitatory effects (*see below*)
  hyperexcitability, 61, 96
  inhibition, 22
  inhibitory feedback system, 50
  pain, 65
    excitation, 66
Central excitatory effects, 97, 105, 113, 130
  of arthralgic pain, inflammatory, 226
  of carotidynia, 255
  dental pain and, 119–120, 134–135
  in "dry-socket" pain, 232
  of ear pain, 270
  of nasal mucosa pain, 261
  in reflex sympathetic dystrophy, 306
  in temporomandibular joint pain, 184
    capsular, 201
    retrodiscal, 199
  in tic douloureux, 281
  of vascular pain, 242
  of visceral pain, 238
    mucosa, 259

Centric position: of teeth, 188
Cephalalgia: histamine, 243
Cerebellopontine angle tumors, 85
Cerebral cortex, 22
Cervical
  ganglion, superior, 42
  nerves
    spinal, 39–40, 41
    upper, superficial sensory distribution of, 38
  sympathetic chain, 42, 237, 259
Chemoceptive pain receptors, 21
Cholecystokinin, 82, 380
Chorda tympani nerve, 39
Christian Science, 367
Chronic pain
  antidepressants for, 378
  behavior, 318–320
  diagnosis, differential, 385
  of face, 317, 320
  functional, 311, 316–317, 320, 359
    psychotherapy in, formal, 371
  nerve stimulation in, 362
  physical activity in, 366
  structural, 311–316, 320, 359
  syndrome, 311
    of face, 318
  therapeutic options, 385
  vs. acute pain, 7–8
Chronicity, 57, 311–324, 370
  symptoms of, 317–318
Ciliary ganglion, 41
Clinical pain vs. experimental pain, 7
Closed-lock, 189
Colchicine, 354, 375
Cold laser, 362
Compensation pain, 315
Compresses: hot and cold, 55
Condyle
  displacement, radiographic evidence of, 194, 195
  fixation, radiographic evidence, 193
  hyperplasia, 209
    cross-bite malocclusion due to, 223
  mandibular
    enlargement of, 220
    hyperplasia, 222
    radiography of, 213

movement
  capsular restraint on,
    radiographic evidence of, 203
  restriction by fibrosis,
    contracture or adhesions, 213
Confidence, 57
Connective tissue (see Soft
  connective tissue)
Conscious volition: and masticatory
  function, 32
Consciousness: oral, 106, 148
Consultation, 353
  medical, indications for, 338
Contingency management, 371
Continuous pain, 6
Contraception: oral, and
  mucogingival pain, 110
Contracture
  myostatic, 365
  restricting condylar movement,
    213
Convergence, 61
  of neurons, 18
Conversion hysteria (see Hysteria,
  conversion)
Coping strategies, 371
Coronary vasodilators, 379
Corpuscles
  Krause's, 19
  Meissner's, 19
  Merkel's, 19
  pacinian, 19
  Ruffini's, 19
Corticosteroids, 374
Cough reflex, 259
Counseling, 370
Counterirritants, 55
Counterirritation, 360
Cranium
  arteritis, 255
  nerves of, 36
  pain, 84
    primary, 84
  parasympathetic afferent fibers, 34
Cross-bite malocclusion: due to
  condylar hyperplasia, 223
"Cross talk," 24
Cryocautery, 372
Cutaneous
  (See also Skin)
  pain, 18, 95, 100, 102–115

diagnosis, differential, 113–114,
  381
of face, 102–104
therapeutic options, 381
stimulation, 359–360, 365
  nonnoxious, modulating effect,
    54–55
symptoms, 332
Cyclic myospasm, 71
Cyclo-oxygenase, 26
  aspirin and, 374
Cyst, 232, 234
  epidermoid, 291
  glandular pain and, 266
  radicular, 123

D

Deafferentation
  effects, of ethyl alcohol, 377
  of neurogenous pain, 78
  pain, 82–83, 99, 101, 115
    diagnosis, differential, 384
    peripheral, 83
    therapeutic options, 384
  therapy, 359
  peripheral, 141
  of peripheral nerves, 372
  syndromes, 98, 304
    expressed as mandibular
      toothache, 307
    expressed as reflex sympathetic
      dystrophy, 308
Decompression, 372–373
Decubital ulcer, 111
  denture causing, 112
Deep pain (see Pain, deep)
Deflection: of temporomandibular
  joint, 226
Delta fibers, 18
Delusional pain, 99, 101, 321–323
  psychiatric complication in, 371
Demyelination, 78–79, 274
Dendrites, 16
Dental
  abscess, 138
  origin of pain, 116–143
    as somatic pain, deep, 118
  pain
    analgesic blocking of, 120
    anesthetic for, topical, 120

Dental (cont.)
　autonomic effects, 120, 134
　behavior of, 118–120
　central excitatory effects and, 119–120
　diagnosis, differential, 382
　localization of, 118–119
　neuritic, 141
　periodontal, 100
　pulpal, 100
　quality of, 118
　relationship to initiating stimulus, 119
　relationship to other orofacial pain syndromes, 117
　secondary effects of, 134–135
　summation effects, 119
　therapeutic options, 382
　vertical laminated pattern and, 134
Dentist: responsibility of, 1
Denture
　decubital ulcer due to, 112
　stomatitis venenata due to, 108
Depression, 7, 57, 316, 318
　agitated, tricyclics in, 378
　retardant, 378
　signs of, 318
Dermal segmentation, 62
Dermatome, 62
　arrangement of, 63
Despair, 57
Diabetes, 110
Diagnosis, 325–355
　analgesic blocking for, 348–352
　clinical, confirmation of, 348–354
　confirmed working, 343, 354
　drugs for, 352–353
　objective of, 325
　tentative clinical, 334
Diathermy, 365
Dietary supplement therapy, 358, 379–380
Digastric muscle, anterior, 155
　referred pain of, 155
　trigger point in, 155
Diphtheria, 260
Disc
　articular, degenerative change in, radiographic evidence, 194, 195

　attachment pain, 100
　jamming, 165
　temporomandibular joint (see Temporomandibular joint, disc)
Discitis, 189, 217
　disc attachment pain due to, 191
Dislocation
　spontaneous, 175
　temporomandibular joint, 186
D-leucine, 380
Doctor-patient relationship, 326
Dopamine, 26, 55, 242, 379
Dorsal root
　entry zone, 24
　ganglion cells, 24
D-phenylalanine, 380
Drugs, 358, 373–379
　anti-inflammatory, 374–375
　for diagnosis, 352–353
　morphinelike, 374
　neuroactive, 377
　neurolytic, 377
"Dry-socket" pain, 232
　central excitatory effects, 232
Dull pain, 6
Dysesthesia, 82, 372, 373
　absent after glycerol, 377
Dyskinesia: tardive, after phenothiazines, 378
Dystrophy (see Reflex sympathetic dystrophy)

E

Eagle's syndrome, 255, 298
　diagnosis, differential, 227, 261
Ear (See also Auricular)
Earache, 11, 268
　elevator muscle spasm and, 164
　masseter muscle and, 150
　muscles of facial expression and, 157
　sternocleidomastoid muscle and, 155
Edema: angioneurotic, 298
Effector neuron, 17
Efferent(s)
　circuits, descending, 49
　neural circuits, 22–23
　neuron, 17

parasympathetic, 41
sympathetic, 42
Electric
　pulp test, 128
　pulp tester, 339
　pulp testing, 296
　stimulation
　　nerve, transcutaneous, 53–54, 361
　　of periosteum, 363
Electroacupuncture, 54, 361–362
　discussion of, 56
Elevator muscle
　inflammation, 176, 178
　masticatory, in pain-dysfunction syndrome, 165
　spasm, 167, 170–172, 173
　　increase in passive interarticular pressure, 165
Emergency nature: of pain, 9–10
EMG silent period, 147
Emotional significance: of conversion hysteria, 321
Emotional stress, 76, 104, 243, 304
Emotional tension, 106, 242, 248, 250
Emotional value: of pain, 11–12
End-net, 21, 42
Endoneurium, 16
Endorphin, 23, 54, 55, 361, 369, 370
　alpha-, 55
　analgesia, 27
　beta-, 55
　gamma-, 55
　system, 320
Enkephalin, 55
　leucine-, 55
　methionine-, 55
Enlarging pain, 6
Ephapse, 17, 78
Ephaptic transfer, 24
Epidermoid cyst, 291
Epinephrine, 242, 377
Epineurium, 16
Episode: of pain, 6
Ergotamine tartrate, 77, 108, 140, 238, 247, 252, 352, 354, 379
Erythema multiforme: stomatitis medicamentosa expressed as, 109
Esophagitis, 237

Esophagus: spasm, 259
Ethyl alcohol, 377
Ethyl chloride spray, 360
Eugenol, 375
Evaluation
　objective, 5
　subjective, 5
Examination, 325–355
　chart, 327–328,
　charting of, 327–329
　clinical, 338–345
　masticatory system, 340–344
　of mouth, 338–340
　of musculature, regional, 344–345
　radiographic, 342–343
　radiography of facial structures in, 341
　of teeth, 338–340
Exanthematous diseases, 110
Excitatory effects
　central (*see* Central excitatory effects)
　secondary, 128
Exercise, 365
　muscle, do's and don'ts of therapy, 386
　range-of-motion, 366
　reciprocal inhibition in, 365
Expectancy, 57, 314
Experimental pain vs. clinical pain, 7
Exteroceptive
　nociceptors, 3
　stimuli, 35
Exteroceptors, 19
Extraoral injection: technique for, 350–351
Eye (*see* Ocular)

F

Face
　chronic pain syndrome of, 318
　cutaneous pains of, 102–104
　lamination, significance of, 68–70
　muscles of facial expression, 157–159
　　pain patterns of, 158
　　trigger points of, 158
　nerve, 39, 40
　neuralgia, atypical, 243, 245, 247, 248–249

Face (cont.)
 pain chronicity in, 317
 neuritis, 298
 pain
  atypical, 319
  chronic, 101, 317, 320
  deafferentation, 301–309
  glandular, 266
  neuropathic, 271–274
  syndrome, chronic, 99
  vascular, 238, 243
 paralysis, 298
 structures, radiography of, in pain examination, 341
Facilitation: of neuron, 18
Fasciitis, 175
Fatigue, 76
Fear, 57
 assurance in, 370
Feedback
 central inhibitory feedback system, 50,
 reflex feedback control, 32
Fibers
 alpha, 18
 beta, 18
 delta, 18
 gamma, 18
 type A, 18
 type B, 18
 type C, 18
Fibrosis
 capsular, of temporomandibular joint, 200
  inflamed, 204
  restricting condylar movement, 213
Fibrositis, 75, 148
Filling: recurrent caries beneath, 127
Fluoride-resistant acid phosphatase, 82
Fluori-Methane, 365
Fossa tumors: middle, 85
Fracture
 of articular disc, 190
 styloid process, causing neuritic neuralgia, 299
FRAP, 82, 83
Fungoid infection, 111
 of oral mucosa, 112

G

GABA, 56, 380
Gag reflex, 259, 337
Gamma aminobutyric acid, 56, 380
Gamma-endorphin, 55
Gamma fibers, 18
Gangliolysis, 372–373
Ganglion
 cells, dorsal root, 24
 cervical, superior, 42
 ciliary, 41
 gasserian, 23
 otic, 41
 pterygopalatine, 41
 stellate, 42, 237
  blocking of, 259, 306, 349, 364
  submandibular, 41
Gangrene: pulpal, 123
Gasserian ganglion, 23
Gastric symptoms, 332
Gate control theory, 45–53, 81, 273, 359, 360–361
 action system, 51
 central control trigger, 49–50
 critical firing level, 48–49
 presetting the gate, 47
 resetting the gate, 47–48
 schematic diagram of, 46
 summary of, 51–53
 in tic douloureux, 281
Gelatinosa
 neurons, 25
 substantia, 25
Gelation, 200
Genesis of pain, 73–90
 inflammation, 73–74
 muscular, 74–77
 neural, 78–80
 vascular, 77–78
Gingivitis
 necrotizing ulcerative, 111
 during pregnancy, 110
Glandular pain, 100
 diagnosis, differential, 384
 therapeutic options, 384
Glossodynia, 106–107, 113, 319
Glossopharyngeal
 nerve, 39, 40
  neuralgia of, neuritic, 299
  neuralgia of, paroxysmal, 287

neuralgia (see Neuralgia, glossopharyngeal)
neuritis, 286, 298–299
Glossopyrosis, 319
Glutamic acid, 380
Glycine, 56, 377, 380
Golgi tendon organs, 20, 76
Gomphosis, 116
Granuloma: periapical, 123
Gray matter
　periaqueductal, 26
　spinal cord, lamination of, 24–25
Gray nerves, 16
Gray: periaqueductal, 54
Grinding: selective, in malocclusion, 162
Guaiacol, 375
Guanethidine, 377

H

Hallucinations, 85
　schizophrenic, 321
Hallucinatory pain, 320
Head
　autonomic nerves of, 37
　pain, primary intracranial, 84
Headache, 12, 84
　cluster, 243, 379
　dental pain and, 134
　during depression, 378
　elevator muscle spasm and, 164
　examination, 253
　with eye pain, 266
　frontal, and sternocleidomastoid muscle, 155
　Horton's, 243
　lower-half, 243
　menstrual, 253
　migraine (see Migraine)
　Monday-morning, 253
　muscle contraction, 78, 156
　　biofeedback training in, 367
　muscles of facial expression and, 157
　nasal mucosa pain and, 261, 262
　occlusal disengagement in, 368
　pharyngitis and, 260
　postocular, 157
　post-traumatic, 243

　sick, 253
　sinus, 262, 264
　sinus headache toothache, 140
　Sluder's, 243
　Sunday, 253
　temporalis muscle and, 150
　temporomandibular arthralgia in, 184
　tension, 78, 243, 247, 268
　　nerve stimulation in, 362
　　occipitofrontalis muscle and, 157
　　sternocleidomastoid muscle and, 155
　　trapezius muscle and, 156
　vascular
　　aura phase, 243
　　headache phase, 243
　wash-day, 253
Heart (see Cardiac)
"Heartburn," 237
Heat: infrared, 360
Heat therapy: deep, 365
Hemarthrosis, 197
Hemolyzed red blood cells, 358
Herpes
　lesions of, 115
　postherpetic neuralgia (see Neuralgia, postherpetic)
　simplex, 111
　　acyclovir in, 376
　zoster, 65, 81, 98, 99, 101, 103, 292, 300–301
　　discussion of, 115
　　herpetic eruptions of, 300
　　of mandibular nerve, 302
　　trigeminal, 300–301
Heterotopic pain, 64–66, 113, 348
　referred
　　from cardiac muscle, 139
　　from masseter muscle, 137
　　from nasal mucosa, inflamed, 264
　　from submandibular gland, inflamed, 267
　　trigger point pain of sternocleidomastoid muscle causing, 269
　　vascular pain syndrome causing, 246
High-altitude toothache, 126

Histamine, 28, 77, 238, 242, 352, 358, 379
  cephalalgia, 243
Historical note: on pain, 2–3
History, 329–333
  chronological, 332–333
  description of patient's complaint, 329–332
  -taking, 329
HoKu acupoint, 362
Horner's syndrome, 336
Horton's headache, 243
Hydrotherapy, 55, 360, 365
Hyperalgesia, 67, 82
  primary, 67, 105
  prostaglandin, 27, 74
  secondary, 65, 67–68, 113–114, 130, 149
    deep, 68
    dental pain and, 134
    superficial, 68
    in temporomandibular arthralgia, 184
    tooth pain from, 142
    vertical lamination pattern, 119
Hyperemia: and gate control theory, 47
Hyperesthesia, 82, 265
Hyperexcitability: central, 61, 96
Hypernociceptors, 77
Hyperplasia of condyle, 209
  cross-bite malocclusion due to, 223
  mandibular, 222
Hyperuricemia, 209, 227, 354
Hypnoanalgesia, 56
Hypnosis, 57, 370
Hypnotherapy, 370
Hypoesthesia, 265
Hysteria, conversion, 85
  pain of, 99, 101, 320–321
  psychiatric consultation in, 371
  psychogenic pain expressed as, 322

I

Iatrogenic pains, 86
Identifying the proper pain category, 345–348
  as deep, 347
  as functional, 345–347
  as musculoskeletal, 348
  as neurogenous, 347
  as primary, 347
  as secondary, 347
  as somatic, 347
  as structural, 345–347
  as superficial, 347
  as visceral, 348
Image: body, 12, 313
Imipramine, 376
Incisor: maxillary central, 125
Induced pain, 6
Infectious mononucleosis, 260, 266
Inflammation, 358
  of elevator muscles, 176, 178
  exudate of, 175
  gate control theory and, 47
  muscle pain due to, 172–177, 180, 385
  of nasal mucosa, 264
  pain of (see Inflammatory pain)
  periarticular, of temporomandibular joint, 209
  pulpal, 132
  of submandibular gland, 267
  in vascular pain, 243, 254–255
Inflammatory arthritis, 359
Inflammatory neuritis, 359
Inflammatory pain, 239
  deep heat in, 365
  of temporomandibular joint, 183
  vs. noninflammatory pain, 9
Infra-auricular pain, 152
Infrared heat, 360
Inhibition
  central, 22
  of neuron, 18
Inhibitory system: descending, 26, 54
Injection: extraoral, technique for, 350–351
Innervation: alien, 83
Interarticular pressure, 188
Interdisciplinary management, 2
Intermittent pain, 6
Interneurons, 17
Internuncial neuron, 17
Interocclusal devices, 368
Interoceptive stimuli, 35

INDEX

Interoceptors, 19
Intersegmental spreading, 71
Interview: preliminary, 326–327
Intoxications, 110
Intracranial pain, 84
   primary, 84
Intractable pain, 6
Ischemia, 76, 358
   compression, 366
   myocardial, 352
Isometric contraction, 77
   of muscle, 72
Isotonic contraction, 77
   of muscle, 72
Itching, 6
   pricking, 331

J

Joint (*see* Temporomandibular joint)

K

Krause's corpuscles, 19

L

Lacrimal glands: and glandular pain, 266
Lamina, retrodiscal
   inferior, 196
   superior, 196
Lamination: of spinal cord gray substance, 24–25
Lancinating pain, 332
Laryngitis: in streptococcal pharyngitis, 260
Laser: cold, 362
Learning: to cope with pain, 370
Leucine-enkephalin, 55
D-Leucine, 380
Ligaments
   discal, of temporomandibular joint, 184
   periodontal, 129
   stylohyoid, 227
   temporomandibular (*see* Temporomandibular ligament)
Limb pain, phantom, 379
   nerve stimulation in, 362

Limb: phantom, biofeedback training in, 367
Limbic system, 15
β-Lipotropin, 55
Low-intensity pain, 5
L-tryptophan, 27, 380
Lymph glands: and glandular pain, 266
Lymphadenitis, 175, 234, 266
   in streptococcal pharyngitis, 260
Lymphadenopathy, 266

M

Malignant tumors, 85, 359
   of temporomandibular joint, 217
     arthralgia due to, 224
Malingered pain, 314
Malingering, 12
Malocclusion
   acute, 153, 163
   capsular pain and, 200
   cross-bite, due to condylar hyperplasia, 223
   elevator muscle spasm and, 165
   retrodiscal pain and, 196
   temporomandibular joint arthritis causing, 206
Management, 356–392
   contingency, 371
   interdisciplinary, 2
Mandible
   condyle (*see* Condyle, mandibular)
   hypomobility, 212
Mandibular
   incisal path, 163
   nerve
     herpes zoster of, 302
     neuralgia of, paroxysmal, 285
   repositioning splint, 368
   toothache, deafferentation syndrome expressed as, 307
Massage, 54, 365
   deep, 365
   superficial, 359
Masseter muscle, 150
   referred pain from, 137
   spasm, 164
   technique for extraoral injection, 350

Masseter muscle (cont.)
  trigger points in, 152
Masticatory
  dysfunction, 162
  function, regional character of, 32–33
  muscle pain, schematic drawing, 161
  myalgia, 167, 171, 173, 176, 178, 385–386
  myositis, 175, 176, 178
  myospasm, reciprocal inhibition in, 365
Masticatory pain, 157, 162, 185, 242, 247, 252, 268, 282, 340
  chronicity of pain in, 317
  confirmed working diagnosis before therapy in, 343
  diagnosis, differential, 289
  differentiated
    from glossopharyngeal neuralgia, 286
    from reflex sympathetic dystrophy, 306
  -dysfunction syndrome, 134, 164, 270
    elevator masticatory muscles in, 165
  migrainous neuralgia mistaken for, 251
  muscle
    diagnosis, differential, 382
    therapeutic options, 382
  of muscle origin, 177–180
  myospasm, secondary to migrainous neuralgia, 249
  in neuritis, glossopharyngeal, 298
  neuritis mistaken for, auriculotemporal, 293
  recalcitrant, 319
  splints in, 369
Masticatory system: examination of, 340–344
Maxillary nerve: paroxysmal neuralgia of, 284
Maxillary sinusitis, 140, 262, 294, 296
Maximum-intensity pain, 5
McGill Pain Questionnaire, 13, 333–334

Mechanoreceptors, 116, 130
  periodontal, 147
Medical consultation: indications for, 338
Medical screening: form for, 339
Medicinal therapy, 358, 373–379
Meditation, 367
Meissner's corpuscles, 19
Meningioma, 291
Menstrual headache, 253
Menstrual toothache, 126
Mentation, 313
Merkels's corpuscles, 19
Mesencephalic nucleus, 22
Methionine-enkephalin, 55
Methocarbamol, 378
  in muscle spasm, 353
Microsurgical repair, 372
Migraine, 317
  biofeedback training in, 367
  classic, 78, 100, 241, 243, 248, 253–254
  common, 78, 100, 243
    discussion of, 253
    prodromal phase, 253
  typical, 239
  variants, 138, 243
Migrainous neuralgia (see Neuralgia, migrainous)
Migrating pain, 6
Model: of pain determinants, 52
Modulation (see Pain, modulation)
Molar
  first
    mandibular, periodontal lesion, 132
    mandibular, pulpal pain, 124
    mandibular, in traumatic occlusion, 131
    with pulpal and periodontal pain, 127
  second
    mandibular, abscess of, 126
    mandibular, with recurrent caries, 127
    maxillary, caries of, 128
    pulpal pain from, 129
  third
    mandibular, abscess of, 296
    maxillary impacted, 129

Index

Monday-morning headache, 253
Monitor: myo-monitor, 362
Monoamine(s), 26
   oxidase inhibitors, 376, 379
Mononucleosis: infectious, 266
Morphine, 380
   receptors, 55
   sulphate, 376
Morphinelike drugs, 374
Motivational-affective property: of pain, 4, 52
Motor
   changes, 332
   function, checking of, 335
   nerve pain, 65
   neuron, 17
   points, 150
Mouth
   (*See also* Oral)
   burning, 106–107
   examination of, 338–340
   mucogingival pain of, 104–113
   opening, extracapsular restriction, 166
   pain
      deafferentation, 301–309
      glandular, 266
      neuropathic, 271–274
      vascular, 238–243
Mucogingival pain, 95, 100, 102–115
   allergic responses and, 107–110
   diagnosis, differential, 113–115, 381
   from injury, massive superficial, 107
   isolated pain, 111–113
   local infections and, 110–111
   of mouth, 104–113
   oral contraception and, 110
   pregnancy and, 110
   systemic disease and, 110–111
   therapeutic options, 381
   without local cause, 113
Mucogingival scars, 275
Mucosa, nasal (*see* Nasal mucosa)
Mucosa pain
   diagnosis, differential, 384
   nasal, 237
   ostium maxillare, 237
   therapeutic options, 384

Mucous glands: and glandular pain, 266
Multiple sclerosis, 79, 291
   neuralgia in, symptomatic, 274
Muscle
   activity, normal, 365
   antagonists, 147
   atrophy, 149
   cardiac, pain referred from, 139
   contraction
      headache, 78, 156
      headache, biofeedback training in, 367
      isometric, 72, 77
      isotonic, 72, 77
   contracture, 175
   digastric, anterior, 155
   elevator (*see* Elevator muscle)
   exercise therapy, do's and don'ts of, 386
   of facial expression (*see* Face, muscles of facial expression)
   inflammation, pain of, 100
   manipulation, functional, 169
   masseter (*see* Masseter muscle)
   occipitofrontalis (*see* Occipitofrontalis muscle)
   orbicularis oculi, 157
   origin of pain, 144–181
      masticatory, 177–180
   pain, 98, 100, 144, 354
      analgesic blocking, 146
      central excitatory effects of, 144
      as deep somatic pain, 144
      diagnosis, differential, 382
      general features of, 146–147
      graduated response, 144
      inflammation, 100, 146, 180, 385
      inflammation causing, 172–177
      masticatory, distribution of, 161
      origin, 144–181
      relationship to orofacial pain syndromes, 145
      splinting, 146, 148
      splinting, protective, 178–179
      therapeutic options, 382
   in pain genesis, 74–77
   platysma, 157
   relaxants, 354, 377–378
   spasm (*see* Spasm, muscle)

Muscle (*cont.*)
  spindles, 20, 76, 168
  splinting, 86, 185, 226, 369
    pain, 74–75
    pain, protective, 385
  sternocleidomastoid (*see*
      Sternocleidomastoid muscle)
  temporalis (*see* Temporalis
      muscle)
  toothache referred from, 136–137
  trapezius (*see* Trapezius muscle)
  zygomaticus major, 157
Musculature: regional, examination
    of, 344–345
Musculoskeletal pain, 97, 100, 144,
    236
  as deep somatic pain, 229
  identification of, 348
  vs. visceral pain, 9
Mustard plaster, 55
Myalgia: masticatory, 167, 171, 173,
    176, 178, 385–386
Myelin sheath, 16
Myelination, 21, 78
Myocardial ischemia, 352
Myofascial
  genesis of pain, 145, 148
  pain, 75
    -dysfunction syndrome, 162, 362
    -dysfunction syndrome,
        biofeedback training in, 367
    reference zones of, 151
  syndrome, 242, 364
Myofascial trigger point, 66, 75, 134,
    148, 150
  mechanism, 71
  pain, 100, 146, 148–159, 179, 227,
      232, 364, 365, 385
    central excitatory effects, 149
    therapeutic trial in, 150
  stretch and spray for, 365
Myofasciitis, 175–176
Myogenous pain, 74, 144, 378
Myo-monitor, 362
Myoneural junction, 76, 150
Myositis, 86
  masticatory, 175, 176, 178
Myospasm, 86, 130, 364
  cyclic, 71
  cycling, 134

masticatory pain, secondary to
    migrainous neuralgia, 249
masticatory, reciprocal inhibition
    in, 365
Myospastic activity, 369
Myostatic contracture, 365
Myotatic reflex, 20, 34
Myotoxicity, 349

N

Naloxone, 54, 55, 147, 362, 369
Nasal mucosa
  inflamed, 264
  pain, 237, 261–264
    central excitatory effects, 261
Nasal symptoms, 332
Necrotizing ulcerative gingivitis,
    111
Neocortex, 15
Neocortical processes, 3
Neoplasia (*see* Tumors)
Neospinothalamic tract, 25
Nerve(s)
  abducent, 40
  accessory, 40–41
  alien innervation, 83
  alveolar, neuritic neuralgia of, 295
    inferior nerve, 297
  auriculotemporal, paroxysmal
      neuralgia of, 283
  autonomic, of head, 37
  carotid, internal, 42
  cell, 16–18
    body, 16, 23
  cervical
    pain, 159
    upper, superficial sensory
        distribution of, 38
  chorda tympani, 39
  compression, 79
  cranial, 36
  endings, free, 19
  entrapment, 79
  facial, 39, 40
  function in maxillofacial area,
      neurologic survey for, 336
  glossopharyngeal (*see*
      Glossopharyngeal nerve)
  gray, 16

injury pain, nerve stimulation in, 362
intermediate, of Wrisberg, 39
mandibular
  herpes zoster of, 302
  neuralgia of, paroxysmal, 285
maxillary, paroxysmal neuralgia of, 284
motor, pain, 65
ninth, neuralgia, 286–288
oculomotor, 40
pain, sensory, 65
peripheral
  deafferentation of, 372
  injury, 83
somatic
  motor, 40–41
  sensory, 35–40
spinal
  cervical, 39–40, 41
  thoracic, 34
stimulation
  cutaneous, 359–360
  percutaneous, 362–363
  subcutaneous, 362
  transcutaneous, 360–362
  transcutaneous electrical, 53–54, 361
thoracic, pain, 159
transmission of afferent impulses, 21–23
trigeminal, 35–39, 40
  distribution of, superficial sensory, 38
  herpes zoster of, 300
  mandibular division, 35–39
  maxillary division, 35
  opthalmic division, 35
  unmyelinated fibers and myelinated fibers in, 80
trochlear, 40
vagus, 39, 40
vidian, neuralgia, 243
visceral, afferent, 34
white, 16
Nervous intermedius, 39
Nervous system
  autonomic, 35
  somatic, 35
  visceral, 35, 41–42

Neural
  circuits, efferent, 22–23
  genesis of pain, 78–80
  mechanisms of pain, 15–31
    phylogenic considerations, 15
  pathways, peripheral, 32–43
  structures, 16–23
Neuralgia
  atypical, differential diagnosis, 252
  facial, atypical, 243, 245, 247, 248–249
    pain chronicity in, 317
  geniculate, 282, 286, 288–289
    differential diagnosis, 261
  glossopharyngeal, 228, 268, 282, 286
    anticonvulsants in, 377
    differential diagnosis, 261, 289–290
  idiopathic, 101, 273, 279–280, 317, 359
  major, 273
  migrainous, 34, 100, 138, 240, 241, 243–252, 288, 364
    masticatory myospasm pain secondary to, 249
    mistaken for masticatory pain, 251
  minor, 274
  neuritic, 65, 79–80, 98, 99, 101, 114–115, 244, 265, 292–298
    of alveolar nerve, 295
    of alveolar nerve, inferior, 297
    of glossopharyngeal nerve, 299
  ninth nerve, 286–288
  pain, 275
    paroxysmal, 79
    phenytoin for, 376
  paroxysmal, 65, 79, 99, 100, 114, 244, 273, 279–291
    of auriculotemporal nerve, 283
    of glossopharyngeal nerve, 287
    of mandibular nerve, 285
    of maxillary nerve, 284
    pain of, 289
    phenytoin in diagnosis of, 353
  postherpetic, 65, 99, 101, 115, 292, 300, 301, 373
    cryocautery in, 372

Neuralgia (*cont.*)
  placebo therapy in, 369
  primary, 273
  secondary, 274
  sphenopalatine, 243
  symptomatic, 101, 273–274, 281, 290–291, 359
  trigeminal, 280, 364
    anticonvulsants in, 377
    atypical, 291, 298
    idiopathic, on examination chart, 329
    myelinated fiber changes in, 81
    symptomatic, 79
    thermolysis in, radiofrequency, 372
    tympanic plexus, 286
  typical, 273, 280
  vascular, 245
  vidian nerve, 243
Neurectomy: peripheral, 372
Neuritic
  dental pain, 141
  neuralgia (*see* Neuralgia, neuritic)
Neuritic pain, 140, 273, 286, 292
  chronicity of, 317
  differential diagnosis, 252
Neuritic toothache, 294
Neuritis, 292
  alveolar
    inferior, 293
    superior, 293
  auriculotemporal, 293
  facial, 298
  glossopharyngeal, 286, 298–299
  inflammatory, 359
  neuroactive drugs and, 377
  peripheral, 99, 101, 292–293
  trigeminal, 293–298
Neuroactive drugs, 377
Neurochemical effects, 26–28
Neurofibrils, 16
Neurogenous pain, 78, 93, 114–115, 265, 271–310
  classification, 100–101
  of deafferentation origin, relationship to other orofacial pain syndromes, 305
  diagnosis, differential, 289–290, 384
  discussion of, 98–99
  identification of, 347

neuralgias as form of, paroxysmal, 279
of neuroma, traumatic, 228
of neuropathic origin, relationship to other orofacial pain syndromes, 272
summation in, 289
therapeutic options, 384
therapy of, cause-related, 359
vs. somatic pain, 8
Neurogenous toothache, 140–141
Neurolemma, 16
Neurologic survey, 334–337
  of nerve function in maxillofacial area, 336
Neurologic symptoms, 332
Neurolytic block, 372
Neurolytic drug, 377
Neuroma
  pain
    ephaptic transfer, 275
    traumatic, 81–82, 98, 99, 100, 274–279
    traumatic, in temporomandibular joint, 277
    traumatic, 79, 114, 273, 359
    neurogenous pain of, 228
Neuromodulators: endogenous opiates as, 55
Neuron, 16–18
  afferent, 17
    primary, 23–24
  convergence, 18
  effector, 17
  efferent, 17
  facilitation of, 18
  gelatinosa, 25
  inhibition of, 18
  internuncial, 17
  motor, 17
  nociceptive, 24
  postganglionic, 17
  preganglionic, 17
  receptor, 17
  sensory, 17
  summation of, 18
Neuropathic pain, 99, 100
  diagnosis, differential, 384
  of mouth and face, 271–273
  therapeutic options, 384
Neuropathy, 78
Neurosis, 313

INDEX   **409**

Neurosurgery, 358, 371–373
Neuroticism, 57, 317
Neurotransmitters, 55
  excitatory, substance P 23, 27–28
Nitroglycerin, 352
Nociceptive
  neurons, 24
  pain receptors, 21
  pathways, peripheral, 33–35
  reflex, 20
Nociceptors: exteroceptive, 3
Nodes of Ranvier, 16, 21
Norepinephrine, 26, 55, 83, 242, 303, 378, 379
Nose (see Nasal)
Nucleotomy: trigeminal, 373
Nucleus, 16
  caudalis, 22
  mesencephalic, 22
  proprius, 25
  raphe
    magnus, 27, 54
    medullary, 26
  trigeminal spinal tract, 22, 25
  schema of, 69
Nutritional deficiencies, 110

O

Obscure pain, 10, 11
Occipitofrontalis muscle, 157, 267
  referred pain of, 157
  trigger points in, 157
Occlusal disengagement, 368–369, 378
Occlusal overstressing, 131
Occlusal reconstruction, 162
Occlusal splints, 368–369
Occlusion
  correcting splint, 368
  disharmony, radiographic evidence of, 195
  traumatic, molar in, 131
Ocular pain, 100, 266–268
  diagnosis, differential, 384
  therapeutic options, 384
Oculomotor nerves, 40
Odontalgia
  atypical, 100, 139, 243, 252–253
  pulpal, 253
Odontogenous pain, 119, 136, 296
  examination in, 339

Oil gland: and glandular pain, 266
Open-bite: progressive anterior, and temporomandibular joint rheumatoid arthritis, 206, 207
Open-lock, 189
Opiates, endogenous, 55
Opioid analgesics, 374
Opioid: endogenous, 79
Opioid peptides, 55, 242, 274, 304, 361, 362, 374
Oral
  (See also Mouth)
  consciousness, 106, 148
  contraception, and mucogingival pain, 110
  mucosa, fungoid infection of, 112
Orbicularis oculi muscle, 157
Organic structural cause: of pain, 358
Orofacial pain
  categories of, 93–101
  syndrome(s)
    classification of, 91–101, 103, 346
    relationship to dental pain, 117
    relationship to muscle pain, 145
Orthodromic propagation, 24
Osseous infection: spreading, 133
Osseous pain, 100, 229–232
  diagnosis, differential, 383
  relationship to other orofacial pain syndromes, 230
  therapeutic options, 383
Osteitis, 231, 239
Osteoarthritis, 206
Osteomyelitis, 231, 232, 233
Ostium maxillare, 261, 265
  mucosa pain, 237
  stimulation causing referred pain, 263
Otic ganglion, 41
Otitis
  externa, 268
  media, 162, 212, 270

P

Pacinian corpuscles, 19
Pain
  aching, 7, 331
  acute, vs. chronic pain, 7–8
  arthritic (see Arthritic pain)

410 INDEX

Pain (cont.)
  attention to, 4
  auricular (see Auricular pain)
  autonomic reflex, 303
  bright, 6, 331
  burning, 7, 18, 331
  capsular, 100
  causalgic, 303, 377
  of cellulitis, 229
  central, 65
    excitation, 66
  chronic (see Chronic pain)
  chronicity, 7, 57, 85
  classifications, 91–92
  clinical, vs. experimental pain, 7
  compensation, 315
  concepts of, changing, 3–5
  consequences of, 4, 57
  continuous, 6, 331
  controlled by consequences in environment, 371
  cutaneous (see Cutaneous, pain)
  cycling, interruption with analgesic blocking, 363–364
  deafferentation (see Deafferentation, pain)
  deep
    autonomic effects of, 70
    central excitatory effects of, 61–64
    identification of, 347
    motor effects of, 70–71
    myospastic activity in, 71
    secondary effects of, 61–72
    sensory effects of, 64–70
  deep somatic, 34, 95–98, 100
    muscle pain as, 144
    musculoskeletal pain as, 229
    pain of dental origin as, 118
    of temporomandibular joint, 182
    of visceral mucosa pain, 257
    vs. superficial pain, 8
  definition, 3, 4, 91
  delusional, 99, 101, 321–323
    psychiatric consultation in, 371
  dental (see Dental pain)
  of dental origin (see Dental, origin of pain)
  descending pain inhibitory mechanism, 361
  descriptors, 13
  determinants, model of, 52
  diagnosis (see Diagnosis)
  differences in pains, 7
  diffuse, 332
  disc attachment, 100
  "dry-socket," 232
    central excitatory effects, 232
  dull, 6, 331
  dysfunction syndrome, 160–163, 179, 247, 251
    masticatory, 134, 146, 270
    masticatory, elevator masticatory muscles in, 165
    myofascial, 162, 362
    myofascial, biofeedback training in, 367
    secondary to migrainous neuralgia, 249
    spasm of elevator muscle in, 167, 171, 173
  effect of functional activities on, 332
  emergency nature of, 9–10
  emotional value of, 11–12
  enlarging, 6, 332
  episode of, 6
  evaluation (see Evaluation)
  examination in (see Examination)
  experimental, vs. clinical pain, 7
  face (see Face, pain)
  gate control theory of (see Gate control theory)
  genesis (see Genesis of pain)
  glandular (see Glandular pain)
  hallucinatory, 320
  head, primary intracranial, 84
  heterotopic (see Heterotopic pain)
  historical note on, 2–3
  history (see History)
  of hysteria, conversion, 99, 101, 320–321
  iatrogenic, 86
  identifying the proper pain category (see Identifying the proper pain category)
  induced, 6, 330
  inflammatory (see Inflammatory pain)
  infra-auricular, 152
  inhibition, 163, 169
  inhibitory influence of, 231

INDEX 411

of injury
   attention given to, 73
   consequences of, 73
intensity, 330
intermittent, 6, 331
intracranial, 84
   of head, primary, 84
intractable, 6
lancinating, 332
learning to cope with, 370
localization behavior, 332
localized, 332
low-intensity, 5
malingered, 314
management (see Management)
manner of flow, 330
masticatory (see Masticatory pain)
maximum-intensity, 5
McGill Pain Questionnaire, 13, 333–334
migrating, 6, 332
mild, 5, 330
modulation, 44–60, 73, 315
   concept of, 44–45
   excitatory factors, 57
   inhibitory factors, 57
   nonnoxious cutaneous stimulation, 54–55
   psychological effects, 56–57
momentary, 331
motivational-affective property, 4, 52
mouth (see Mouth, pain)
mucogingival (see Mucogingival pain)
mucosa (see Mucosa pain)
muscle (see Muscle, pain)
musculoskeletal (see Musculoskeletal pain)
myofascial (see Myofascial pain)
myogenous, 74, 144, 378
nasal mucosa, 261–264
   central excitatory effects, 261
nerve
   cervical, 159
   injury, nerve stimulation in, 362
   motor, 65
   sensory, 65
   thoracic, 159
neural mechanisms, 15–31
   phylogenic considerations, 15

of neuralgia (see Neuralgia)
neuritic (see Neuritic pain)
neurogenous (see Neurogenous pain)
neurologic survey, 334–337
   of nerve function in maxillofacial area, 336
neuroma (see Neuroma pain)
neuropathic (see Neuropathic pain)
obscure, 10, 11
ocular (see Ocular pain)
odontogenous, 119, 136, 296
onset mode, 330
organic structural cause of, 358
orofacial (see Orofacial pain)
osseous (see Osseous pain)
paranasal sinus, 264
paroxysmal, 6, 274, 330
pathologic, 7
pathways, peripheral, 33
perception of, 313
   gate control theory and, 51
   -reaction hypothesis, 44
periapical, 130
periodic, 6
periodontal (see Periodontal pain)
of periodontal origin, 130–133
periosteal (see Periosteal pain)
phantom (see Phantom pain)
pharyngeal mucosa, 260–261
   differential diagnosis, 260–261
post-traumatic pain syndrome, 291
preauricular (see Preauricular pain)
preliminary interview in, 326–327
pressure pain syndrome, 131–132
pricking, 6, 18
primary, vs. secondary pain, 8
projected, 65–66
protracted, 6, 332
psychogenesis of, 311
psychogenic (see Psychogenic pain)
psychologic survey, 337–338
psychoneurotic, 44, 101
pulpal (see Pulpal pain)
pulsatile, 7
pulsating, 331
quality of, 331
radiating, 332

Pain (cont.)
  reaction, 313
    gate control theory and, 51
  receptors
    as chemoceptive, 21
    as nociceptive, 21
  recurrent, 6, 331
  referred (see Referred pain)
  refractory period, 280
  remission of, 6
  retrodiscal, 100
  retro-orbital, 266
  salivary gland, 266
  of scar tissue, differential diagnosis, 228
  secondary, 332
    vs. primary pain, 8
  sensation, quality of, 6–7
  sensory-discriminative dimension of, 4, 51–52
  severe, 330
  severity, 5
  signal detection theory, 7
  silent, 146
  site of, 10–11, 68, 94, 325
  soft connective tissue (see Soft connective tissue pain)
  somatic (see Somatic pain)
  somatic-generated, therapy of, 358–359
  source of, 10–11, 68, 169, 325, 348
    of temporomandibular joint, 185
  splinting, protective, 100
  spontaneous, 5–6, 330
    vs. stimulus-evoked pain, 9
  spreading, 6, 71, 332
  steady, 6, 330
  stimulus-evoked, vs. spontaneous pain, 9
  stinging, 6–7
  superficial, vs. deep somatic pain, 8
  as symptom, 5–6
    clinical, 1–14
  temporal behavior of, 5–6, 331
  temporomandibular joint (see Temporomandibular joint, pain)
  therapy, trials, 353–354
  thresholds, 27, 55
  throbbing, 7
  tolerance, 55, 380
  tooth (see Toothache)
  trigger point (see Trigger point, pain)
  triggered, 6, 330
  from tumors, 85
  vascular (see Vascular pain)
  visceral (see Visceral pain)
  zones of reference, 75
Palatal cellulitis, 234
Palatal reflex, 337
Paleospinothalamic tract, 25
Papilledema, 85
Paralysis: facial, 298
Paranasal sinus pain, 264–266
Paranasal sinusitis, 265
Parasympathetic(s), 35
  afferent
    fibers, cranial, 34
    sacral, 34
  afferents, 41
  autonomics, 35
  efferents, 41
Paresthesia, 82, 265, 372
Paroxysmal pain, 6
Pathologic pain, 7
Pellagra, 110
Pemphigus, 110
Perception-reaction hypothesis: in pain, 44
Periapical abscess, 123, 124, 131
Periapical pain, 130
Periaqueductal gray, 54
Perineurium, 16
Periodic pain, 6
Periodontal
  abscess, 123, 126
    lateral, 131
  disease, 121
  ligaments, 129
  mechanoreceptors, 20, 147
  origin of pain, 130–133
  pain, 120, 124
    cause, 131–132
    cause for, reasonable, 127
    dental, 100
    stimulus-evoked, 129–130
  pocket, 132
Periodontoclasia, 132
Periosteal pain, 100, 229, 232–233
  diagnosis, differential, 383

INDEX

relationship to other orofacial pain syndromes, 230
therapeutic options, 383
Periosteitis, 233, 239
Peripheral therapy, 372
Periventricular structure, 26
Perostium: electric stimulation of, 363
Personality disintegration, 370
Phantom limb: biofeedback training in, 367
Phantom pain, 82, 99, 101, 141, 303, 309
  limb, 379
    nerve stimulation in, 362
Phantom toothache, 309
Pharyngeal mucosa pain, 260–261
  differential diagnosis, 260–261
Pharyngeal reflex, 337
Pharyngitis, 237, 260
  streptococcal, 260
Phenol, 377
Phenolphthalein: and stomatitis medicamentosa, 109
Phenothiazines, 377
  extrapyramidal effects of, 378
D-Phenylalanine, 380
Phenytoin, 353, 376
Phosphates, 358
Physical activity, 366
Physiotherapy, 354, 357, 365–366
  manipulation in, functional, 365
Placebo effect, 316, 367, 369, 378
Placebo therapy, 358, 369
  trial, 337
Platelets, 359
Platysma muscle, 157
Postherpetic (*see* Neuralgia, postherpetic)
Post-traumatic pain syndrome, 291
Potassium, 28, 358
Preauricular pain
  heterotopic pain felt as, 267, 269
  masseter muscle and, 150
Preganglionic neuron, 17
Pregnancy
  gingivitis during, 110
  mucogingival pain and, 110
Preliminary interview, 326–327
Pressure pain syndrome, 131–132
Pricking itching, 331

Pricking pain, 6, 18
Primary pain vs. secondary pain, 8
Probenecid, 354, 375
Professional rapport, 326
Projected pain, 65–66
Proprioceptive stimuli, 35
Proprioceptors, 19–20, 182
Prostaglandin, 26–27, 74, 242, 358
  aspirin and, 374
  biosynthesis, 374
  hyperalgesia, 27, 74
Protracted pain, 6
Pseudoparalysis, 148
Psychiatric screening, 370
Psychogenesis, 141
  of pain, 311
Psychogenic
  intensification, 7
    of pain, 311, 314, 315, 316, 370
    of psychoneurosis, 99
  toothache, 141
Psychogenic pain, 85, 93, 311–324, 337, 338, 359
  classification, 101
  diagnosis, differential, 385
  discussion of, 99–100
  expressed as conversion hysteria, 322
  regional, 321
  relationship to other orofacial pain syndromes, 312
  therapeutic options, 385
Psychologic survey, 337–338
Psychological modulating effects, 56–57
Psychoneurosis: psychogenic intensification in, 99
Psychoneurotic pain, 44, 101
Psychosis, 85
Psychotherapy, 358, 369–371
  formal, 371
Pterygoid muscle
  lateral, 20
    inferior, 153
    inferior, spasm of, 165–170
    referred pain and trigger points of, 154
    spasm, 170–172
    superior, 153–155
    technique for extraoral injection, 351

Pterygoid muscle (*cont.*)
  medial, 152
    referred pain of, 154
    technique for extraoral injection, 351
    trigger point of, 154
Pterygopalatine ganglia, 41
Pulp
  (*See also* Pulpal pain)
  gangrene, 123
  inflammation, 132
  odontalgia, 253
  test, electric, 128
  tester, 133, 339
  testing, electric, 296
Pulpal origin
  of pain, 121–129
  of toothache, clinical characteristics, 135–136
Pulpal pain, 120, 306
  (*See also* Pulp)
  acute, 121–124
    without evident cause, 128
  cause for, reasonable, 127
  chronic, 124–125
  dental, 100
  identification of, criteria for, 127–129
  mixed, 126
  in molar, first, mandibular, 124
  from molar, second, 129
  obscure causes of, 129
  recurrent, 126
  stimulus-induced, 120–121
  after trauma, 124
Pulpitis, 239
  acute, 124
    dental pain and, 134
  chronic, 124
  of molar, mandibular second, 126
Pulsatile pain, 7
Pulsating pain, 331

R

Radicular cyst, 123
Radiography, 342–343
  of facial structures in pain examination, 341
  of mandibular condyle, 213
    hyperplasia, 222
  of temporomandibular joint (*see* Temporomandibular joint, radiography)
Ramsay Hunt syndrome, 301
  differential diagnosis, 261
Rapport: professional, 326
Receptor neuron, 17
Recurrent pain, 6
Red blood cells: hemolyzed, 358
Reference zones, 66, 75, 150
  of myofascial pain, 151
Referred pain, 11, 65, 66–67, 113–114, 119, 130, 146
  dental pain and, 134
  of digastric muscle, anterior, 155
  felt in joint area, differential diagnosis, 227
  from masseter muscle, 137
  from nasal mucosa, inflamed, 264
  of occipitofrontalis muscle, 157
  ostium maxillare stimulation causing, 263
  of pterygoid muscle, 154
  spontaneous, 149
  of sternocleidomastoid muscle, 156
  from submandibular gland inflammation, 267
  from temporalis muscle, 153
  of temporomandibular joint, 184
  toothache referred from muscles, 136
  of trapezius muscle, 156
Reflex
  arc, 17
  autonomic, pain, 303
  axon, 68
  carotid sinus, 336
  cough, 259
  feedback control, 32
  gag, 259, 337
  myotatic, 20, 34
  nociceptive, 20
  palatal, 337
  pharyngeal, 337
  sneeze, 259
  stretch, 20
    inverse, 21
  superficial, checking of, 336–337
  sympathetic dystrophy, 82, 99, 303–308
    (*See also* Causalgia)

analgesic blocking in, 364
central excitatory effects, 306
chronicity and pain in, 317
classification of, 101
deafferentation syndrome expressed as, 308
differential diagnosis, 252
Refractory period, 280
in tic douloureux, 281
Relaxation, 366–369
techniques, 366–367
training, 358
Remission of pain, 6
Resorption: of tooth, internal, 125
Respiratory infection: upper, and nasal mucosa pain, 262–263
Reticular formation, 25
Retrodiscal pain, 100
Retrodiscitis, 196, 217
Retro-orbital pain, 266
Rheumatoid arthralgia, 206
Rheumatoid arthritis, 209, 227
open-bite due to, progressive anterior, 207
of temporomandibular joint, 205
advanced, 208
early, radiography, 207
Rhinitis, allergic, 245, 247, 252, 262
in nasal mucosa pain, 261
Rhizotomy, 372–373
Ruffini's corpuscles, 19

S

Sacral parasympathetic afferents, 34
Saliva, 104
Salivary glands
major, and glandular pain, 266
pain, 266
Scalding, 107
Scar tissue: painful, differential diagnosis, 228
Scars
mucogingival, 275
painful, 275
Schizophrenia, 85
Schizophrenic hallucination, 321
Sclerosis, multiple, 79, 291
neuralgia in, symptomatic, 274
Screening
medical, form for, 339
psychiatric, 370

Sebaceous glands: and glandular pain, 266
Secondary pain vs. primary pain, 8
Sensation: quality of pain, 6–7
Sensations, 332
Senses, special, 332
checking of, 335
Sensor-tranducers, 19
Sensory
descriptors, 333
-discriminative dimension of pain, 4, 51–52
function, checking of, 335
neuron, 17
receptive field, 82, 83
receptors, 19–23
stimulation, 357
Serenity, 57
Serotonin, 27, 54, 55, 77, 243, 358, 378, 379
Sialolithiais, 266
Sick headache, 253
Signal detection theory, 7
Sinus
carotid, reflex, 336
headache, 262, 264
toothache, 140
of Morgagni syndrome, 219
paranasal, pain, 264–266
Sinusitis, 134, 138, 245, 247, 252, 265
chronic, 265
maxillary, 140, 262, 294, 296
obstructive, 265
paranasal, 265
source of, 264–265
Site
of origin of pain, 94
of pain, 10–11, 68, 94, 325
Sjögren's syndrome, 106
Skeletal pain
(See also Musculoskeletal pain)
as deep somatic pain, 229
Skin
(See also Cutaneous)
pressing, 359
rubbing, 359
Sluder's headache, 243
Sneeze reflex, 259
Soft connective tissue pain, 100, 229, 233–235
diagnosis, differential, 383

INDEX

Soft connective tissue pain (*cont.*)
  relationship to other orofacial pain syndromes, 230
  therapeutic options, 383
Soma, 23
Somatic
  nerves (*see* Nerves, somatic)
  nervous system, 35
Somatic pain, 93
  classification, 100
  deep (*see* Pain, deep somatic)
  discussion of, 93–94
  superficial, 3, 93–95, 100, 102
  vs. neurogenous pain, 8
Somatostatin, 379
Spasm
  esophageal, 259
  increasing passive interarticular pressure, 163
  muscle, 71–72, 76, 119, 129, 149, 353
    elevator muscles, 163–165, 167, 170–172, 173
    masseter, 164
    pain, 76–77, 100, 146, 160–172, 179, 385
    pain, analgesic blocking in, 363
    pterygoid, 165–170
    pterygoid, lateral, 170–172
  myospasm (*see* Myospasm)
Spatial summation, 49
Special senses, 332
  checking of, 335
Sphenopalatine neuralgia, 243
Spine
  cord, gray substance lamination, 24–25
  effects of noxious impulses on, 64
  nerves (*see* Nerves, spinal)
  trigeminal nucleus, 22, 25
    schema of, 69
Spinoreticulothalamic system, 25
Splenius cervicis, 267
Splint
  disengaging, 368
  mandibular repositioning, 368
  occlusal, 368–369
  occlusion correcting, 368
Splinting
  muscle (*see* Muscle, splinting)

pain, protective, 100
Spontaneous pain, 5–6
  vs. stimulus-evoked pain, 9
Spreading pain, 6, 71
Sprouts, 83
Steady pain, 6
Stellate ganglion, 42, 237
  blocking of, 259, 306, 349, 364
Sternocleidomastoid muscle, 155, 267
  referred pain of, 156
  trigger point in, 156
  trigger point pain affecting, 269
Stevens-Johnson syndrome, 108
Stimulation (*see* Nerve, stimulation)
Stimulus-evoked pain vs. spontaneous pain, 9
Stinging pain, 6–7
Stomach symptoms, 332
Stomatitis
  aphthous, 111, 301
  desquamative, 108
  medicamentosa, 108
    expressed as erythema multiforme, 109
  venenata due to denture, 108
Streptococcal pharyngitis, 260
Stress: emotional, 76, 104, 243, 304
Stretch reflex, 20
  inverse, 21
Stylohyoid ligament, 227
Styloid process, 227
  fracture causing neuritic neuralgia, 299
Submandibular ganglia, 41
Submandibular gland: inflammation, heterotopic pain referred from, 267
Subnucleus
  caudalis, 24–25, 117, 121
  oralis, 117, 121
Subperiosteal abscess, 233
Substance P, 24, 27–28, 82, 83, 374, 379
Substantia gelatinosa, 25, 45, 83
Succinylcholine: chlorida, 353, 378
Summation
  effects, 96, 98
  of neurons, 18
Sunday headache, 253

INDEX

Superficial pain vs. deep somatic pain, 8
Surface massage, 365
Swallowing, 259
Sympathectomy, 42
Sympathetic(s), 35
  afferents, 34, 41–42
  autonomics, 35
  blockade, 364
  chain, cervical, 42, 237, 259
  change, 34
  dystrophy, reflex (*see* Reflex, sympathetic dystrophy)
  efferents, 42
Synapse, 17, 78
Synaptic junction, 17
Syncope, 286

T

Taste fibers, 39
Teeth
  (*See also* Tooth)
  centric position of, 188
  examination of, 338–340
  tender, 142
Temporal arteritis, 239, 254
Temporal behavior: of pain, 5–6, 331
Temporal summation, 48
Temporalis muscle, 150–152
  referred pain from, 153
  technique for injecting, 350
  trigger points in, 153
Temporomandibular arthralgia, 182
  central excitatory effects, 226
  expressed as arthritic pain
    due to cancer, 224
    due to degenerative joint disease, 214
    due to fibrous ankylosis, 218
    due to hyperuricemia, 216
  expressed as capsular pain
    due to capsular fibrosis, 204
    due to trauma, 201
  expressed as disc attachment pain
    due to discitis, 191
  expressed as retrodiscal pain due to trauma, 198
  pain, inflammatory, 226
    differential diagnosis, 226
Temporomandibular joint
  ankylosis, fibrous, 206
  arthralgia (*see* Temporomandibular arthralgia)
  arthritis, 200
    pain of (*see* Arthritic pain of temporomandibular joint)
    rheumatoid (*see* Rheumatoid arthritis, of temporomandibular joint)
    traumatic, radiography of, 212
  cancer, 217, 224
  capsular fibrosis, 200
    inflamed, 204
  condyles (*see* Condyle)
  deflection, 226
  degenerative disease, 210, 211
  degenerative joint disease, 206
  deviation, 226
  disc
    articular, fracture, 190
    interference disorders, 189
    jamming, 189
  discal ligaments, 184
  dislocation, 186
  displacement
    anterior, 188
    functional, 189
    posterior, 188
  inflammation, periarticular, 209
  ligament (*see* Temporomandibular ligament)
  luxation, 186
  neuroma pain in, 277
  pain, 98, 100, 182–229
    arthritic (*see* Arthritic pain of temporomandibular joint)
    capsular, 182, 200–205
    capsular, central excitatory effects, 201
    central excitatory effects, 184
    as deep somatic pain, 182
    diagnosis, differential, 225–226, 382–383
    disc-attachment, 182, 186–196
    -dysfunction syndrome (*see* Pain, -dysfunction syndrome)

Temporomandibular joint (cont.)
   inflammatory, 183
   referred, differential diagnosis, 227
   relationship to other orofacial pain syndromes, 183
   retrodiscal, 182, 196–200
   retrodiscal, central excitatory effects of, 199
   source of, 185
   sternocleidomastoid muscle and, 155
   therapeutic options, 383
   radiographic evidence
      of articular disc degeneration, 194, 195
      of capsular restraint on condylar movement, 203
      of condylar displacement, 194, 195
      of condylar fixation, 193
      of occlusal disharmony, 195
   radiography of, 168, 170, 172, 174, 177, 179, 192–195, 199, 202, 203, 205, 215, 217, 219, 225, 250, 268
      of arthritis, traumatic, 212
      of deformation, marked, 211
      of degenerative change, 209
      of degenerative disease, advanced, 210, 211
      with lack of structural harmony, 221
      of osseous change, 210, 211
      of rheumatoid arthritis, advanced, 208
      of rheumatoid arthritis, early, 207
      series of films needed to satisfactorily visualize the temporomandibular joint, 344
   retrodiscal tissue, 184
Temporomandibular, ligament
   inner horizontal, 185
   outer oblique, 185
Tender teeth, 142
Tendinitis, 175
Tendon: Golgi tendon organs, 20, 76
Tension
   emotional, 106, 242, 248, 250
   headache (see Headache, tension)

Tentorium cerebelli, 39, 84
Thalamus, 22
   projection to, 25–26
Theory (see Gate control theory)
Therapy
   (See also Treatment)
   cause-related, 357, 358–359
   dietary supplement, 358, 379–380
   guidelines for, 380–381
   heat, deep, 365
   hypnotherapy, 370
   medicinal, 358, 373–379
   peripheral, 372
   placebo, 358, 369
   physiotherapy, 365–366
      functional manipulation in, 365
   psychotherapy, 358, 369–371
      formal, 371
   thermal, 360, 365
   trigger point, 364, 365–366
Thermal therapy, 360, 365
Thermocoagulation, 373
Thermolysis: radiofrequency, in trigeminal neuralgia, 372
Thoracic spinal nerves, 34
Throbbing pain, 7
Tic convulsif, 281
Tic douloureux, 5, 141, 174, 247, 280–286, 290
   auriculotemporal branch in, 282
   central excitatory effects, 281
   on examination chart, 329
   idiopathic, 79
   not responding to nerve stimulation, 362
   refractory period, 281
   summation in, 281
   triggering, 281
Tickle, 6
Tinnitus, 150
Tongue: burning, 106–107
Tonsillitis, 260
Tooth
   (See also Teeth)
   pain (see Toothache)
   resorption, internal, 125
   tender teeth, 142
Toothache, 11, 135, 245
   of cardiac origin, 137–138
   facial neuralgia occuring as, atypical, 247

heterotopic pain felt as, 246, 264
high-altitude, 126
from hyperalgesia, secondary, 142
mandibular, deafferentation syndrome expressed as, 307
masseter muscle and, 150
menstrual, 126
muscles of facial expression and, 157
myogenous, 136
nasal mucosa pain and, 261, 262
neuritic, 294
neuritis and, trigeminal, 293
neurogenous, 140–141
of nondental origin, 135–142
  cardinal warning signs, 141–142
odontogenous, 294, 306
phantom, 309
psychogenic intensification, 141
of pulpal origin, clinical characteristics of, 135–136
referred from muscles, 136–137
reflex sympathetic dystrophy causing, 306
sinus headache, 140
tic douloureux and, 282
vascular, 139–140, 252
of vascular origin, 138–140
Topical anesthesia, 97
Tractotomy: trigeminal, 373
Training
  biofeedback, 367–369
  relaxation, 358
Tranquilizers, 377–378
  major, 377
  minor, 378
Transport substances, 83
Trapezius muscle, 155–157
  referred pain of, 156
  trigger points of, 156
Trauma
  arthritis due to, 205, 209, 212
  post-traumatic pain syndrome, 291
  pulpal pain after, 124
Traumatic
  neuroma, 79, 114, 273, 359
  neuroma pain (*see* Neuroma pain, traumatic)
Treatment
  occlusion, molar in, 131
  (*See also* Therapy)

modalities, 357–358
Tricyclics (*see* Antidepressants, tricyclics)
Trigeminal
  herpes zoster, 300–301
  nerve (*see* Nerve, trigeminal)
  neuralgia (*see* Neuralgia, trigeminal)
  neuritis, 293–298
  nucleotomy, 373
  spinal tract nucleus, 22, 25
  tractotomy, 373
Trigger point
  active, 149
  central excitatory effect, 76
  of digastric muscle, anterior, 155
  latent, 149
  in masseter muscle, 152
  mechanism, 71
  of muscles of facial expression, 158
  myofascial (*see* Myofascial trigger point)
  of occipitofrontalis muscle, 157
  pain, 75–76
    myofascial (*see* Myofascial, trigger point pain)
    of sternocleidomastoid muscle, 269
  of pterygoid muscle, 154
  satellite, 149
  secondary, 149
  of sternocleidomastoid muscle, 156
  in temporalis muscle, 153
  therapy, 364, 365–366
  of trapezius muscle, 156
Triggered pain, 6, 330
Triptyline, 376
Trismus, 175, 219, 234
Trochlear nerves, 40
Trotter's syndrome, 219
L-Tryptophan, 27, 380
Tumors, 232, 234
  benign, 85
  brain, 85
  cerebellopontine angle, 85
  extracranial, 85
  glandular pain and, 266
  malignant, 85
  of temporomandibular joint, 217, 224

Tumors (cont.)
  middle fossa, 85
  neuralgia in, symptomatic, 274
  pain from, 85
Turbinates: points stimulated on, 262
Tympanic plexus neuralgia, 286

U

Ulcer
  aphthous, 115
  decubital, 111
    denture causing, 112
Ulcerative gingivitis: necrotizing, 111
Ultrasound, 365

V

Vagus nerve, 39, 40
Vapocoolant therapy, 55, 360
  intermittency in, 360
Vapocoolants, 354
Varicella, 81
Vascular genesis: of pain, 77–78
Vascular headache (see Headache, vascular)
Vascular neuralgia, 245
Vascular origin: of toothache, 138–140
Vascular pain, 77, 98, 100, 138, 236–237, 379
  antidepressants for, 378
  central excitatory effects, 242
  diagnosis, differential, 383
  of face, 238–243
  of inflammation, 243, 254–255
  of mouth, 238–243
  relationship to other orofacial pain syndromes, 244
  syndrome, 253, 352
    heterotopic pain due to, 246
  therapeutic options, 383–384
  therapy of, 353–354
Vascular toothache, 139–140, 252

Vasoactive agents, 379
Vasodilators: coronary, 379
Vertigo: postural, 155
Vessels (see Vascular)
Vibration, 55
  mechanical, 360, 365
Vidian nerve neuralgia, 243
Vincent's angina, 260
Vincent's infection, 111
Viral infection: causing nasal mucosa pain, 261
Visceral
  afferents, high threshold receptors of, 237
  nerve, afferent, 34
  nervous system, 35, 41–42
Visceral pain, 98, 100, 236, 257–270
  behavior of, 237–238
  central excitatory effects, 238
  identification of, 348
  of mucosa, 100, 257–260
    central excitatory effects, 259
    deep somatic, 257
    relationship to other orofacial pain syndromes, 258
  vs. musculoskeletal pain, 9

W

Warning signs: cardinal, in toothache of nondental origin, 141–142
White nerves, 16
Withdrawal reaction, 95
Wrisberg intermediate nerves, 39

X

Xerostomia, 106

Z

Zones of reference (see Reference zones)
Zoster (see Herpes zoster)
Zygomaticus major muscle, 157